Practical Laparoscopic Surgery for General Surgeons

Edited by

I. M. C. Macintyre MD, FRCS
Consultant Surgeon, Western General Hospital, Edinburgh, UK

With a Foreword by Professor D. C. Carter MD, FRCS (Ed), FRCS (Glas)
Regius Professor of Clinical Surgery, University of Edinburgh, UK

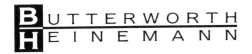

Butterworth-Heinemann Ltd
Linacre House, Jordan Hill, Oxford OX2 8DP

 A member of the Reed Elsevier plc group

OXFORD LONDON BOSTON
MUNICH NEW DELHI SINGAPORE SYDNEY
TOKYO TORONTO WELLINGTON

First published 1994

British Library Cataloguing in Publication Data
Practical Laparoscopic Surgery for
General Surgeons
  I. MacIntyre, I. M. C.
  617.4

ISBN 0 7506 0742 4

Composition by Scribe Design, Gillingham, Kent, UK
Printed and bound in Great Britain by Martins the Printers, Berwick upon Tweed

Contents

Contributors

Mohan C. Airan MD, FACS
Associate Chairman, Department of Surgery
Mount Sinai Hospital Medical Center;
Clinical Professor of Surgery, Chicago
Medical School, USA

H.D. Becker MD
Eberhard-Karls-Universität Tübingen
Klinikum Schnarrenberg
Chirugische Klinik
Tübingen, Germany

G. Bell ChM, FRCS
Consultant Surgeon
Inverclyde Royal Hospital
Greenock, Renfrewshire
UK

Brock M. Bordelon MD
Department of Surgery
University of Utah School of Medicine
USA

A.W. Bradbury BSc, MD, FRCS (Ed)
Lecturer
University Department of Surgery
Royal Infirmary
Edinburgh, UK

G. Buess MD
Eberhard-Karls-Universität Tübingen
Klinikum Schnarrenberg
Chirugische Klinik
Tübingen, Germany

D.S. Byrne MB, ChB, FRCS
Surgical Registrar
Stobhill General Hospital
Glasgow, UK

Sarah Cheslyn-Curtis MS, FRCS, FRCS (Gen)
Consultant Surgeon
Luton and Dunstable Hospital
Luton, UK

S.C. Sydney Chung MD, MRCP, FRCS
Reader in Surgery and Chief
of the Combined Endoscopy Unit, Chinese
University of Hong Kong

John D. Corbitt Jr MD, FACS
Diplomates American Board of Surgery
JFK Medical Center
Palm Beach County, Florida, USA

R.J. Donnelly FRCS
The Cardiothoracic Centre
Liverpool, UK

H.J. Espiner MB, FRCS, ChM
Consultant Surgeon
Bristol Royal Infirmary
Bristol, UK

Charles J. Filipi MD
Assistant Professor of Surgery
Department of Surgery
Creighton University
Omaha, Nebraska, USA

J. Fowler FRCS
Department of Urology
Western General Hospital
Edinburgh, UK

J.G. Geraghty FRCS
Department of Surgery
Meath and Adelaide Hospitals
Dublin, Ireland

Ronald A. Hinder MD, PhD
Professor, Department of Surgery
Creighton University
Omaha, Nebraska, USA

John G. Hunter MD, FACS
Assistant Professor of Surgery
Department of Surgery
University of Utah School of Medicine
USA

I.M.C. Macintyre MD, FRCS
Consultant Surgeon
Western General Hospital
Edinburgh, UK

B. Mentges MD
Eberhard-Karls-Universität Tübingen
Klinikum Schnarrenberg
Chirugische Klinik
Tübingen, Germany

Simon Patersen-Brown MS, MPhil, FRCS
Consultant Surgeon
Royal Infirmary
Edinburgh, UK

J.B. Rainey ChM, FRCS (Ed)
Consultant Surgeon
Department of Surgery, St John's Hospital at
Howden Livingston, West Lothian, Scotland,
UK

R.C.G. Russell MS, FRCS
Consultant Surgeon
Pancreatobiliary Unit
The Middlesex Hospital, London, UK

R.J.C. Steele MD, FRCS
Senior Lecturer in Surgery
University of Nottingham, UK

Sung-Tao Ko MD, FACS, FRCS (C)
Chief of Surgical Endoscopy, Mount Sinai
Hospital Medical Center; Associate Clinical
Professor of Surgery, Chicago Medical School,
Chicago, USA

W.A. Tanner MD, FRCS (I)
Consultant Surgeon
Department of Clinical Surgery
Meath and Adelaide Hospitals
Dublin, Ireland

J.E.A. Wickham MS, MB, BSc, FRCS,
FRCP, FRCR
Director of the Academic Unit
Institute of Urology, University of London;
President of the International Society of
Minimally Invasive Therapy

R.G. Wilson ChM, FRCS (Ed)
Consultant Surgeon
Western General Hospital
Edinburgh, UK

Foreword

Minimally-invasive techniques are a revolution in surgery and continue to develop since the first laparoscopic cholecystectomy was performed in 1988, making this the fastest growing area of general surgery. *Practical Laparoscopic Surgery for General Surgeons* gives a practical and pragmatic explanation of laparoscopic procedures, providing a valuable guide for surgeons experienced in the techniques and for those learning them.

Macintyre has brought together a group of respected surgeons in the field from Europe and North America. Each chapter describes surgical procedures where patients benefit more from laparoscopy than from traditional open surgery. Chapters are enhanced with very clear figures, not only of the techniques involved for procedures such as appendicectomy, oesophageal resection or pulmonary surgery, but also of the equipment which is vital for such procedures.

For all general surgeons, *Practical Laparoscopic Surgery for General Surgeons* is essential reading, illuminating this interesting, albeit controversial, subject and giving confidence to use techniques often perceived as being complicated.

Professor D.C. Carter
MD FRCS (Ed) FRCS (Glas)
Regius Professor of Clinical Surgery,
University of Edinburgh

Preface

It is no exaggeration to claim that minimally invasive surgery is the greatest change in general surgical practice this century. The advent of the chip camera has allowed the development of laparoscopy from a diagnostic procedure performed by a single operator into a sub-specialty where many of the commonly performed intra-abdominal and intra-thoracic procedures can be performed by a surgical team. Laparoscopic cholecystectomy demonstrated to surgeons, patients and managers the enormous benefits which laparoscopic techniques could achieve and over a few short years laparoscopic cholecystectomy replaced open cholecystectomy as the procedure of choice. It was inevitable that laparoscopic techniques should be applied to a wide variety of other general surgical procedures to see if similar benefits could be obtained.

The general surgeon has witnessed a revolution—laparoscopic techniques now touch virtually every facet of his work. For a group traditionally cautious about adopting new procedures, the pace of change has been exciting if at times almost alarming. In this text we have attempted to describe the instruments and the techniques which are in common usage. The rate of change was such that it was inevitable that a text such as this would be dated at the time of publication. The fundamental equipment, the basic techniques and many of the more specialised techniques, however, form a core of knowledge which every general surgeon today must acquire.

We have tried to produce a text which will be valuable not only to the surgeon in training but also to the surgeon already practising these techniques whether in developed countries or in the developing world.

If this text provides clarification, understanding and insight into the equipment and techniques of this exciting new area of general surgery then its aim will have been amply fulfilled.

I.M.C. Macintyre
Edinburgh

1

An introduction to minimally invasive therapy

J.E.A. Wickham

The development of the concept of minimally invasive therapy

As little as 10 years ago a patient presenting for treatment of a 1 cm calculus in a kidney was likely to have been subjected to a major operative procedure. The kidney was approached through a 10 inch loin incision disrupting much muscle. The kidney was mobilized and if necessary the parenchyma was incised to obtain access to the calculus which was then removed. The wound was closed with compressive suturing which quite often damaged the blood supply and nerves to the abdominal wall.

In 1979 my radiological colleagues and I at the Institute of Urology decided to explore the possibility of the removal of small calculi from the kidney by an endoscopic procedure. The method adopted was to perform a direct percutaneous puncture into kidney with a fine spinal needle under radiological control. Once the collecting system had been accessed a guide wire was passed down the sheath of the needle and then over the guide wire graduated dilators were introduced to dilate up a track of approximately 26 French. Over the last dilator a hollow plastic sleeve was passed and the dilator removed. We were therefore left with a hollow conduit into the kidney down which suitable endoscopes could be passed to identify the contained calculus and hopefully remove it.

Our first attempts at removing calculi by this method were quite successful. Obviously the size of the stones that could be removed were limited by the dimensions of the access track and the initial endoscopes used were conventional cystoscopes. The calculi were secured in endoscopic baskets and removed, but it soon became apparent that the instruments we were using were totally unsuitable for this type of work. I therefore contacted the instrument manufacturers and laid down a user's specification for purpose-built nephroscopes, the main feature being a large, straight, direct access operating channel and an oblique optic. These instruments became available very quickly and we were then able to pass a series of grabbing alligator forceps of fairly robust construction to secure the stones and remove them.

It also became apparent that we would need some method of tackling larger stones by disintegrating them *in situ* and then removing the pieces. It was again the manufacturers, mainly in West Germany, who had already produced instruments for fragmenting bladder calculi by ultrasound or electrohydraulic discharge, who converted these latter into a suitable form that we could use through our new nephroscopes.

With this instrumentation we were then able to tackle all types of calculi (even up to staghorn configurations), fragment them and remove them satisfactorily. While this new method of removing calculi was possibly more demanding and time consuming, the lack of morbidity experienced by these patients when compared with the previous open surgical techniques was remarkable. Patients who would normally have remained in hospital at least 10–14 days after a nephrolithotomy were able to leave hospital after 3 days and resume their normal activities within 5–7 days. There was no need for the usual lengthy convalescence of about 6 weeks after open surgery.

Using these methods we were able to treat at least 98% of all renal calculi satisfactorily and it was only in 1982 when the first commercially available extracorporeal lithotripters became available from the Dornier company in Munich, West Germany, that we again needed to revise our technique of nephrolithotomy.

The concept of extracorporeally disintegrating calculi by shockwaves, so brilliantly conceived by Professor Eisenberger, then changed the whole face of renal stone surgery. The first Dornier lithotripter in England was installed in the Welbeck Clinic in 1983 and during the course of 2 1/2 years over 1,200 patients were treated on this machine with a stone clearance rate of 92%. This method of extracorporeal lithotripsy with no trauma of access to the patient resulted in an even greater reduction in therapeutic complications. Patients were hospitalized for 3 days and then able to leave almost immediately. The Dornier lithotripter had one disadvantage – it was painful therapy which required general anaesthesia.

In 1984 when the second generation Piezolithotripters became available from Germany lithotripsy advanced further. The great advantage of the Piezolith was pain-free treatment. The device induced shockwaves by an array of Piezoelectric elements each producing a small shockwave which passed through an individual path into the body. The shockwaves were focused at a 2 mm area on the surface of the stone and the Piezolith units activated simultaneously. A pressure of 150 kilobars was induced at the site of impact, thus crumbling the stone. The patient was not able to appreciate the passage of the shockwaves and the procedure became painless and reduced treatment to the status of a 'walk in/walk out' therapy. Patients needed no hospitalization, no period of convalescence and the results of therapy after close follow-up over several years demonstrated that this machine was as effective in removing renal calculi as previous methods. Because this machine was 'gentler', – staged treatments were sometimes required to fragment the stones – on average about three attendances in a totally unselected series of stones of all types and sizes. The patients, however, were quite happy to accede to this method of treatment as they were not undergoing any significant trauma.

At about this time we reviewed our results of open surgery, percutaneous nephrolithotomy by endoscope and Dornier lithotripsy in nearly matched groups of 350 patients. We found that our complication rate had fallen from a level of 132 quite major complications for open surgery to that of only 37 relatively minor complications for Dornier lithotripsy. This series was later updated to second generation lithotripsy to include 350 patients treated by Piezolithotripsy when the complication rate had dropped even further to 15, again with fairly minor problems (Table 1.1).

In 1984/1985 my colleagues and I at the Institute of Urology began to focus our attention on the significance of these results and it

Table 1.1   Stone surgery

Complication (350 patients)	Open surgery	PCN	ESWL 1	ESWL 2
Cardiac	10	10	11	–
Pulmonary	43	1	1	–
Gastrointestinal	4	–	–	–
Renal failure	11	–	1	–
Septicaemia	11	34	5	2
Upper tract obstruction	6	12	15	13
Leaking fistulae	21	5	–	–
Wound infection	26	–	–	–
More than one complication	43	4	4	1
Total complication	132	62	37	15

became rapidly apparent that a sequence of events of some significance was taking place. Clearly the events we were witnessing appeared to result entirely from the lack of iatrogenic surgical trauma inflicted on patients to achieve the same therapeutic result, i.e. removal of their stones. We as surgeons had obviously been inflicting considerable trauma on these patients which, by the introduction of suitable technology, could be avoided. We therefore began to look at other areas of surgical practice and an examination of the literature of other specialities revealed that we were certainly not unique within urology and that analogous changes were rapidly taking place in other areas. One immediate example was the substitution of the dangerous and often difficult open exploration of the common bile duct by retrograde endoscopic sphincterotomy for gallstone removal and the simple endoscopic diathermy ablation of the endometrium instead of hysterectomy for menorrhagia. These considerations encouraged me to write editorials for the *British Medical Bulletin* on endoscopic surgery in 1986 and the *British Medical Journal* in 1987 entitled 'The New Surgery'. It also seemed to us at the Institute of Urology that a new terminology was required to encapsulate this concept, and the best that we could suggest at this time was the term 'minimally invasive surgery'. This title, although clumsy, appears to have been adopted worldwide in the last few years.

In pursuit of our thinking we set up the first Department of Minimally Invasive Surgery at the Institute of Urology in 1985 with the express purpose of developing techniques of urological surgery devoted to the elimination of iatrogenic trauma as far as was possible. In this area we achieved some success. For example, my colleague Graham Watson was intimately concerned with the development of the pulsed dye laser and the miniureteroscope for the atraumatic treatment of difficult ureteric calculi. This technique, coupled with extracorporeal lithotripsy and percutaneous nephrolithotomy, totally eliminated the need for any open surgery for the treatment of ureteric or renal calculi. With my radiological colleague, Michael Kellett, we developed the operation of endoscopic pyelolysis for the treatment of pelvi-ureteric junction obstruction which again eliminated the need for any open surgery for this condition and removed

another open operation from the surgical repertoire.

Further discussion with colleagues in other disciplines followed and it became apparent that there was much to learn from these various fields of activity. Among these was the pioneering work of Palmer and Semm in the field of laparoscopic gynaecology, and of Dubois and Perissat in endoscopic cholecystectomy. Also in interventional radiology entirely new concepts of therapy were being pursued with intravascular embolization and organ stenting, removing the need of recourse to open surgery.

It appeared that we were now entering an entirely new phase of cold interventional therapy and that the open surgery of the scalpel and the operating table were rapidly being replaced by the far less traumatic techniques of the endoscope and the radiologically placed guide wire and catheter. Advances in surgery have not necessarily progressed in a smooth continuum but often in a series of quantum leaps in technology which can be easily defined. From prehistoric times to the middle of the last century, in the pre-anaesthetic era of surgery, procedures were limited to crude amputation, drainage of abscesses and the occasional removal of bladder stones with severe trauma and morbidity, frequently resulting in death.

From 1846, following the introduction of anaesthesia, conventional open surgery as we know it developed, and by careful and meticulous operative procedures many organ systems were accessed and treated though with some considerable limitations due primarily to the risk of sepsis and blood loss.

From 1945 to the mid 1970s, however, with the introduction of antibiotic therapy, blood transfusion and intensive care facilities, surgery was able to expand but occasionally to undesirable levels of iatrogenic trauma. In this period, massive surgical procedures were sometimes undertaken with little thought being given to the ultimate welfare or benefit of the patient. Some of the excesses, particularly of oncological surgery carried out during this period, can only be deplored.

From 1975 onwards there appeared the beginning of a change in attitude to more conservative surgery with more critical thought being given to the reduction of this iatrogenic trauma. In my own speciality of renal stone surgery I began to use vascular arterial occlusion during open surgery with regional hypothermia to protect function, which allowed the operation of nephrolithotomy to become a much more controlled and accurate procedure with minimal blood loss.

From about 1985 a much more conservative approach to surgery developed in a number of specialities. From that time there was increasing awareness of the concept of minimal invasiveness with its very obvious advantage in the reduction of interventional trauma.

It is also interesting to speculate on the nature of iatrogenic surgical traumas that were bringing about the complications that we had become so used to in open surgery. I can identify five obvious areas.

1. The pharmacological trauma of the anaesthetic and the considerable analgesia required post-operatively following massive 'open' surgical procedures.

2. The trauma of access to the target organ which is quite often extensive in procedures such as cardiac, rectal and renal surgery.

3. Haemodynamic trauma engendered by extensive surgical procedures demanding massive blood replacement.

4. The trauma of the definitive therapeutic procedure which when compared to the ones above often appears to be quite minor, i.e. the actual removal of a stone from the kidney once exposed.

5. Equally importantly is the extensive psychological trauma inflicted on a patient both pre- and post-operatively who is scheduled for and undergoes conventional surgery.

These traumas may be conveniently discussed in relation to my own professional interests in nephrolithotomy and can be identified by Figure 1.1.

As one passes from open surgery through percutaneous nephrolithotomy to first and second generation lithotripsy these traumas are seen to be dramatically reduced. For example, second generation lithotripsy requires no anaesthesia and negligible analgesia, and surgical access which previously required a massive loin incision with gross muscle destruction has

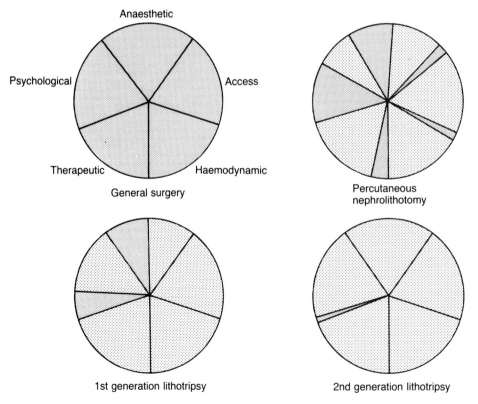

General surgery

Percutaneous nephrolithotomy

1st generation lithotripsy

2nd generation lithotripsy

Fig. 1.1

been obviated. The haemodynamic trauma is ablated with no blood loss during lithotripsy (compared with the 4–6 units frequently required for an open renal stone operation). The trauma of the definitive procedure is negligible when compared with the multiple nephrotomies and parenchymal damage caused to the kidney by extracting stones at open surgery. Finally the psychological trauma is almost ablated and with second generation lithotripsy is removed. Within one decade, therefore, we have progressed from a situation where a patient is exposed to an extensive physical and psychological upheaval to a position where he or she is little inconvenienced and the same therapeutic result has been achieved.

In other fields of surgical therapy similar results are now being obtained. For example, in gynaecology the technique of endometrial ablation for menorrhagia is rapidly replacing conventional hysterectomy, with all its unpleasant sequelae. In gastroenterology the potentially disabling operations of gastrectomy and vagotomy have happily been almost replaced by the pharmacological treatment of peptic ulceration with H2 receptor antagonists. Likewise surgery of the biliary tree has been transformed by the advent of ERCP and laparoscopic cholecystectomy. Treatment of obliterative vascular disease is being increasingly undertaken by the interventional radiologists in both peripheral and coronary arteries. Perhaps before long the vastly invasive operation of coronary artery bypass surgery will be superseded by intravascular balloon dilatation, laser disobliteration or similar techniques. In orthopaedics endoscopy of most large joints is now being achieved and it will probably not be long before total hip replacement will be substituted by the endoscopic relining of joint surfaces with chondrocyte grafts or artificial materials. In ear, nose and throat surgery, endoscopic laser therapy of tumours of the larynx, pharynx and base of the skull is reducing the need for mutilating operations.

It appears therefore that enormous changes are rapidly taking place in the whole of the surgical and radiological environment, the mainspring of which is the desire to reduce therapeutic trauma by the increasing application of physical technology. It is in this regard that the instrument engineers are assuming an increasingly important role in the furtherance of our work.

The consequences of minimally invasive therapy

It is rapidly becoming obvious that the emergence of these minimally invasive techniques is beginning to have a profound effect in several important areas of patient management.

Hospital design

Rapid recovery and speed of passage of these patients during their treatment reduce the requirement for prolonged inpatient hospital care. Many of these procedures can be carried out as a day case or more usually on a one night stay basis and the need for the 'large hotel' type of hospital accommodation will surely recede rapidly. In the United States over 60% of all elective surgery is carried out as a day case procedure. Although Europe is at present lagging behind, I am sure that within the next 5 years similar figures will be achieved on this side of the Atlantic.

In terms of hospital design it would seem that stand alone, single storey, 'production line units' in areas with good car parking and good transport access will replace the old type of 500–1500 bed 'mega institutions'. For the overnight stay following the surgical procedure, hostel accommodation only will be required. Thus minimally invasive therapy or day surgery is economically advantageous to both patients and society in general. There is far less use of hospital resources and greater flexibility for the patient to make his or her own choice as to timing of therapy.

Nurses involved in minimally invasive therapy will have to deal with more patients and will require specialist training for the increasing variety of new treatments becoming available. This type of practice has considerable psychological advantages, particularly for children, but also for adults because of the early return to work or other activities, earlier access to treatment and reduction of hospital-acquired infections. With better organization and co-operation between hospital, clinic and community care organizations, monitoring of the rapidly discharged patient should gradually be improved but it will inevitably lead to a larger workload for community practitioners.

Within these centres operating room design will also change radically from the simple concept of the operating table and scalpel to the purpose-built and designed interventional suite containing radiological, ultrasonic and endoscopic facilities, multiple monitor displays and other ancillary instrumentation. Increasingly with MIT, surgery is becoming endoscopic but the operator no longer looks directly through the eyepiece of the endoscope but, with suitable camera attachments, watches and performs the procedure by directly observing the television screen. This has the enormous advantage that everybody in the operating theatre can see exactly what is being undertaken by the surgeon. In this way they not only maintain their interest but also actively intervene to assist in the operative process. Mechanisms for the rapid delivery of patients to and their removal from the operating theatre are already in train.

A total reappraisal of the mechanisms of achieving asepsis during the operative process will have to be undertaken and for many procedures it would seem totally unnecessary for the operator to 'gown up' and wear a cap and mask. As with interventional radiology it is quite often sufficient for the operator to wear just a simple scrub suit and a pair of sterile gloves. A vast amount of saving could be made in the reduction of the supply of sterile operating clothing. This saving may, however, be outweighed by the need for more complicated methods of sterilization of endoscopes so that this can be performed rapidly between larger numbers of cases passing quickly through the units.

The type of doctor

Even more major changes seem certain in surgery in the next decade. With increasing input from other disciplines into the interventional process it is now computed that there are no less than 200 groups of allied health personnel other than doctors currently involved in the therapeutic process. Obviously, not all of these are associated with intervention but a number of specialities are already assuming the therapeutic role dominated until recently by conventional surgeons. The most important group is, of course, the interventional radiologists who are performing such operations as intrabiliary stenting and therapeutic embolization. Also of considerable importance are the physician–gastroenterologists who are now doing most of the ERCPs, procedures for biliary tract stones and therapeutic colonoscopy that used to be the province of the general surgeon.

It also seems very likely that new groups will form and a team approach to therapy will emerge with the conventional surgeon comprising a much smaller element of the group which may be under the control of a director of interventional therapy who will in all probability be a physician (Figure 1.2). It seems inevitable that no one person can acquire expertise in all these various disciplines. So surgeons appear almost destined to become pure technologists despite the hope that they might remain the all-encompassing 'physician who operates'. I am sure that the descriptive title for such an interventionist is of little consequence to the patient as long as the

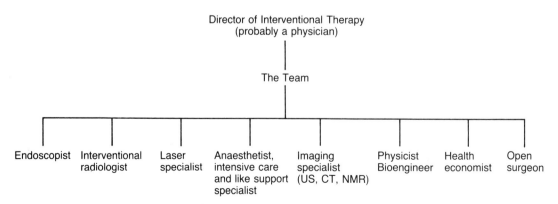

Fig. 1.2

treatment is expeditious, atraumatic and efficient. Whether this is carried out by a surgeon, physician or interventional radiologist is quite immaterial. It would therefore seem that surgeons are reluctantly going to have to accept the changing status whereby they will only be one member of a group of interventionists and not necessarily as at present 'the leader of the pack'.

Changes in speciality boundaries

As a result of the changes described above, the speciality boundaries will also become realigned. A skilled endoscopist can now encompass the therapy of various organ systems such as endoscopic nephrolithotomy, endoscopic cholecystectomy, endoscopic endometrial ablation, endoscopic appendicectomy, endoscopic hernia repair, etc. Professor Roy Calne has posed the pertinent question: 'Is there any reason why an expert arthroscopist needs to be trained as a general physician?' It may well be that specific physicians will after diagnosis direct the patient to the most efficient 'subcontractor interventionist'. As long as he or she is expert at their task they need not have an extensive medical knowledge.

The long-held concept that the surgeon needs to be expert in pre-operative and particularly post-operative patient care and resuscitation is likewise being rapidly eroded by the anaesthetists and intensive care physicians who are far more skilled in the metabolic and biochemical management of the patient in the post-operative period than the average surgeon. This is perhaps a further reason why technical therapy could probably be carried out by less generally trained interventionists.

These changing concepts will obviously have a profound effect on surgical training. It would seem possible that increasingly large amounts of surgical interventional therapy are going to be undertaken by endoscopy and it would seem somewhat illogical primarily to train a surgeon as a butcher or an anatomical dissector as is now the case. Surely he should have a primary training as a microendoscopist and possibly as a bioengineer with much less emphasis on open surgery as the key discipline in interventional therapy. In fact when one regards the whole spectrum of advancing surgical therapy it seems that even in a fall

back situation it will be increasingly unnecessary to revert to an open operating technique. Many situations such as haemorrhage in practically any organ in the body can be managed by the interventional radiologist using selective embolization. Again collections of biological fluids can be drained quite often percutaneously under local anaesthesia by interventional radiology rather than open drainage procedures, a particularly valuable alternative for the unfit patient.

Health economists

These radically changing techniques are inevitably going to alter the whole attitude of the health economist to interventional therapy. Whether health care continues to be funded by government centrally or by individual insurance policies it is important to impress upon the suppliers of such funds that these new techniques are going to require a shift of resource from long-stay hospital accommodation to short-stay treatment requiring the use of expensive high technology. Money will have to be diverted to develop and purchase more complex instrumentation with less money being required for hotel services. In many countries it has proved difficult to get this message across and to persuade the financiers of this need to transfer budgeting from one area to another. Insurance companies in particular seem happy to ride on the back of the success of the minimal interventionist whose techniques result in reduced expenditure on inpatient hospital care. The interventionist, however, continues to be rewarded as if the patient had had conventional open surgery with little account of the increased cost of technology used and no recognition of the skill involved in new procedures.

The Society of Minimally Invasive Therapy

Following the considerations expressed above it was felt in 1989 that attempts should be made to bring together these diverse strands of interest into one recognizable society. It was thought that this society should comprise of those surgeons particularly interested in minimally invasive techniques, the interventional radiologists who are attacking the problem from a slightly different direction and finally, and even more importantly, the instrument manufacturers upon whom the success of all these procedures vitally depends.

With this aim in mind a number of interested parties inaugurated the first meeting of the Society of Minimally Invasive Therapy at the Royal Institution, London, in December 1989. As discussion progressed through the first morning of the meeting, the feeling was very much expressed by one of the leaders of the radiologists that they did not wish to be constrained under the banner of 'surgery'. It was therefore suggested that the term 'minimally invasive surgery' should be substituted by the term 'minimally invasive therapy' to encompass all disciplines and this was agreed by the society. Since this inaugural meeting the society has progressed rapidly and has had four further international meetings – one in Vienna, Austria, in 1990, Boston, USA, in 1991, Dublin in 1992 and Orlando in 1993. The society now has its own *Journal of Minimally Invasive Therapy* and the aim of both the society and the journal is to provide a forum for any clinicians, medical ancillary workers or manufacturers to present and discuss speculative and innovate techniques which would be of interest to all specialities. Under the umbrella of 'minimally invasive therapy' we have the interests of general surgeons, vascular surgeons, neurosurgeons, otorhinolaryngologists, gynaecologists, urologists, orthopaedic surgeons, ophthalmologists, interventional radiologists, health economists, lawyers and, most importantly, excellent contributions from industry and the instrument manufacturers. At our meeting in Boston in 1991 over 500 delegates attended and presented papers both on innovations and on larger series of already established minimally invasive techniques. We look forward to even larger gatherings in the future.

Conclusion

It is apparent that the ultimate consequences of these changes in interventional therapy are likely to be profound. Paramount in our thinking is the reduction in mortality and morbidity that is being experienced by our patients from the development of these techniques and this must remain our guiding purpose. Changes deriving from this seminal shift in philosophy are considerable and are only just beginning to be appreciated by those in the medical profession who do not yet practise interventional therapy and by those who administer health services.

The pace of change is rapid and the changes are radical. At the fall of the Bastille in 1789 King Louis XVI asked the Duke de Rochfoucald 'C'est une revolt?'; the Duke replied 'Non sire, est une revolution.' There is little doubt that we are in the throes of a revolution, more importantly for our patients and only a little less so for ourselves the physicians.

Further reading

Calne, R.Y. (1991). OK surgical technology. *British Medical Journal*, **301**, 1479–80.

Dubois, F., Icaro, P., Berthelot, G. and Levard, H. (1990). Coelioscopic cholecystectomy. Preliminary report of 36 cases. *Annals of Surgery*, **211**, 60–2.

Wickham, J.E.A. (1987). The new surgery *British Medical Journal*, **295**, 1581–2.

2

Equipment and instruments for laparoscopic surgery

I.M.C. Macintyre

Advances in laparoscopic surgery have been made possible by improvements in video technology and instruments. There is little doubt that forthcoming years will see further developments and innovations in both instruments and electronic technology which will allow continuing expansion of endoscopic surgery. The equipment for laparoscopic surgery can be classified under four headings:

1. Equipment for visualization.
2. Equipment to establish and maintain pneumoperitoneum.
3. Power sources.
4. Surgical instruments.

Video equipment

Video equipment for endoscopic surgery can be considered under the following headings:

1. Light course.
2. Telescopes.
3. Video camera system.
4. Monitors.
5. Video recorder.

Light source (Figure 2.1)

Light is conducted to the endoscope by a fibre-optic cable. Modern light sources provide cold light. It is important to appreciate that this refers to the spectrum of light delivered and that the light produced from the end of the fibre-optic cable and from the end of the telescope has sufficient heat to scorch the

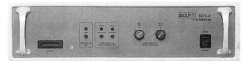

Fig. 2.1 Light source.

drapes or the patient. The power of the light source varies from 100 watts to 300–400 watts and uses a xenon, halogen or tungsten lamp. Modern light sources are fitted with automatic brightness controls which vary the light strength delivered according to the light strength of the incoming video signal, thereby providing greater illumination for long-distance shots and reducing glare when the telescope is close to the subject being illuminated. Light sources are also fitted with an emergency lamp which will automatically cut-in in case of failure of the primary lamp.

Telescopes

Modern laparoscopes (Figure 2.2) use the Hopkins lens system which gives better definition of the image. Instead of the traditional lens–air–lens system, the Hopkins optical system uses a series of glass rods with lenses placed at appropriate intervals along the shaft of the instrument. This provides better resolution and contrast, a wider viewing angle in a single viewing field, fibre-optic light transmission and allows the use of smaller instruments with a smaller outside diameter. The telescope allows the illumination and magnification

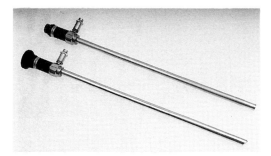

Fig. 2.2 The modern laparoscope.

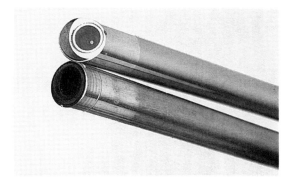

Fig. 2.3 Laparoscope showing 0° and 30° angulation.

which enhance laparoscopic surgery. Telescopes can be either forward viewing (or 0°) or fore-oblique (either 25° or 30°) (Figure 2.3). For laparoscopic cholecystectomy most surgeons use a 0° forward viewing instrument. For other operative procedures a 30° instrument may be preferable where the ability to 'see round corners' is an advantage.

Both 5 mm and 10 mm telescopes are required for therapeutic laparoscopy. The 5 mm instrument may be used at an alternative entry site (usually in the upper quadrant of the abdomen) where standard subumbilical trocar entry is contraindicated, usually because of a midline scar.

Misting of telescopes, which is common in the abdominal cavity, can be overcome in several ways. The telescope may be warmed before insertion either by placing in a water bath or by holding it in warm hands. Fogging during the procedure may be reduced by cleaning the lens with a dry swab and treating it with a demisting agent such as Ultrastop. Alternatively the lens may be wiped by a sponge which has been impregnated with such a solution (FRED, Dexide Inc., Fort Worth).

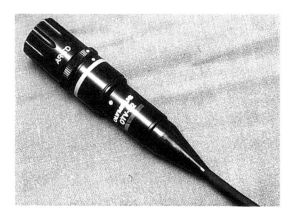

Fig. 2.4 A single CCD camera.

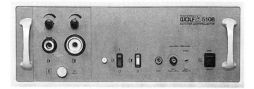

Fig. 2.5 Camera unit.

Video camera system

Video cameras are becoming progressively smaller and lighter with improvements in electronic optics. The development of the CCD (charge-couple device) or 'chip' camera in 1986 (Figure 2.4) paved the way for the wider use of therapeutic laparoscopy. Most video cameras used for laparoscopy will couple onto a standard optical eyepiece using an adapter without much loss of definition and without loss of light. The camera systems can be sterilized by immersion in solutions like

activated gluteraldehyde, although it is preferable to use a sterile plastic sleeve to avoid this and prevent the need for immersion (Figure 2.5). The camera system will also include automatic adjustment of white balance and allow manual adjustment of red and blue colours. Automatic measurement of the light from the subject provides an automatic increase in the light to the subject usually down to a minimum of 15 lux. Standard video cameras operate on a single 'chip' or CCD. A

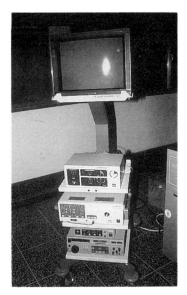

Fig. 2.6 A 'stack' for minimally invasive surgery showing monitor, insufflator, light source/camera unit and video tape recorder.

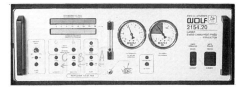

Fig. 2.7 CO_2 insufflator.

typical camera CCD contains up to 300,000 pixels giving high definition with a horizontal resolution of more than 400 lines. Three-CCD cameras are now available with a total of over 1 million pixels giving a horizontal resolution of more than 600 lines. Whether the greater cost of such cameras can be justified by significantly enhanced visualization remains to be seen.

Monitors

High resolution television monitors are available, the size depending on the particular procedure (Figure 2.6). For laparoscopic work two 19 inch or 21 inch monitors are recommended. These monitors are most conveniently mounted on a trolley at eye level for the surgeon and assistant. Medium or high

resolution monitors should be used for laparoscopic surgery giving more than 400 lines of horizontal resolution. High definition monitors giving 600–700 lines of resolution are now available and those giving 1,100 lines of resolution will soon be available.

Video recorder

A video recorder, while not essential, is highly desirable for endoscopic surgery. Review of recorded procedures can be a valuable contribution to training, in assessing intra-operative reasons for subsequent complications and, of course, for teaching and demonstrations. Archive recordings of the procedure may, in future, be of value in defence against litigation.

The choice of VHS, SVHS or U-matic depends upon the prevailing local system and the funding available. High band U-matic gives high quality reproduction and is close to a world standard at present. VHS, even more widely available, gives lesser quality reproduction and SVHS is not as yet widely available.

Equipment for pneumoperitoneum

Insufflator

Pneumoperitoneum for laparoscopic surgery should be established and maintained using an appropriate insufflator (Figure 2.7). Ideally the insufflator should run from a 1 litre CO_2 cylinder (which will provide approximately 350 litres of carbon dioxide gas). Visual displays must show the pressure of CO_2 in the cylinder, the volume of CO_2 which has been insufflated into the patient and the intra-abdominal pressure. There should be a control to preset the selected intra-abdominal pressure – usually 13–15 mm of mercury but in some instances as low as 7 mm of mercury. The insufflator should be able to deliver preset gas flows of 1 litre per minute for initial filling and 3–4 litres per minute for the second stage of filling. There should also be an automatic high flow setting to maintain intraperitoneal pressure constant at the preset level during the operation. CO_2 is delivered to the patient via an Luer-lock connector to which standard plastic tubing is connected. This tubing is connected to the Veress needle.

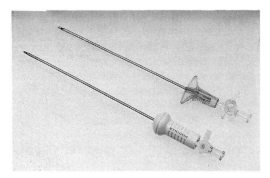

Fig. 2.8. Disposable Veress needles.

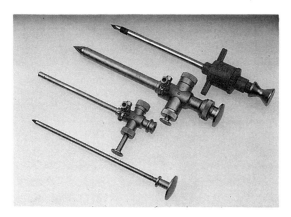

Fig. 2.9 Reusable trocar and cannulae.

Veress needle (Figure 2.8)

The Veress needle was originally designed to induce pneumoperitoneum in the treatment of pulmonary tuberculosis. With minimal modification it has become the standard way to induce the pneumoperitoneum. The needle has a spring-loaded obturator which retracts as the needle passes through the anterior abdominal wall and springs forward to cover the tip when resistance drops as the peritoneal cavity is entered. Reusable and disposable varieties are available.

Hassan valve

The Hassan valve was designed to induce a safe pneumoperitoneum in patients where multiple previous abdominal scars contraindicate the passage of a Veress needle. A small incision is made through the skin and anterior abdominal wall and the peritoneum is entered under direct vision. The Hassan valve is placed into the peritoneal cavity so as to create a gas-tight seal and is held in place by sutures through the skin of the anterior abdominal wall. CO_c insufflation is then carried out in the usual way.

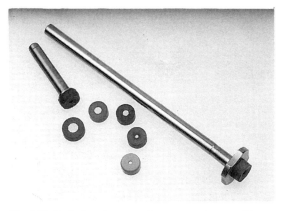

Fig. 2.10 Reducing sleeves and grommets for reusable cannulae.

Trocar and cannula

Trocars and cannulae provide access into the peritoneal cavity for laparoscopes and ˌinstruments. They are available in a variety of external diameters. For laparoscopic cholecystectomy 5 mm and 10 mm trocars are used. For larger instruments 12 mm and 18 mm cannulae are available and for extraction of bulky tissue 30 mm and 40 mm cannulae have been used.

Traditional trocars and canulae are stainless steel and reusable (Figure 2.9). The trocar requires to be resharpened at regular intervals. The cannula has a bevelled end to reduce the possibility of the end being occluded by tissue. A gas-tight seal is provided by a spring-loaded trumpet valve which allows passage of instruments with minimal loss of gas. Incorporated into each cannula is a stopcock with a tap to allow continued insufflation of CO_2 through the cannula.

An air-tight seal at the top end of the cannula is provided by rubber grommets.

By using 5 mm adapters or downsizers (Figure 2.10) 10/11 mm cannulae may be converted to accept 5 mm instruments. For reusable cannulae these adapters or converters are 5 mm metal cylinders which pass through

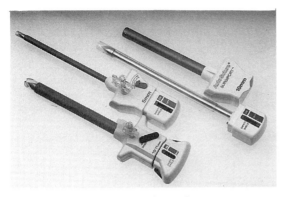

Fig. 2.11 Disposable trocar and cannulae.

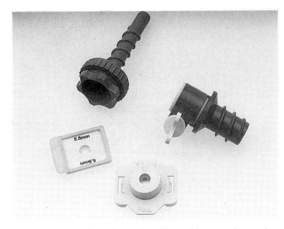

Fig. 2.12 Reducing adapter for disposable cannulae and Surgigrip for USSC cannulae.

the trumpet valve holding it open, the gas-tight seal being provided by a 5 mm bung at the top of the adapter tube. Adapters for disposable trocars (Figure 2.11) are rectangular plates which form a gas-tight seal against the rectangular top of the cannula. A 5 mm aperture provides a gas-tight seal around the instruments.

Some disposable cannulae (Endopath Ethicon Ltd) incorporate a mechanism to prevent the cannula slipping out of the anterior abdominal wall after insertion (Figure 2.12). This takes the form of a plastic corkscrew incorporated into the shaft of the cannula. Other types have a detachable corkscrew device which may be fitted over the cannula before placement into the anterior abdominal wall (Surgigrip, Autosuture).

Power sources

Power sources for laparoscopic surgery are required to coagulate and to cut tissue. Two principal sources are commonly used:
1. Electrosurgery.
2. Laser.

Electrosurgery

Modern electrosurgical generators (or diathermy units) produce an electrical current with a radio frequency between 500 and 750 kilohertz. The frequency is too rapid to produce cell depolarization so that no electrical shock is produced but the tissues are heated. The current from modern electrosurgical generators can produce three types of waveform. In cutting mode the waveform is a pure high frequency alternating current which produces highest tissue heating. Tissue may be heated to over 100°C at which temperature it is vaporized. The energy does not pass deeply into the tissue which limits both the thermal injury and the coagulating effect.

In coagulating mode the current is also a pure sine wave but is produced in short bursts. This has the effect of slowing and limiting the heating effect thereby producing a greater coagulating effect.

Blended current, as the name suggests, is a combination of the above modes and the waveform consists of bursts of high amplitude sine wave passing the cutting current but interspersed with low voltage current. Many electrosurgical units allow the surgeon to modify the ratio of cutting to coagulating current enabling him to define accurately the current in a spectrum between pure cutting and pure coagulating.

In laparoscopic surgery monopolar rather than bipolar systems are used. In such systems the electrical energy is delivered to the tissue through a wire connected to the dissecting or coagulating instrument, the circuit being completed by the earthing (grounding) pad attached to the patient, usually on the thigh.

A recent modification of standard electrosurgical coagulation is the argon beam coagulation system (Beacon Laboratories Inc., Colorado, USA). This system can be used in conjunction with many standard electrosurgical units. A stream of argon gas conducts the coagulating current to the target tissue, providing a more uniform flow of energy with less tissue damage. The tip may be held up to a centimetre away from the target tissue and the inert argon gas, which flows at 2 litres per minute, clears bleeding to allow better visualization and more precise coagulation of bleeding vessels. The argon beam produces a 2–3 mm eschar on the surface of the bleeding tissue.

Thermal lasers

Laser is an acronym for *l*ight *a*mplification by *s*timulated *e*mission of *r*adiation. The lasers used as a power source for laparoscopic surgery are thermal lasers. A pure laser produces light that is coherent (i.e. the wavelengths are always in phase), monochromatic (the light is all of one wavelength) and collimated (the paths of the photons and thus the laser beam remain perfectly parallel throughout its path). In practice, although surgical lasers are monochromatic some produce more than one colour. Collimation is not absolute and coherence is lost when the laser beam passes through a wave guide or fibre-optic cable. Laser power output is measured in watts but it is the power density (measured in watts per square centimetre) which is more relevant to the surgeon as this directly determines the thermal effect. This power density depends upon both the total output of the laser and also the spot size, the surface area on which the laser beam is concentrated. The spot size in turn depends upon how the laser beam is delivered and how it is focused.

Another important phenomenon which alters the efficacy of the laser is its interaction with the target tissue. For greatest efficacy the laser should be absorbed by the tissue which results in the laser power being converted into thermal energy. The efficacy may be reduced by reflection of the laser from the surface of the tissue, transmission through the tissue without absorption or scattering of the laser beam energy within the tissue. Absorption depends upon the wavelength of the tissue; thus the argon laser will be absorbed by haemoglobin and the Nd:YAG laser absorbed by tissue protein.

Three lasers have been commonly used in laparoscopic surgery. The Nd:YAG laser

produces light in the infrared part of the spectrum; the KTP/YAG laser (in which the Nd:YAG laser wavelength is halved by a KTP (potassium–titanyl–phosphate) crystal allowing the operator to switch between a wavelength of 1064 and 532 nm); the KTP/532 laser which produces light of wavelength 532 nm; and the argon laser which produces light from the blue part of the electromagnetic spectrum.

Laser energy may be delivered by contact or non-contact methods. In contact methods a variety of contact laser probes made of sapphire crystal (which has low thermal conductivity and high melting temperature) are fixed to the end of the probe and contact the tissues directly. These come in a variety of shapes for cutting or coagulation. In the non-contact technique the bare fibre is used to cut or coagulate. This has the disadvantage that only the tip of the fibre rather than the side is active and past pointing injuries to distant tissues may occur accidentally. The disadvantage of the contact technique is that the contact probe remains hot for up to 10 seconds after activation with the theoretical risk of injury of contact burn of adjacent tissues. It is also more expensive.

Instruments for laparoscopic surgery

The development of instruments for laparoscopic surgery is in its infancy. Continuing and increasing development of these instruments will result in the application of laparoscopic therapeutic techniques to an ever-wider range of therapeutic procedures.

Forceps

Grasping forceps have a wide variety of uses. These may be traumatic 'or atraumatic. Traumatic forceps should be applied only to tissue which is to be resected, while atraumatic forceps are applied to tissue which is not to be resected. Atraumatic grasping forceps may be smooth or serrated. Traumatic forceps have coarser serration or may be toothed (Figure 2.13). Commonly used general grasping forceps include the Reddick-Olsen (Storz) and the Semm claw grasping forceps (Storz). Spring-loaded forceps with two, three or four grasping limbs are available (Weck).

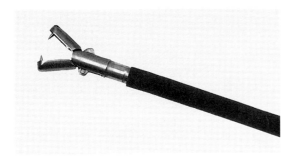

Fig. 2.13 Toothed grasping forceps.

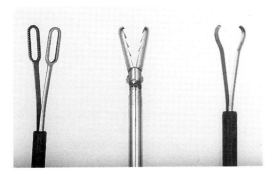

Fig. 2.14 Atraumatic graspers.

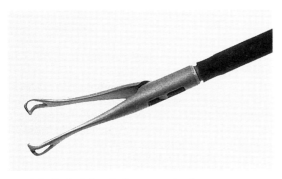

Fig. 2.15 Endo Babcock tissue grasping forceps.

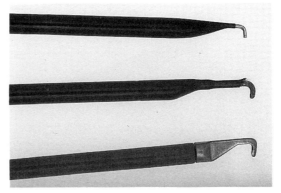

Fig. 2.16 Dissecting hook.

most appropriate. Bowel grasping forceps such as the Dorsey are used to grasp and retract bowel which is not to be resected. Variations on the theme have been developed by Micro France. These include the Meyer directional jaw forceps which allow the jaws of the forceps to be moved through 90°.

Disposable forceps designed for single use are also now available – Endograsp (USSC).

Tissue forceps, based on the tissue forceps used in conventional open surgery, are used for similar indications in laparoscopic surgery (Figures 2.14 and 2.15). The Congreve–Allis and the Congreve–Babcock have been developed by Mueller (Baxter Healthcare). Biopsy forceps are used primarily to biopsy peritoneal lesions but are used increasingly to biopsy lesions on viscera. The double-spoon design is

Dissecting instruments

Dissection in laparoscopic surgery, as in conventional surgery, may be sharp or blunt. For blunt dissection the curved dissector (Micro-France) is of particular use when dissecting around large curved structures such as the oesophagus or major vascular pedicles. The Maryland dissector is similar with straight jaws. Dissection where a plane of cleavage between tissues (e.g. between liver and gallbladder) can be established using the spatula dissector.

For sharp dissection the hook electrode initially developed by Dubois is available from several companies (Storz, Wolf) (Figure 2.16). This is used to divide tissues (which have been put under tension by appropriate retraction) by passing a coagulating or cutting current across the top. These, combined with suction (Storz) and disposable hook electrode–sucker–irrigators, are also now available (Valleylab). Sharp dissection may also be carried out by scissors (Figure 2.17). Dissecting scissors based on the conventional Metzenbaum or Macindoe have been designed by Hugh (Standard Instant Pty). Scissors with a single moving blade and with blades curved to a hook at the tip (hook scissors) are used to divide tissues.

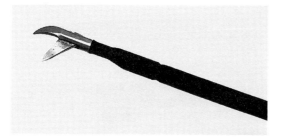

Fig. 2.17 Endoscopic scissors – single moving blade.

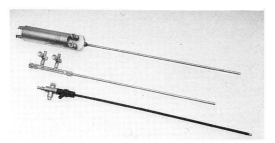

Fig. 2.18 Suction/irrigation devices.

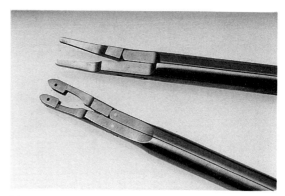

Fig. 2.19 Reusable clip appliers.

Suction irrigation instruments

Suction/irrigation devices (Figure 2.18) combine conventional suction with irrigation of saline or antibiotic solution. These can be controlled either by trumpet valves (Wolf) or by a tap (Storz). These are also available combined with a dissecting hook (Valleylab) or with a coagulating tip.

Clip appliers

Blood vessels which are too large to coagulate may be clipped before division. Available clip appliers include the Ligaclip range (Ethicon). The 10 mm diameter clip applier may be used to apply 9 mm or 5 mm titanium or stainless steel clips. The Absolok clip applier (Ethicon) applies self-locking clips made of PDS which are absorbable. Of the disposable clip appliers (Figure 2.19) the Endoclip Applier (USSC) delivers 15 (9 mm) clips. All of these instruments can be turned on their long axis through 360° to enable the angled jaws to be placed in the most appropriate position for application of the clip.

Cholangiography equipment

Operative cholangiography may be performed using a cholangiogram clamp (Reddick–Olsen,

Storz). This enables a fine (3F or 4F) catheter to be clamped securely within the cystic duct allowing a water-tight seal. Alternatively a cholangiogram catheter such as the Arrow–Karlan may be used. This is inserted into the cystic duct where it is held in place by a 0.6 ml balloon which also prevents backflow of blood and bile.

Needle holders

Laparoscopic suturing is becoming increasingly used. A variety of sutures have been designed with straight, curved and ski-shaped needles. These needles can be triangular in cross section to prevent twisting of the needle in the jaws of the needle holder. According to the size of the needle 3 mm, 5 mm and 10 mm needle holders may be used. While these are of conventional design other needle holders (Cook) are designed so that the needle is held in a spring-loaded piston.

Retractors (Figures 2.20 and 2.21)

Of the retractors available the Cuschieri Endoretractor (Storz) is designed for use with a 30° forward oblique telescope. The tip of the instrument can be moved through 60° enabling the lever action to retract the liver out of the field of vision. The Desplantez retractor (Micro France) and the Nouaille liver retractor (Micro France) opens into a twin diamond shape and a kite shape respectively. Although designed primarily as liver retractors they can be used to retract a variety of tissues within the peritoneal cavity such as omentum and bowel.

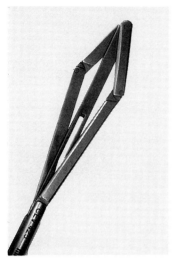

Fig. 2.20 'Kite' endoscopic retractor.

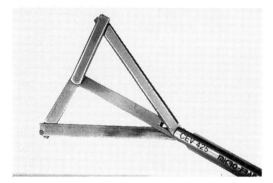

Fig. 2.21 Triangular endoscopic retractor.

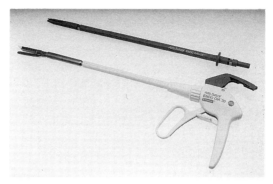

Fig. 2.22 Endo GIA stapling device.

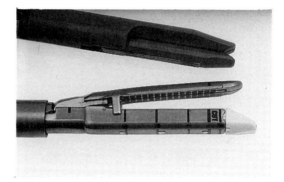

Fig. 2.23 Endo GIA stapling device – close-up of jaws.

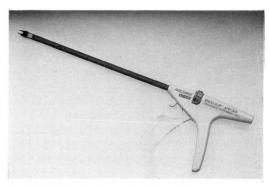

Fig. 2.24 Endoclip disposable clip applier.

Stapling instruments (Figures 2.22–2.24)

Stapling instruments are now available for laparoscopic use. The Endo GIA (USSC) is an endoscopic variant of the GIA (USSC) which staples and divides the bowel. This instrument requires a 13 mm cannula for its insertion. The instrument will divide and staple over a length of 3 cm but instruments which divide a 6 mm length of tissue are being developed. Although a disposable instrument, this can be reloaded with different cartridges during the same procedure to enable the division of bowel using the cartridge and the division of blood vessels using the vascular cartridge.

Extraction bags to facilitate the removal of resected tissues through a small stab wound have been developed. The Espiner bag and the BERT bag (Vernon Caris Ltd) are examples. Devices which ease the extraction of the gallbladder loaded with multiple calculi include the laprolith (Baxter). This device mechanically fragments gallstones to allow their extraction before the gallbladder is extracted.

3

Pneumoperitoneum – induction and complications

S. Paterson-Brown

Introduction

The ability to perform safe and efficient laparoscopic surgery relies first and foremost on the production of a safe pneumoperitoneum and the careful insertion of trocars. Failure to do this puts the remainder of the procedure in jeopardy and introduces unnecessary morbidity to a 'minimally invasive' procedure. By and large laparoscopy is a relatively new technique to many general surgeons, who may have only come across it in the context of instrumental injury incurred during gynaecological procedures. Although the potential for injury is real, the incidence of overall complications from purely diagnostic laparoscopy should be less than 4% with very few major complications (Chamberlain and Brown 1978). The principles of safe laparoscopy rely on familiarity with the Veress needle, confidence in recognizing the position of the Veress needle, and the insertion of all but the first trocar under direct vision. Patients who have had previous surgery and those who are obese pose additional problems to the laparoscopist but the basic principles remain the same.

Technique

Anaesthesia

In general, laparoscopy is best performed in the operating theatre, although it can be done in the accident department or by the bedside in special circumstances. Therapeutic laparoscopy is almost always performed under general anaesthesia with the patient intubated, paralysed and ventilated. Diagnostic laparoscopy also is usually performed under general anaesthetic although the use of local anaesthesia and intravenous sedation is a well-recognized technique for the elective investigation of patients with suspected widespread intra-abdominal malignancy who often present with ascites and/or abdominal masses (Hall et al. 1980). Because CO_2 insufflation is irritant to the peritoneum N_2O has been used as an alternative (Salky et al. 1985). In the investigation of acute abdominal pain laparoscopy is better tolerated under general anaesthesia because of the probable presence of inflammation of the parietes (Udwadia 1986). The recent introduction of a minilaparoscope, which has been used successfully under local anaesthesia to evaluate blunt abdominal trauma (Cuschieri et al. 1988), may yet prove to be useful in patients with abdominal pain although the difficulties posed by parietal peritoneal inflammation remain.

General anaesthesia

Diagnostic laparoscopy under general anaesthesia is often performed without muscle relaxation, particularly in the gynaecological patient. For longer therapeutic procedures, however, the production of the pneumoperitoneum and maintenance of a constant intraperitoneal pressure during surgery are greatly facilitated by relaxant anaesthesia. Propofol is a popular agent for induction and appears to be associated with much lower post-operative side effects than other commonly used agents such as thiopentone and etomidate (de Grood *et al.* 1987). Muscle relaxation with either atracurium or vecuronium is preferable to suxamethonium in order to prevent the 'suxamethonium pains' which can be observed in the early post-operative period and may impede early discharge following laparoscopic surgery. Anaesthesia is maintained using a combination of oxygen, nitrous oxide and a volatile agent such as enflurane or isoflurane. Intermittent boluses, or alternatively a continuous infusion, of the muscle relaxant will be required in order to maintain satisfactory relaxation of the abdominal musculature. This will help to prevent intermittent rises in intraperitoneal pressure occurring during the procedure caused by contraction of the abdominal wall muscles with associated alarming of the insufflator. Additional peri-operative analgesia may be achieved with modest opiate supplements, such as fentanyl, or the pre-operative administration of non-steroidal anti-inflammatory suppositories such as diclofenac. Excessive administration of strong opiates, either during laparoscopy or in the immediate post-operative period, should be avoided if the side effects of nausea and vomiting are to be kept to a minimum. Diclofenac given rectally by suppository is a useful alternative. Infiltration of the laparoscopic incisions with a long-acting local anaesthetic agent such as bupivicaine (0.25%) can help reduce post-operative analgesic requirements.

Local anaesthesia

Patients undergoing laparoscopy under local anaesthesia usually require intravenous sedation. The sites for insertion of the needle and trocars should be infiltrated with long-acting local anaesthetic agents, with care being taken to infiltrate down to and including the parietal peritoneum.

Patient preparation

It is important that the bladder is empty before inserting the Veress needle. Whether the patient is asked to void urine before arriving in the operating room, or whether a urinary catheter is inserted after anaesthesia, depends on the surgeon's preference. In gynaecological patients prophylactic catheterization before laparoscopy is associated with a significantly higher incidence of urinary tract infection compared to patients who are not catheterized (Akhtar *et al.* 1985). Whichever method is chosen the surgeon should percuss the suprapubic region before inserting the Veress needle to confirm the bladder has been emptied. Routine use of a nasogastric tube is unnecessary during insufflation and also for diagnostic laparoscopy, although it may be inserted to improve access to the upper abdomen during laparoscopic surgery if the stomach and duodenum are distended.

Insufflation using the Veress needle

Once the patient is on the operating table the whole abdomen is prepared and draped. Wide access may be necessary for insertion of additional ports for retraction and should not be compromised by inadequate skin preparation. A small incision is then made at the selected point for insertion of the Veress needle down to the fascia using a fine scalpel blade. In patients without previous surgery this point is either in the subumbilical or supraumbilical region as the peritoneum is closely adherent to the undersurface of the umbilicus at this point and therefore provides a natural anatomical weakness through which the Veress needle can be passed. For this reason the supraumbilical site is probably associated with less insufflation of the rectus sheath then the subumbilical route (if the Veress needle is inserted towards the pelvis) but there are no data to support this opinion. Although the transverse incision is probably more common, longitudinal incisions have been shown to heal better in the subumbilical region (East and Steele 1988).

In patients who have undergone previous abdominal surgery insufflation should be performed at a site distant to the abdominal scar and may necessitate insertion of the Veress needle at an oblique angle or through either the right or left iliac fossa. If these sites are used care must be taken to avoid the inferior epigastric vessels.

Many surgeons prefer to place the patient in the Trendelenberg position before inserting

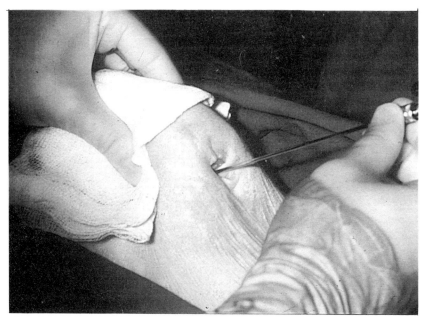

Fig. 3.1 Insertion of the Veress needle towards the pelvis with the surgeon's left hand elevating the infraumbilical abdominal wall.

the Veress needle as this allows the viscera to fall out of the pelvis away from the needle. Elevation of the adjacent abdominal wall with the surgeon's left hand helps to 'steady' the tissues for the needle to traverse but is not essential provided the surgeon is aware of the proximity of the underlying viscera and insertion is performed in a slow, controlled manner. The Veress needle is then inserted at an angle of around 45° towards the pelvic hollow (Figure 3.1), although in obese patients the needle may need to be inserted at a more vertical angle in order to reach the peritoneal cavity. The spring-loaded central trocar is pushed back as the needle traverses the abdominal wall and springs back to cover the sharp point once the peritoneal cavity has been entered (Figures 3.2a, b and c). When the procedure is being performed under local anaesthesia it is difficult to elevate the lower abdominal wall and instead the patient should be asked to tense the abdominal muscles as the needle is inserted. A small cough from the patient during this stage of the procedure will often assist the Veress needle to enter the peritoneal cavity.

Confirmation of position of the Veress needle

Two clicks can be heard from the Veress needle before it enters the peritoneal cavity. The first as it traverses the rectus sheath and the second as it traverses the peritoneum. The closer the Veress needle is to the umbilicus the closer the two clicks will become and may merge into one. Similarly if the linea alba has been incised with the initial skin incision only one click will be heard. Confirmation of the position of the needle is useful and can be demonstrated by a number of methods:

Hanging drop technique. A drop of saline is placed over the hub of the Veress needle. Once the peritoneal cavity has been entered the drop will be drawn down into the needle by the negative intraperitoneal pressure.

Injection of saline. Failure to aspirate a small volume of saline injected through the Veress needle suggests that the tip lies within the peritoneal cavity, whereas reaspiration indicates that the tip remains in the extraperitoneal space.

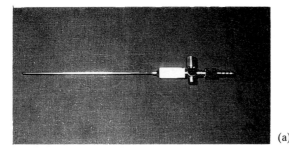
(a)

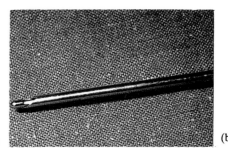
(b)

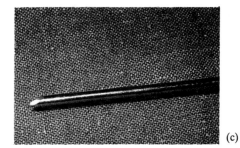
(c)

Fig. 3.2 (a) The Veress needle; (b) the tip of the needle with the internal blunt trocar forward; (c) the tip with the internal blunt trocar withdrawn as would occur whilst the needle traverses the abdominal wall.

Insufflation flow pressure. The flow pressure through the needle should be the same after insertion as before (usually 8–10 mmHg with a flow of 1 litre/min). This is displayed on the insufflator and free flow of gas confirmed by viewing the ball in the flow chamber (Figure 3.3).

Needle movement. Insufflation pressure and flow rate should not be affected by needle movement and the needle should be able to move freely from side to side. Occasionally at the start of insufflation needle movement may help to improve flow if the needle abuts against adjacent structures such as the omentum. Once some gas has been introduced this problem usually resolves.

Insufflation under direct vision

Patients who have undergone several previous abdominal operations are likely to have widespread intraperitoneal adhesions. In such patients an alternative insufflation site may be used or insufflation performed under direct vision. For the latter technique the laparo-scopic port is inserted without the sharp-tipped central introducer, the site of insertion being encircled by a purse-string suture. A specially adapted trocar has been designed for this purpose through which the insufflation can proceed (Hassan trocar – see Figure 3.4). The peritoneum is approached by sharp dissection under direct vision. 'Stay' sutures are placed through the peritoneum and linea alba on each side and once the cone-shaped tip of the Hassan trocar has been inserted into this opening, the sutures are locked over the 'wings' on each side of the port. This technique prevents the port slipping in and out and minimizes the air leak which often escapes despite the simple purse-string suture. The length of port within the peritoneal cavity can be altered by moving the 'wings' up and down the shaft of the port.

Type and volume of gas for insufflation

Carbon dioxide is the gas most commonly used for insufflation. It is relatively inert, permitting the use of electrocoagulation, and is readily absorbed by the peritoneal membrane.

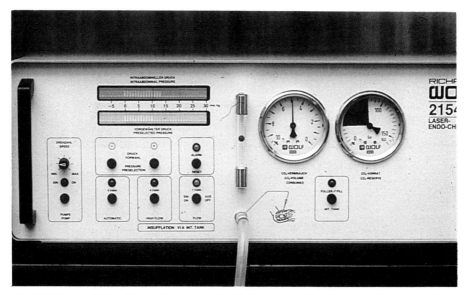

Fig. 3.3 The insufflator. The readings shown in this figure were taken from a patient who had just undergone insufflation and before the laparoscopic trocars had been inserted. The pressure is 'set' at 10 mmHg (yellow light), the flow rate is 1 litre/min which produces an intra-abdominal pressure of 13 mmHg in this patient. Good flow is confirmed by the ball in the chamber. A total of 5 litres has been insufflated in this patient (left-hand dial) which is why the intra-abdominal pressure has begun to rise above the 10 mmHg expected.

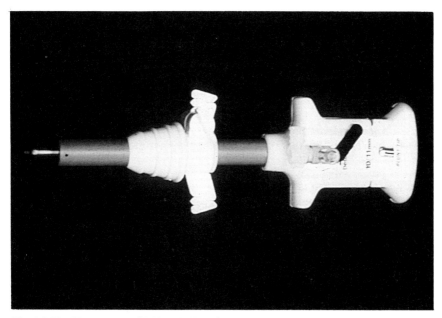

Fig. 3.4 The Hassan trocar (Ethicon Ltd, UK). The internal introducer is blunt and the position of the 'wings' for attachment of the sutures is adjustable.

However, for diagnostic laparoscopy it is even possible to use room air and, in developing countries some surgeons insufflate using a hand-held sigmoidoscope balloon (Udwadia 1986). When laparoscopy is being performed under local anaesthesia it may be preferable to insufflate with nitrous oxide to reduce the pain from peritoneal irritation and distension associated with the pneumoperitoneum. However, this is obviously not suitable if surgical intervention is needed as electrocoagulation cannot be used.

The volume of gas used for insufflation varies from patient to patient and no fixed figure should be quoted. In the author's experience complications from the introduction of the trocars are much more likely when an inadequate volume of gas has been insufflated. It is essential that the abdomen is tense before the trocar for the laparoscope is inserted. This ensures that an adequate cushion of CO_2 exists into which the laparoscopic trocar can be inserted, with as much room as possible between the abdominal wall and the underlying viscera. The volume of pneumoperitoneum may vary between 3 and 6 litres depending on the shape and build of the patient.

Removal of gas at the end of the procedure is important if post-operative pain and in particular shoulder tip pain is to be reduced. The mechanism is thought to be due to the formation of carbonic acid from the carbon dioxide insufflated, and insertion of a suction drain at the end of the laparoscopy results in decreased severity and frequency of pain (Alexander and Hull 1987).

Insertion of trocars

Insertion of the first trocar is undoubtedly associated with the greatest potential for injury for diagnostic laparoscopy. As already discussed the volume of pneumoperitoneum is important, but so is the technique of insertion. The trocar should be inserted using the right hand with the left being used to prevent any sudden and excessive movement of the trocar in a downward direction. As for insertion of the Veress needle, the trocar should be directed towards the pelvis but kept well clear of the pelvic brim. The gas inlet valve of the trocar may be kept in the 'open' position so that a hiss can be heard on entry into the peritoneal cavity, following which the outer sleeve can be safely advanced over the internal introducer. Laparoscopic inspection of the peritoneal cavity may then take place. This initial insertion of the (in most cases) 'cold' laparoscope will result in steaming of the tip and clouding of vision. The laparoscope may be warmed by hand or warmed in a water bath before insertion. Warming of the tip by pressing it against adjacent viscera such as the uterus, bladder or liver will help remove this condensation and clear the vision. If condensation remains a problem during the laparoscopic procedure, the CO_2 inflow should be taken away from the laparoscopic port and connected to another 10 mm port. This prevents the flow of cold gas around the laparoscope tip from causing repeated condensation and blurring of vision.

Complications

It is undoubtedly the production of the pneumoperitoneum and insertion of the instruments which produce most of the major complications of diagnostic laparoscopy (Chamberlain and Brown 1978). Injury to the vessels around the aortic bifurcation and pelvic brim, in addition to damage to the overlying bowel and mesentery from injudicious insertion of the Veress needle and first trocar, should be kept to a minimum if not eradicated by taking care to pass the trocar in the direction of the pelvis well clear of the posterior wall. The recent introduction of disposable trocars which have an outer sheath which springs forward to cover the sharp tip of the trocar may help to reduce the risks of damage to underlying viscera (Figure 3.5).

Table 3.1 Complications of laparoscopy (Chamberlain and Brown 1978)

Complication	Rate per 1,000 laparoscopies
Failed insufflation	11.0
Haemorrhage	7.2
Trauma to viscera	5.4
Infection	1.7
Anaesthetic related	1.4
Deep vein thrombosis	0.2
Pulmonary embolism	0.2

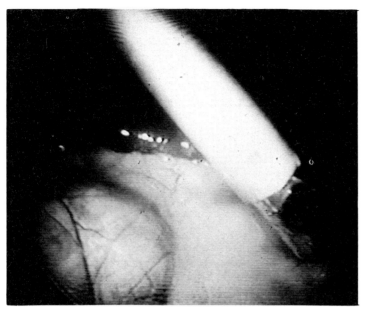

Fig. 3.5 A disposable 5 mm trocar which has been inserted. The outer sleeve which springs forward to cover the sharp tip is clearly seen.

Contraindications to laparoscopy

It must be remembered that laparoscopy is an invasive technique and that not all patients are suitable. Multiple previous abdominal operations or a provisional diagnosis of intestinal obstruction are relative contraindications as is the presence of a large hiatus hernia or irreducible external hernia and severe cardiopulmonary diseases in which the production of a pneumoperitoneum is particularly hazardous (Berci and Cuschieri 1986). Gross obesity may also make laparoscopy difficult due to the length of tissue through which the Veress needle and laparoscopic instruments must travel in order to reach the peritoneal cavity and intra-abdominal structures. The presence of a clotting abnormality is not a contraindication to laparoscopy, although, as with patients who have had previous abdominal surgery, initial insufflation may be made safer by approaching the peritoneum under direct vision.

Complications of the pneumoperitoneum

Complications from the pneumoperitoneum may be divided into two: those which occur during the insertion of instruments and the establishment of the pneumoperitoneum; and those which relate directly to the mechanical and metabolic derangements associated with the raised intra-abdominal pressure and presence of CO_2 within the peritoneal cavity.

A confidential enquiry into gynaecological laparoscopy reported by the Royal College of Obstetricians and Gynaecologists (Chamberlain and Brown 1978) showed that in 50,247 gynaecological patients undergoing laparoscopy there were 1,818 complications (3.6%). There were only four deaths (representing a mortality of 8 per 100,000) and these resulted respectively from gas embolism, perforated bowel and cardiac arrest (two cases). These figures include both diagnostic and operative laparoscopic procedures (most operative laparoscopies being tubal sterilization). Diagnostic laparoscopy was associated with a complication rate of 2.9%, compared to 4% for sterilization procedures. A summary of the type of complications is given in Table 3.1 and what is striking is the number of failed insufflations, none of which appeared to have been associated with an attempt at insufflation under direct vision.

Cardiac arrhythmias and acid-base disturbances have been reported following insufflation of CO_2 (Scott and Julian 1972) but subsequent reports have suggested that these can be reduced if not abolished by paralysing and ventilating the patient rather than allowing them to breathe spontaneously (Morley 1972). However, excessive insufflation of the peritoneal cavity to pressures in excess of 20 mmHg have been shown to lower central venous pressure, pulse pressure and cardiac output, suggesting that venous return has been reduced (Motew *et al.* 1973). Patients should therefore be closely monitored during the procedure for cardiorespiratory complications.

Acknowledgements

I am grateful to Drs Anthony Pollock and Dermot McKeown, Consultant Anaesthetists in the Royal Infirmary, Edinburgh, for their advice regarding anaesthesia for laparoscopy.

References

Akhtar, M.S., Beere, D.M., Wright, J.T. and MacRae, K.D. (1985). Is bladder catheterization really necessary before laparoscopy? *British Journal of Obstetrics and Gynaecology*, **92**, 1176–8.

Alexander, J.I. and Hull, M.G.R. (1987). Abdominal pain after laparoscopy: the value of a gas drain. *British Journal of Obstetrics and Gynaecology*, **94**, 267–9.

Berci, G. and Cuschieri, A. (1986). *Practical Laparoscopy*. Bailliere and Tindall, London, pp. 33–7.

Chamberlain, G.V.P. and Carron Brown, J.A. (1978). Report of the working party of the confidential enquiry into gynaecological laparoscopy. Royal College of Obstetricians and Gynaecologists, London.

Cuschieri, A., Hennessy, T.P.J., Stephens, R. and Berci, G. (1988). Diagnosis of significant abdominal trauma after road traffic accidents: preliminary results of a multicentre trial comparing minilaparoscopy with peritoneal lavage. *Annals of the Royal College of Surgeons of England*, **70**, 153–5.

de Grood, P.M.R.M., Harbers, J.B.M., van Egmond, J. and Crul, J.F. (1987). Anaesthesia for laparoscopy. *Anaesthesia*, **42**, 815–23.

East, M.C. and Steele, P.R.M. (1988). Laparoscopic incisions at the lower umbilical verge. *British Medical Journal*, **296**, 753–4.

Hall, T.J., Donaldson, D.R. and Brennan, T.G. (1980). The value of laparoscopy under local anaesthesia in 250 medical and surgical patients. *British Journal of Surgery*, **67**, 751–3.

Morley, T.R. (1972). Cardiac arrhythmias during laparoscopy (letter). *British Medical Journal*, **ii**, 295–6.

Motew, M., Ivankovitch, A.D., Bieniarz, J. et al. (1973). Cardiovascular effects and acid-base and blood gas changes during laparoscopy. *American Journal of Obstetrics and Gynaecology*, **115**, 1002–12.

Salkey, B., Bauer, J., Gelernt, I. and Kreel, I. (1985). Laparoscopy for gastrointestinal diseases. *Mount Sinai Journal of Medicine*, **52**, 228–32.

Scott, D.B. and Julian, D.G. (1972). Observations on cardiac arrhythmias during laparoscopy. *British Medical Journal*, **i**, 411–13.

Udwadia, T.E. (1986). Peritoneoscopy for surgeons. *Annals of the Royal College of Surgeons of England*, **68**, 125–9.

4

Laparoscopic cholecystectomy – techniques, problems and solutions

H.J. Espiner

Laparoscopic cholecystectomy is now the treatment of choice in all patients with symptomatic gallstone disease who in the recent past would have been offered open cholecystectomy.

The operation is conducted under general anaesthesia with endotracheal intubation, muscle relaxation, and monitoring of end tidal CO_2. Our preferred premedication is temazepam (10–20 mg orally) and diclofenac sodium (100 mg suppository) given 1 1/2 hours pre-operatively and, for short-acting analgesia during the operation, fentanyl (50–100 mg half-hourly) is added. Peri-operative antibiotics, subcutaneous heparin and compression stockings are routine.

Preparation

In planning the operation particular care must be taken to assess the likelihood of stones within the common bile duct. Persistent abnormalities in liver function tests and dilatation of the common duct, as shown on ultrasound, will alert the surgeon to the possibility and arrangements must be made for their management. In many centres a policy of endoscopic clearance of such stones prior to cholecystectomy has been adopted. If clearance is to be completed during the operation appropriate arrangements for increased operating time and available instrumentation must be made.

Nasogastric intubation has been found to be unnecessary as gastric distension is rarely a problem in exposure. Bladder catheterization was considered essential for safety when the umbilicus was chosen as the site for Veress needle insertion, but this is not required routinely. To assist the safe placement of trocars the course of the right superior epigastric artery may be marked out from the costal margin to the level of the umbilicus using a hand-held Doppler (BV102 Vascular Flow Detector – Sonicad, England). This simple step eliminates the risk of direct trocar laceration which may cause serious haemorrhage.

Theatre set-up

Several arrangements have been described for theatre set-up, but these are variants of two basic arrangements each depending on the position of the operating surgeon.

Position one (Figure 4.1)

The surgeon stands on the patient's left with the camera operator to his left and the chief assistant and theatre nurse standing opposite. The 21 inch monitors are placed at eye level on heavy duty mobile stands which are docked against the table at shoulder level and angled at 45°. The insufflator, light source, camera control box and tape recorder are mounted on the stand opposite the surgeon; a clear view of the display panel of the insufflator is essential while raising the pneumoperitoneum. The abdomen from pubis to nipple line is prepared

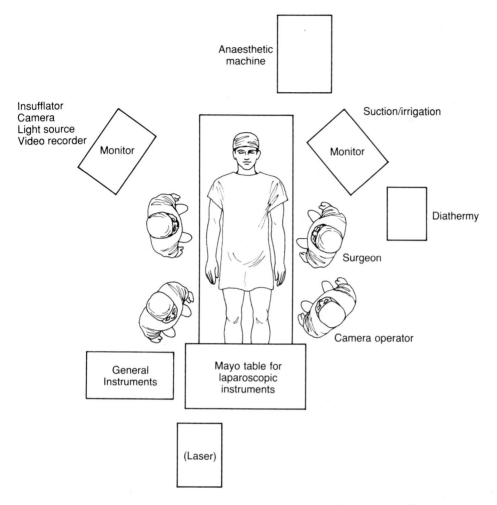

Fig. 4.1. Two monitors are used to give the whole team a clear view of the procedure. They are mounted on stacks which house the video laparoscopic instruments.

and draped, and a screen is placed across the field at the level of the second rib. The camera cable, light cable and insufflation tubing are placed in a fold of the drapes on the right side of the abdomen from just below the anterior superior iliac spine to the level of the 9th rib and thence across to the instrument stand. The diathermy and suction irrigation apparatus are placed to the left of the patient; an instrument quiver is attached to the drapes on the right side of the chest for storage of diathermy forceps, scissors, suction irrigation cannula and diathermy hook and their attached cables and tubing across the chest are placed out of the surgeon's way on his right. A Mayo table holds

all the trocars, cannulae and frequently used laparoscopic instruments plus spare gas seals, small swabs and telescope cleaning fluids. A trolley at the right holds all the other instruments. If a laser is to be used it can be placed across the foot of the table. A general laparotomy set should always be available in the theatre. Retractors which can be attached to the operating table to hold static instruments or the video laparoscope are becoming popular.

With this arrangement the surgeon can operate with a two-handed technique while his assistant provides the retraction necessary for good exposure. The theatre nurse has good access to all the ports for quick instrument change allowing the surgeon to maintain his concentration on the screen throughout. The operation can be conducted with a team of three instead of four; in this formation the assistant holds a static retractor, as well as one of the operating instruments, while the surgeon holds the camera in his left hand and dissects with his right. Although the assistant is more involved with this method, the surgeon is not developing a two-handed technique which will be useful for more complex laparoscopic procedures. A better option is for the assistant or the theatre nurse to hold the camera.

Position 2

This arrangement has gained popularity in continental Europe. The patient's legs are placed on supports and abducted with little flexion at the hip (Lloyd–Davies position). The surgeon stands or sits between the legs while the assistant stands on the patient's left. When reversed Trendelenburg tilt is applied the surgeon is directly facing the operation field. The arrangement of instruments is similar to that described for position 1.

Instruments

Laparoscopic cholecystectomy can be completed with a surprisingly small number of instruments. The basic set should include graspers, scissors, dissecting forceps with diathermy capability and hook electrodes together with a 5 mm suction irrigation cannula, a 10 mm clip applier and micro scissors. Additional instruments of great value in difficult cases are 10 mm crocodile graspers for holding very thick-walled gallbladders; 10 mm scoop morsellating forceps for picking up and crushing gallstones, as well as for blunt entry and re-entry of a 10 mm cannula; 10 mm suction/irrigation system which can cope with thick mucopus, blood clots and small gallstones; and extra telescopes, including 10 mm 30° and 5 mm 0° and 30°. As well as the above reusable instruments, some disposable trocars and cannulae should always be available together with their appropriate reducers.

The telescope should be kept in a warmer to avoid fogging and a camera sleeve will eliminate the misting caused by droplets of steriliz-

ing solution trapped between the lens and the telescope. It will also eliminate the need to retain toxic gluteraldehyde in the theatre area.

Access

The first 10 mm trocar and cannula is inserted in the subumbilical position and the 10 mm 0° telescope with camera attached is introduced. The Veress needle and its tract are inspected before removal and the exit wound observed for undue bleeding. A general laparoscopy is then completed before direct inspection of the gallbladder area. The bowel and omentum directly below the entry site should be inspected carefully for puncture trauma.

Three additional access cannulae are placed: one for static retraction of the liver and the other two for the surgeon to dissect the tissues which he holds under tension using a two-handed technique. The first puncture is made in the region of the midclavicular line below the costal margin and directly over the fundus of the gallbladder as indicated by finger depression of the abdominal wall. Care must be taken to avoid the superior epigastric artery which often lies directly in the path of the 5 mm trocar; if the patient is thin, transillumination with the telescope pushed up to the abdominal wall may show the vessel, but the more certain way is to mark its course pre-operatively, as described above. The fundus is grasped and lifted anteriorly and the inferior surface of the liver and gallbladder inspected for adhesions which might limit rotation of the liver. The second cannula is placed laterally in the anterior axillary line and usually level with the umbilicus; avoid an insertion too low as full rotation may be difficult or even impossible in the obese patient. Ratchet or spring wire forceps with gripping teeth or grooves are best and if handled gently should not tear a thin-walled gallbladder provided its peritoneal covering remains intact. The third cannula is inserted in the midline, below the xiphisternum to be level with the liver when rotated by the fundus holding forceps; it must be sufficiently high for easy dissection, but not too high, or access to the right side of the gallbladder may be difficult. The trocar should pierce the linea alba at an angle so that the peritoneum is entered to the right of the falciform ligament. This avoids minor bleeding which may be a nuisance as it drops from the

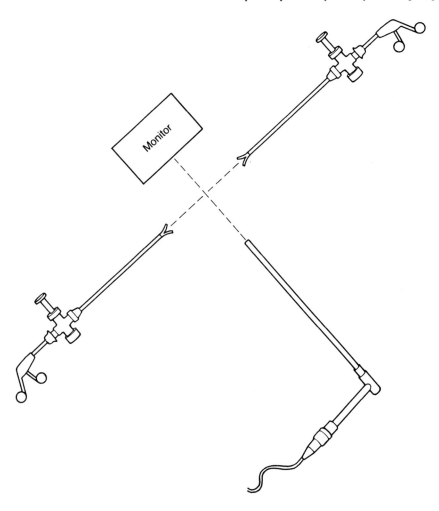

Fig. 4.2. The monitor should be placed at right angles to the visual axis. Dissection is most efficient when the instruments are also at right angles. All placement must be under visual control.

end of the cannula into the operation field. This insertion is best observed with the telescope in the midline and the falciform ligament vertical in the centre of the field of view. A 10 mm cannula is used in this situation so that clip appliers, scoop forceps and large aspiration/irrigation instruments may be introduced. There is a temptation to direct these access cannulae towards the telescope on insertion, but this should be avoided. Instead the line in which the instruments will be used

is chosen; this makes instrument changing much quicker and dissection less tiring.

Exposure

A useful rule for safe laparoscopic surgery is that every movement of every instrument should be visible on the monitor. This may require 'zooming out' with the telescope to give a global view of the whole field as instruments are introduced and 'zooming in' to follow the tips of the instruments to their action points. The camera operator and surgeon should both look along the line of the telescope directly at the monitor which should be placed at right angles to this visual axis (Figure 4.2). The two operating instruments are also used in a plane at right angles to this axis but not too close to it. Other instruments required for exposure must be placed first under visual control and then held static. The surgeon should never hesitate to use additional ports for such static aids to exposure in difficult cases. Additional grasping forceps and laparoscopic retractors may be inserted through these additional ports. By arranging these instruments correctly before starting, the surgeon is free to use both hands to dissect efficiently, the left hand holding the tissue in balanced tension, while the right hand carries out the dissection. The secret is to maintain exactly the correct tension for the particular tissue.

The fundus is grasped by the lateral port forceps and the liver is rotated superiorly, taking care to divide any adhesions to its inferior surface to prevent capsular tears. The body of the gallbladder now comes into view and the midclavicular line forceps grasp the lower third or neck area drawing it anteriorly, inferiorly and to the right. This exposes the left (medial) aspect of Hartmann's pouch and the peritoneal sheet which extends from the gallbladder to the liver and across to the porta hepatis covering the extrahepatic ducts and related vessels. If the transverse colon and omentum obstruct the view, the reverse Trendelenburg position will help as will rotation of the table to bring the right side uppermost.

When the surgeon operates standing between the patients legs a different exposure may be preferred.[1] The midclavicular line puncture is made about 3 cm medial to the position of the gallbladder fundus and a 5 mm irrigation cannula used to elevate gently the inferior surface of the liver into the direct view of the surgeon. Care must be taken not to puncture Glisson's capsule. The anterior axillary line forceps are placed laterally at a site where finger depression of the abdominal wall meets the fundus of the gallbladder before the liver edge is rotated. The grasping forceps applied through this cannula distract the neck of the gallbladder

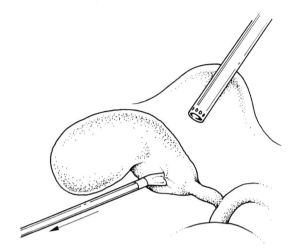

Fig. 4.3. The liver edge is gently elevated with a suction/irrigation instrument while a grasping forceps distracts the gallbladder neck inferiorly and to the right, drawing the cystic duct away from the line of the common duct.

to the right and inferiorly. It is probable that this exposure opens out Calot's triangle more efficiently with greater divergence of the cystic duct from the common bile duct (Figure 4.3).

Dissection

In open cholecystectomy the orthodox technique involves careful dissection in Calot's triangle and demonstration of the junction of the cystic duct with the common bile duct before any structure is divided and this is the method almost universally adopted for laparoscopic cholecystectomy.

Safety rests entirely on adequate identification of the anatomy; the surgeon must be aware of possible anomalies and be able to detect them and deal with the distortion caused by pathological changes. Bile duct injury should not occur yet most authors quote an incidence of 0.1–0.2%[2] and it still remains higher for laparoscopic cholecystectomy.[3] The problem with this approach is that unless the common hepatic duct is identified, the junction of the cystic duct with

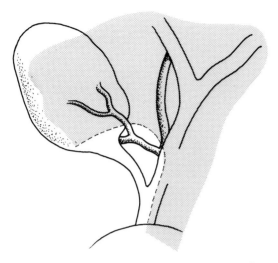

Fig. 4.4. The structures in Calot's triangle must be fully displayed. The junction of the cystic duct with the common duct must be seen before any clips are applied.

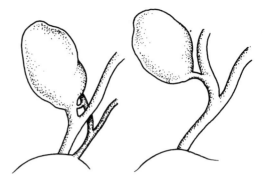

Fig. 4.5. When the gallbladder is grossly inflamed, it may overlie a short cystic duct entering the right hepatic duct. With a low union of left and right ducts, the left duct is easily mistaken for the common hepatic duct, and a serious injury may follow.

the common bile duct has not been properly displayed. Virtually all current texts which deal with techniques of cholecystectomy fail to show this crucial step (Figure 4.4). Nothing is certain unless the duct, assumed to be the common hepatic duct, has been seen to be formed by the union of right and left hepatic ducts outside the liver and until this becomes mandatory in every case, there will always be an irreducible incidence of major duct excision. Variation in ductal anatomy gives rise to further problems. An obvious hazard is the low union of the right and left hepatic ducts combined with the short cystic duct which joins the right hepatic duct: the left hepatic duct is assumed to be the common hepatic duct and the right duct is easily mistaken for the cystic duct and transected (Figure 4.5). In laparoscopic cholecystectomy the risk of injury is increased: it is not always easy to expose the right and left hepatic ducts when using a standard 0° telescope and because 'the line of sight' is at a small angle to the plane of the duct, the common hepatic duct appears foreshortened (Figure 4.6).

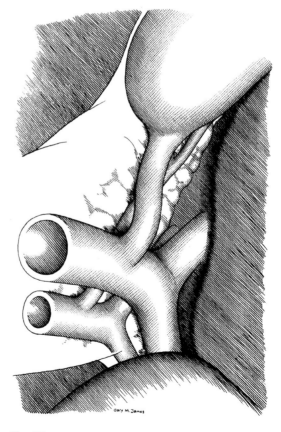

Fig. 4.6.

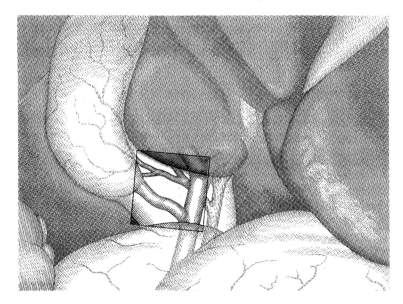

Fig. 4.7. Conventional exposure in Calot's triangle may be difficult in the presence of chronic inflammation

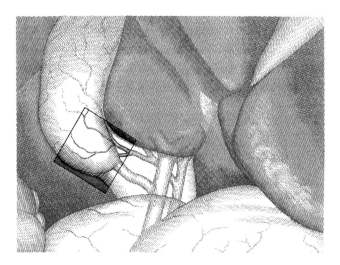

Fig. 4.8. By shifting the focus of attention peripherally, difficult dissection and possible errors of judgement are avoided

The fundus down technique eliminates the risk of bile duct injury simply by freeing the gallbladder from the liver progressively until only the cystic duct remains in continuity with the extrahepatic tract; if the dissection is conducted on the gallbladder wall throughout, damage to adjacent or adherent structures is avoided. Although this approach is possible laparoscopically, it is difficult and best applied using an angled telescope. The advantages, however, can be retained by employing the same close dissection, but on the lower third of the gallbladder as the initial step. This 'close dissection technique' avoids exposure in Calot's triangle and thus eliminates the possibility of confusion concerning the anatomy; it is especially effective when inflammation and fibrosis cause gross distortion and obliteration of tissue planes. The focus of attention is shifted peripherally (Figures 4.7 and 4.8).

Method

Dissection begins at the junction of the middle and lower thirds of the gallbladder on its medial side (Figure 4.9a, b). The peritoneal and vascular attachments are separated along a line from the liver to the free edge and

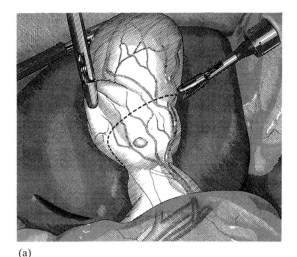

(a)

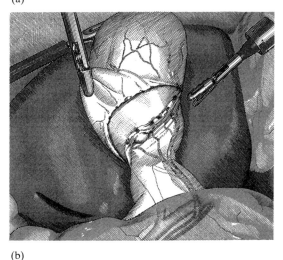

(b)

Fig. 4.9.

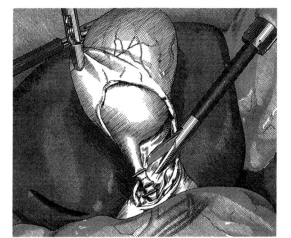

Fig. 4.10.

always above the cystic node. In cases of chronic inflammation this node is always present; by starting the separation above and peripheral to the node it is usually possible to enter a tissue plane free of fibrosis and to expose the underlying wall. Fine-pointed, insulating grasping forceps (5 mm) are used to separate the tissue, and vessels are sealed with short applications of coagulation diathermy; a hook may also be used. Branches of the cystic artery are easily skeletalized and divided without using clips, but it is vitally important that all such divisions are completed *on* the gallbladder – not below it. As the lower border of Hartmann's pouch is reached the gallbladder is rotated medially with the midclavicular line forceps and the peritoneum on the lateral (right) surface is divided easily with the hook from the liver edge to the neck of the gallbladder along the line of the lower border of Hartmann's pouch. The correct positioning of the upper midline cannula will be appreciated during this dissection. This peritoneal division may be carried down onto the cystic duct along its free edge and fibrous and vascular strands in the subperitoneal tissue may be divided before rotating the gallbladder back to present its medial surface again (Figure 4.10). It is now possible to pass a curved 5 mm forceps beneath the freed lower border of the gallbladder and to continue to separate the tissues attached to it as far as the liver edge superiorly. Dissection is then cautiously carried into the angle between Hartmann's pouch and the neck and upper cystic duct inferiorly; great care is taken to seek a posterior branch of the cystic artery which may be adherent in this angle. A good rule is to present all tissue held by the dissecting forceps into the field of view before applying diathermy current to divide it – a large vessel is then seen and can be clipped or formally sealed under direct vision. Dissecting alternately from the left and the right (the 'flag' technique of Jean Mouiel), this clearance is completed expeditiously (Figure 4.11). With the whole lower third of the gallbladder clear from the liver to the upper cystic duct all that remains is to dissect the latter as far centrally as required for safe clipping. The peritoneum is stripped from the duct using forceps or the hook diathermy to divide the delicate strands and when the cystic artery is closely adherent it can be pushed safely away as dissection proceeds. When a

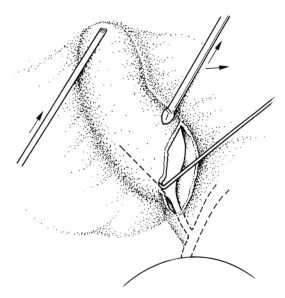

Fig. 4.11. The gallbladder is rotated to the left to expose the right side for division of the peritoneal attachments to the neck and Hartmann's pouch. Note the line of dissection with the hook is kept well up on the gallbladder wall.

prominent cystic node is present in this lower position there are usually quite large branches of the artery in the vicinity and dissection should be conducted with great care. It is not necessary to pursue the cystic duct to the junction with the common bile duct. There is a risk of causing thermal injury if excessive diathermy is used near the main ducts and clips placed very close to the common duct might ulcerate into it with time. It will be noted that formal dissection and division of the cystic artery are avoided with this method; all the small branches are divided *on* the gallbladder wall usually with diathermy. Care is taken to break the sealed small vessels towards the main artery to eliminate any risk of avulsion: all the stripping movements in dissection are directed from the gallbladder towards the porta hepatis medially.

The part played by the left hand in successful dissection cannot be overstated. Correct tension balanced against the firmly elevated fundus gives the surgeon the best exposure of the tissues to be divided by the instrument held in the right hand. When the tension is well maintained small vessels and fibrous strands stand out clearly for division and the correct line of dissection is easily seen. While the surgeon dissects with this two-handed technique the assistant holds the fundus forceps for exposure usually with maximum rotation of the liver superiorly. This technique is very safe, but two rules must be obeyed: the first is that dissection is always *on* the wall of the gallbladder, starting high enough on the body to be certain; the second rule is that as the neck area is freed, direct mural continuity with the duct (identified as the cystic duct) is confirmed. The structure leaving the neck can only be truly identified as the cystic duct if this 'mural continuity' has been shown. The importance of these two rules will be discussed in detail later. A clip is placed across the junction of the cystic duct with the neck of the gallbladder and the duct immediately below is incised. Non-toothed grasping forceps are then used to 'milk' the contents of the cystic duct through this incision so that stones trapped in the segment of duct down towards the junction with the common duct can be removed. Two more clips are placed below the incision making sure the tips of the clip applying forceps are seen projecting beyond the edge of the duct: the proximal clip is placed sufficiently firmly to occlude the lumen, but no more; the peripheral clip is tightly closed. This might reduce the slight risk of necrosis leading to bile leakage post-operatively. If the duct is too wide for clipping a loop ligature may be used. In some patients the neck is long and narrow and may be mistaken for the cystic duct; when it is clipped and divided there is a risk that a segment of devascularized neck will be left below the clip which will necrose and a bile leak will occur when this separates; there is no contraindication to following the neck or the cystic duct itself further centrally, provided the dissection remains precisely on the wall.

Cholangiography

It is generally accepted that all surgeons performing laparoscopic cholecystectomy should master the technique of operative cholangiography and the justification is to be able to define the anatomy and detect possible anomalies of the biliary tree. For those surgeons who prefer to isolate and divide the cystic artery and duct as the initial steps in the operation, routine cholangiography is wise. If a preliminary mistake is made, correct interpretation of the films will prevent escalation to a serious excision. When the 'close dissection technique' described above is followed, a cholangiogram will be required at times in the overall management of common duct stones.

Technique

While there are many instruments and catheters specifically designed for ease of cannulation the most important factor is good exposure, well maintained with the duct in slight tension. The line of the duct is judged and an appropriate site selected for direct puncture of the abdominal wall for independent access for the catheter. A good position is medial to the midclavicular line port bringing the catheter directly over the duct for easy manipulation with the main operating instrument via the upper midline port. An appropriate 14FG cannula will deliver a 4FG catheter without significant loss of gas; the catheter may be prebent or stiffened with a guide wire to facilitate insertion.[4] Sharp micro scissors are used to make a clean cut into the duct which must be free of vascular and areolar tissue; passage of the catheter through the spiral valves may be assisted by injecting saline. A temporary clip is used to hold the catheter in place and to prevent leakage of contents; metal cannulae in the field can be replaced by simple plastic rods while the films are taken.

A water soluble contrast medium with relatively low iodine content (e.g. Hypaque 150) is used and two films are taken. The first exposure is made after injection of 7 ml when the ducts are opacified and any filling defects clearly defined. The second film is taken after 20 ml and gives information regarding flow into the duodenum. A more satisfactory examination is possible with a 'C' arm image intensifier which allows screening during injection and provides direct information regarding flow of contrast across the ampulla.

If the cholangiogram reveals stones there are several options open to the surgeon. Laparoscopic cholecystectomy may be completed and the patient referred for endoscopic cannulation and stone removal with or without papillotomy in the post-operative period. Direct exploration of the common duct can be completed and a 'T' tube sutured in place after the stones have been removed;

alternatively, conversion to open operation may be preferred. Exploration via the cyst duct after dilatation to allow passage of a flexible endoscope of 10 French gauge size has been successful[5] and stones may be retrieved by basket or fragmented by laser or electrohydraulic lithotriptor.

The technique selected will depend on the surgeon's experience and the policy adopted for the management of common duct stones. Now that endoscopic removal is so successful, many prefer a policy of selective cholangiography and reserve exploration for the problem stones persistent after failed endoscopy (e.g. ampullary diverticulum or inflammatory stricture affecting the lower third of the bile duct). Once the surgeon has acquired suturing skills and has become familiar with the angled telescope, laparoscopic choledochotomy should be relatively straightforward, especially as the common duct will already be dilated.

Removal of the gallbladder

The midclavicular line forceps are placed across the neck and the cystic duct divided with scissors just below the outermost clip. With traction maintained the hook electrode or laser is used to divide the peritoneal attachments of the gallbladder from below upwards. The line of division must be at least 1 cm clear of the liver edge to avoid entering its substance and causing troublesome bleeding. On the right lateral side, it is very easy to slip away from the gallbladder wall towards the liver; use the hook to work well up onto the wall beneath the peritoneum before dividing it outwards with the diathermy. Care is needed to avoid large veins often present in the gallbladder fossa; dissection should be through properly tensioned areola tissue just clear of the gallbladder wall. The liver substance should never be entered. It is best to dissect freely with the hook before taking appropriate bundles of tissue for division with the diathermy. Forceps should be used to hold definite vessels for coagulation. The key to easy removal is the correct use of the midclavicular line forceps; traction anteriorly and inferiorly against a firmly held fundus stretches the gallbladder and tenses its peritoneal attachments. Lateral movement exposes the medial surface for division followed by medial movement for lateral separation. After each sequence anterior and superior traction exposes the areolar tissue of the bed for careful division well clear of the liver. As soon as tension is lost more peritoneum is divided as above. When only the upper third remains attached it may be necessary to reapply the midclavicular line forceps nearer the fundus. If the gallbladder is entered during this dissection the contents should be emptied by aspiration and the midclavicular line forceps used to hold the defect closed; a loop ligature may then be placed. If this is not possible spend a little time with the suction irrigation instrument to clear all the bile and small stones before they escape beyond the field of view. The assistant holding the fundus forceps can facilitate the final stages of removal by pushing the fundus laterally or medially to present the relevant peritoneal surface for division under tension. At all times maintain steady traction to tension tissues before proceeding with dissection; use the hook forceps or scissors to define the tissue to be divided, and always divide a little less. In this way the operation continues under full visual control and the risk of unexpected bleeding is greatly reduced.

Any bleeding during removal is a nuisance and should be stopped immediately. Combined suction irrigation instruments which incorporate a diathermy dissecting hook or forceps are useful. A constant flow of fluid over the vessel gives a clear view of the site of bleeding which can be quickly sealed. Before the gallbladder is finally removed, the liver is fully rotated by cephalad traction on the gallbladder to allow a view of the bed to confirm haemostasis and secure occlusion of the cystic duct. Gentle suction irrigation is used to clear the field taking care not to dislodge the clips.

Gallbladder extraction

A thin-walled intact gallbladder with small stones presents no problem. The telescope is taken to the upper midline port and the entry site of the 10 mm cannula at the umbilicus inspected to exclude bowel injury incurred at the initial blind insertion. A 10 mm grasping forceps is then passed through the umbilical cannula and advanced to take the neck of the gallbladder. The fundus holding forceps are released and the gallbladder drawn into the

umbilical cannula under direct vision. As the neck begins to impact on the mouth of the cannula the latter is withdrawn up the shaft of the holding forceps and when clear of the skin the exposed neck can be grasped. A small incision is made to introduce a suction tube, and bile and stones are aspirated before gentle traction is applied for removal.

In the majority of cases such simple removal is not possible; the wall may have been breached during dissection or rendered friable by inflammation; large stones often ulcerate into the wall and cannot be separated easily without risk of rupture and the whole viscus may be just too big. Stretching or incising the puncture site may be a solution, but sutures are then required and a point of weakness introduced if infection follows contamination. There is also a definite and reported risk of strangulation obstruction at the umbilicus. Some surgeons prefer extraction via the upper midline port; the procedure is easily observed without change of camera position and if stones or debris escape they are easily cleared from the anterior surface of the liver. If an incision is necessary there is little risk of serious strangulation obstruction at this site.

A retrieval system provides a more satisfactory solution. A large capacity sac made from strong, impermeable material is deployed through the upper midline cannula and placed on the anterior surface of the liver. The gallbladder is easily placed inside using the fundus forceps. A useful addition is an integral tail which retains the sac through the cannula, but does not impede the simultaneous use of instruments. A 5 mm grasping forceps can be used to take the neck of the gallbladder as it lies within the sac and hold it towards the cannula for easy subsequent access to its contents. Traction on the tail draws the mouth of the sac into the cannula and as the latter is withdrawn through the puncture, the sac impacts on the wound and the mouth of the sac can be developed on the surface. Access to the gallbladder, safely contained within, is simple and it can be quickly cut open and removed. The stones are crushed and aspirated before the sac itself is finally withdrawn. This device is particularly useful in difficult cases where opening the inflamed gallbladder facilitates dissection. The sac is deployed early and large stones and fragments of wall are placed inside and held securely away from the operation field for later removal. When stones greater than 1.5 cm are encountered, it is easy to cut the gallbladder open inside the sac while it is still within the abdominal cavity; the stones are released and crushed under direct vision using suction/irrigation to remove the fragments. The security of containment reduces the risk of wound infection and the small but reported risk of cancer implantation in the umbilicus when an unsuspected carcinoma of the gallbladder is removed by this route.[6]

Closure and drainage

The patient is now placed in the Trendelenburg position and any residual intraperitoneal fluid aspirated by passing the suction/irrigation instrument over the anterior surface of the right lobe of the liver to reach the posterior surface of the diaphragm. If the case has been straightforward and exposure and clipping of the cystic duct has been satisfactorily completed, many surgeons complete the operation without drainage. If, however, there has been any doubt about the closure, or in cases of acute inflammation the duct itself has disintegrated, a soft drain should be placed in the gallbladder bed via the midclavicular line cannula, which is then withdrawn under telescopic control as is the one in the anterior axillary line. When the gallbladder has been removed through the upper midline cannula, the telescope is taken to this site and the umbilical cannula inspected. The peritoneum surrounding the access is carefully examined to exclude adhesions and possible unsuspected bowel laceration and the cannula is then slowly removed with its valve opened to prevent suction of a loop of adjacent bowel into the wound. The upper midline cannula is finally removed with the telescope drawn up its shaft so that the peritoneum can be seen during this final stage. The puncture wounds are irrigated with Savlon (1%) and infiltrated with bupivacaine (0.5%) local anaesthetic. Subcuticular sutures are used for skin closure and the drain is taped in position without suture.

Immediate post-operative care

If possible, opiates are avoided. A nasogastric tube is passed to empty the stomach of any bile and then removed before endotracheal extubation. Maxolon 10 mg is given orally tds for the first 48 hours and coproxamol given as required for pain relief. Some epigastric and shoulder pain is to be expected from the laparoscopy, but this is short-lived and should diminish over the first 12 hours and settle in 4–5 days. Where a drain has been used it may be removed before the local anaesthetic wears off, about 6 hours post-operatively, but if any bile is noted or the volume of serous fluid is in excess of 200 ml, it should be retained for 12 hours for review. Severe abdominal pain, or a pain developing after an initial pain-free interval, must be taken seriously. This operation should have an uneventful course and any deviation from this may be due to a significant potential complication. The two most important conditions to consider in these circumstances are bile peritonitis and a perforated viscus.

Problems and solutions

Access

Previous abdominal surgery and adhesions can make access difficult. In these cases it is wise to have marked out the course of both superior and inferior epigastric arteries pre-operatively. Select a site well away from any scars for insertion of the Veress needle and when a satisfactory pneumoperitoneum has been raised insert a 5 mm trocar and cannula carefully along the tract. Use the 5 mm telescope (without video camera) to inspect the abdominal cavity and note the location of significant adhesions. Suitable sites for additional access ports can be selected for division of adhesions aiming to clear the posterior aspect of the umbilicus for definitive insertion of the laparoscope. There are occasions when it is not possible to establish umbilical access; alternative entry should be made in the left upper abdomen. By applying the principle of static retraction of the gallbladder fundus from anywhere in the right side of the abdomen, good triangulation with 5 mm instruments for dissection can be achieved.

Exposure

When a tongue of liver falls across the field of view, it may be retracted through an additional

5 mm port inserted between the midclavicular line cannula and the midline, just below the costal margin. If a bulky omentum with transverse colon pushes upwards in front of the telescope, in spite of a full head-up tilt and rotation, a 5th port for retraction should be placed midway between umbilicus and xiphisternum and well away from the midline; the left side is often the best. A nasogastric tube may be needed if a distended stomach gets in the way. Difficulty with elevation of the fundus is usually caused by problems with grasping – the wall is too thick for a 5 mm instrument to hold. When gross distension is the problem, aspiration of bile through the midclavicular line port is simple. Direct puncture with the trocar and cannula well into the gallbladder can permit aspiration either directly through the cannula or through a suction tube placed within it. It is important to have the anterior axillary line forceps handy to take hold of the gallbladder as it collapses, so that it does not slip off the cannula; when the cannula has been withdrawn, the forceps are used to close the puncture site as they grasp the fundus. Alternatively, a needle may be passed directly through the abdominal wall, but it must be wide bore to cope with thick bile or mucopus. If the difficulty is inflammatory thickening, a large grasper will be needed; the 5 mm cannula is changed to a 10 mm one and large crocodile forceps are used. Should these be required later to hold the gallbladder at the level of Hartmann's pouch, a small cut may be made into the fundus and a 5 mm spring wire grasper used instead to hold the wall with one of its arms in the lumen. In resolving acute obstructive cholecystitis, gross omental wrapping usually obscures the initial view; careful separation is necessary to avoid quite severe bleeding. Because the adhesions are inflammatory and held only by exudate in the early days after an attack, blunt teasing away from the wall is easy; later when fibrosis supervenes, a site must be carefully chosen to begin dissection – often just adjacent to the liver on the medial side. The omentum is held gently with the left hand while fine grasping forceps in the right hand tease the adhesions down to the gallbladder wall using diathermy to keep a bloodless field. Separation will take time, but a dry field is essential. The stiffened shell of omentum, when freed, may make access awkward – do not hesitate to create an extra

10 mm port well to the right to bring in a 10 mm suction/irrigation instrument to act as an omental retractor and to aspirate fluid which accumulates in the 'well' created as dissection proceeds to expose the gallbladder neck. It is essential to have an experienced assistant in these circumstances.

Problems with dissection and the risk of bile duct injury

The most difficult cases are those of chronic obstructive cholecystitis often presenting as chronic indigestion. The pre-operative ultrasound shows a thick-walled gallbladder containing stones with one impacted in the neck. When the initial episode fails to resolve and repeated attacks follow, the chronic inflammatory tissue obliterates the tissue planes and progressive fibrosis with consequent contracture pulls the structures in Calot's triangle together. The cystic duct is 'taken up' in this process resulting in the adherence of the common hepatic and common bile ducts to the apex of the inflammatory mass which replaces the neck of the gallbladder. Similarly the cystic and right hepatic arteries are tethered onto Hartmann's pouch. These changes present the surgeon with serious problems when the orthodox technique is adopted, because the important landmarks are either displaced or encased in woody oedematous inflammatory tissue (Figure 4.12). It is easy to understand how the common bile duct may be mistaken for the cystic duct in these circumstances. The surgeon expects to identify the cystic duct as the first structure encountered below and central to the gallbladder neck in the free edge of the hepatoduodenal ligament, but the traction and elevation necessary for exposure align the adherent common bile duct into just the course expected for the cystic duct; the hepatic artery, running medial to the common bile duct, is easily mistaken for the duct itself – the stage is thus set for a major bile duct injury. If the common bile duct (which in young women is often quite small) is now clipped and divided, the dissection for removal of the gallbladder readily leads onto the common hepatic duct – which can now be easily misidentified as an 'accessory cystic duct' or 'cysticohepatic duct' and divided. There can be no doubt that operative cholangiography

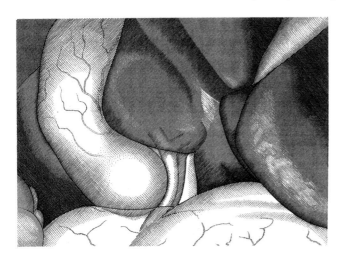

Fig. 4.12. Repeated attacks of cholecystitis in the presence of a stone impacted in the neck of the gallbladder may lead to obliteration of Calot's triangle. The cystic duct is often very short

should prevent the disaster of a major duct excision in these circumstances provided the films are interpreted correctly. However, the common duct still sustains an injury, albeit a less serious one, simply to obtain this information.

In these difficult cases, the safest way to proceed is to apply the 'close dissection technique' described above. The cystic node invariably marks the upper extent of the chronic inflammatory process even if it is obscured by fatty infiltration beneath the peritoneum. The gallbladder above this is usually pliable and a dissection plane can be found working down onto the wall and then onto Hartmann's pouch. The tissues may become more fibrous at the junction of the pouch with the neck and here the cystic node is frequently seen. The branches of the cystic artery are gathered together in the inflammatory tissue and the surgeon must be alert for a large posterior branch adherent to the undersurface of the neck of the gallbladder where it is firmly held in fibrous tissue. Very short teasing movements with fine dissecting forceps will free the vessel intact and its division will open up the angle between the neck and Hartmann's pouch. The peritoneal division on the right side is carried down on the free edge of the neck of the gallbladder, peeling it back on either side to show that the neck is clear. This area is often distended by the impacted stone and it is here that the adherence of the common bile duct will be found. Peeling the inferior surface of the swelling will lead back

up to the shortened cystic duct and the common bile duct will fall away. The 'mural continuity' between the gallbladder and the cystic duct is now confirmed and it is usually possible to free sufficient duct to divide it with confidence. There is no technique of operative cholangiography which can help in these cases; the cystic duct is virtually always obliterated and the outflow from the gallbladder is obstructed by stone. Direct needle puncture of the common bile duct would be the only possible approach. When the impacted stone is large there may be no mobility of the lower third of the gallbladder and access to the left side may be difficult. Dissection in these cases should start high and move down the lateral surface (Figure 4.13a and b); if the duodenum is lightly adherent it may be gently swept away. If fibrosis is encountered beware a cholecystoduodenal fistula and go no further. There are two options, one is to expose the duodenum from the pylorus down to the opposite side of the adherence and to consider if freedom behind the gallbladder can be achieved sufficiently for the passage of a stapling instrument to close the fistula without compromising the duodenal lumen. The second is to make a transverse cut with the diathermy hook in Hartmann's pouch directly onto the stone which is then released and placed in a retrieval sac for later extraction; the gallbladder contents are cleared by suction/irrigation. Hartmann's pouch is then transected, the surgeon working within its wall if there is no easy plane outside. It may be possible to work down to the narrow cystic

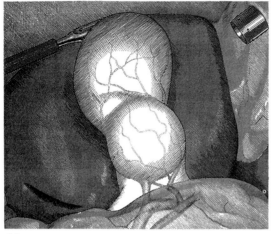

(a)

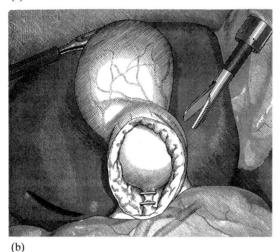

(b)

Fig. 4.13(a),(b).

found in the common bile duct or drainage volume remains high, endoscopic removal or temporary stenting may be required. This subtotal cholecystectomy has been described for open cholecystectomy[7] and has been used with success in a patient with the Mirizzi syndrome diagnosed pre-operatively and treated laparoscopically.[8] In a very small number of cases the above method may not be possible because there is no clear indication where to cut onto Hartmann's pouch; the fundus down method should then be employed. If the gallbladder seems to be very small the fundus down technique is the safest option; the excision can be abandoned at any point and in a case of virtual or congenital absence of the gallbladder, the common duct would not be at risk.

Problems in removal

Sometimes the gallbladder is too rigid to move and no easy plane can be found at the liver edge. An abscess may have destroyed the wall and the viscus disrupts spilling stones into the field. This situation is best solved by piecemeal excision, using laser or cautery. The gallbladder is cut along a line 1 cm from the liver edge until the fundus is reached, a segment of which is preserved to allow continued elevation. The gallbladder fragments and larger stones are placed in a retrieval sac for safe keeping and small stones and debris aspirated after copious irrigation. The options at this stage are either to excise the wall retained in the gallbladder fossa by cutting it into strips, to cauterize the remaining mucosa, or simply to leave the remnant alone after haemostasis is secured. The region should be drained at the end of the operation.

Lost gallstones

It may not be possible to remove all the stones which escape when the gallbladder is opened. A loop ligature placed on a thin-walled gallbladder opened during dissection from the liver bed will limit the problem and deliberate suction irrigation clearance (described elsewhere) is the best approach when the wall is too thick or friable to close. Stones lost when the gallbladder ruptures on removal through the abdominal wall may be very difficult to trace. There are anecdotal reports of late

duct below, but when dense adhesions to the duodenum or common hepatic duct persist, the excision is best terminated and the cavity aspirated and inspected for bile regurgitation. If bile accumulates either the cystic duct is patent or there is a communication between Hartmann's pouch and the right or common hepatic duct (Mirizzi syndrome). A soft tube drain should be placed carefully in the cavity and secured by suture closure of the cuff of gallbladder wall. Provided there is no ductal obstruction, any bile drainage post-operatively will steadily decrease; a tube cholangiogram should then confirm free flow into the duodenum before the tube is removed. If stones are septic complications[9] and although experimental work suggests the problem may be small,[10] the total experience is too short to be sure. It is better to use a retrieval sac routinely to eliminate this problem. Cut gloves and condoms have been used as makeshift pouches, but they are unreliable and carry the risk of starch contamination of the peritoneum or even latex shock.

Bleeding

A bloodless field is essential for safe laparoscopic surgery in any situation and all vessels should be sealed before division. Even minor oozing must be stopped before dissection moves on; not only are tissue planes obscured by blood clot, but the clarity of view is lost as light is absorbed. If heparin (4,000 units per litre) is added to the irrigating field and some is instilled before dissection starts, clotting will be avoided and suction will be effective. Irrigation will show a bleeding point for accurate occlusion. If the small branches of the cystic artery are taken on the gallbladder wall there is no need to dissect the main vessel and there is then no risk of haemorrhage from slipped clips. Bleeding in the gallbladder bed is usually venous and occurs when tension is not well maintained to show the correct areolar plane for dissection. If real haemorrhage is encountered immediately place an open forceps over the site to apply pressure for temporary control. If the gallbladder is mobile push the freed section onto the liver bed. Once initial control is achieved check the CO_2 cylinder and pneumoperitoneum to make certain there will be no sudden loss of exposure; freeze the position of all instruments and clean the telescope. Next assess the best angle for access for clips or loop ligature and if necessary place an extra port. Select the best site for suction irrigation and agree a plan of action. When the instruments are in place inspect the site, determine the line of the vessel and take the necessary steps to achieve haemostasis. When applying clips hold the instrument in place after closure and observe the result; bring another forceps alongside ready to be placed over the vessel if bleeding persists when the applier is removed. A steady flow of irrigating fluid will usually give the surgeon an opportunity to see the breach in the vessel wall. There is no place for packing with

omentum or drainage in this situation. Conversion or reoperation within hours will be required if direct closure is not achieved.

Wound problems

Infection

Wound infection, although potentially less serious than in open cholecystectomy, occurs with the same frequency (0.5–1% of cases)[11] and the most common site is the umbilicus. Gallbladder extraction is a likely factor especially if forceful traction is employed or clean tissue incised in the presence of infected bile. An impermeable retrieval sac eliminates this risk by avoiding direct contamination or the need to enlarge the puncture site.

Herniation

If a cannula larger than 10 mm is used at the umbilicus or a wound dilator is employed to ease extraction of the gallbladder, there is a definite risk of herniation with the possibility of obstruction and strangulation of the small bowel.[12] The clinical presentation of this complication may be misleading, suggesting a simple ileus which might settle; careful examination, however, will reveal a small, slightly tender swelling in the region of the umbilicus and the surgeon should not hesitate to explore. Suture of the fascia has been recommended, but there is a case report of strangulation in spite of suture of the rectus sheath.[13] It is important to withdraw the cannula with the gas valve open to eliminate any suction effect and extraction of the umbilical cannula must be completed under direct vision from the telescope in the upper midline port.

Stone extraction

Incision of the linea alba is frequently advised when the gallbladder is obviously enlarged with a heavy load of stones or one huge calculus. A better solution is to use a retrieval sac and preserve all the advantages of minimal access surgery. If the large stones are freely mobile in the gallbladder, the method described above is effective, i.e. removal of the gallbladder first leaving the stones free in the sac. The 10 mm morsellating forceps are then used to crush the soft cholesterol stones by nibbling from the edge to break them and remove scoopfuls of the debris. Frequent washing assists the procedure which can be observed on camera. A single very hard calculus may be shattered by an electrohydraulic lithotriptor – a simple device usually available in any urological operating theatre. With the stone pulled into the depths of the wound and covered with saline, a few shocks break the shell and the soft centre is easily extracted. When the large stones are embedded in the wall of the gallbladder it is better to cut the wall away while the sac is still inside the abdomen held over the anterior surface of the liver. Once the stone is free it can be crushed with the morsellating forceps and a little time spent reducing the fragments progressively and washing them clear is well worthwhile. The thick wall of the gallbladder can then be cut into smaller pieces to make their removal easier when the sac is drawn up into the wound.

Unexpected cancer implantation

Cancer of the gallbladder is rare and is often diagnosed only on histological examination of the specimen received after the operation. Cases have been reported of nodules appearing in the umbilicus some months after laparoscopic cholecystectomy and it has been suggested that implantation occurs during extraction.[6] If the prognosis is judged to be favourable, wide, local excision of the site is recommended; local radiotherapy has also been suggested. Extraction in a protective sac would probably prevent this unusual complication.

Duodenal perforation

Although this is not yet recognized as a complication specific to laparoscopic cholecystectomy, some of the larger series have included isolated instances in their lists of complications. The mechanism is probably an unsuspected diathermy injury occurring off screen so that the surgeon is completely unaware of the risk. Great care must be taken to be sure there is no shorting onto a metal cannula or suction/irrigation instrument during dissection and if such exposed metal is in contact with the duodenal wall, it should be withdrawn clear before the application of any current. All diathermy instruments must be regularly inspected for the integrity of their insulation.

Biliary leak and bile peritonitis

A bile leak post-operatively is a potentially serious complication demanding urgent assessment. If a drain has been well placed in the gallbladder bed, the presence of bile in the drain gives the diagnosis and if drainage is effective the patient may be free of pain. If the abdomen has not been drained, there will always be some right upper quadrant pain which may be severe. A little seepage of bile through a puncture site should be regarded as diagnostic. The surgeon must always suspect that more bile is leaking than is recovered externally and any persistent pain must be assumed to be due to a slowly progressive bile peritonitis. This is an insidious condition which if treated quickly is a minor setback, but if left untreated or inadequately so, may be disastrous. The most likely causes are failure of cystic duct closure, division of a minor duct in the liver bed or a breach of a major extrahepatic duct.

Failure of cystic duct closure is probably the most common cause, usually from a slipped clip. Another cause is inadequate closure of a duct which is too wide to be completely closed by standard clips (or even larger ones) – a situation best managed by using a loop ligature. Further possible causes include necrosis of the duct at the site of clipping or a long, narrow neck being mistaken for the cystic duct and the clip being placed on which is in effect devascularized stump tissue. Ducts in the liver bed are divided during removal; those entering the gallbladder directly from the liver are usually small and if seen can be safely ligated. If they are not seen transection leads to free bile leakage. Dissection in a plane too deep in the liver bed risks the lateral injury of a duct very close to the surface, an event not recognized as excision proceeds. Bile leakage and peritonitis due to a breach in a major duct represents a failure of technique and will invariably require intervention.

Initial management involves endoscopic cholangiography. This will both establish the diagnosis and offer immediate treatment options. Whatever the source or severity of the leakage, if common duct stones are found

these must be removed or free drainage insti-
tuted either by stenting or by the nasobiliary
route. For small leaks in the liver bed, if
drainage is free no further action will be
required. If there is no drain a tube should be
placed, possibly through the midclavicular line
puncture site under radiological control.
Similar management is acceptable for a small
cystic duct stump leak, but if the clips are seen
to be well clear of the site of the leak,
relaparoscopy and replacement is the better
option. The management of more major
leakage requires good internal drainage; papillotomy or stenting are now accepted practice.
Major extrahepatic duct injury calls for early
reconstruction by hepaticojejunostomy; this
may seem drastic, but the long-established,
good results of this procedure for severe ductal
injuries are the justification. Some radiologists
are recommending long-term stenting, but
judgement must be reserved until the late
results are known; it would seem likely that
severe stricturing will be an unavoidable
problem however late. There is a strong
temptation to rely on ultrasound and CT
scanning in the early assessment of a complication and to accept guided drainage in the
management. This might be acceptable when
the patient's condition is stable and the
features point to a well-localized collection.
The disadvantage of this approach, however, is
that the anatomy and dynamics of the leak
remain unknown and the opportunity to solve
the problem within a few hours of its presentation is lost.

References

1. Perissat, J. (1993). Laparoscopic cholecystectomy: the
   European experience. *American Journal of Surgery*,
   165: 444–9.

2. Raute, M. and Schaupp, W. (1988). Iatrogenic damage
   of the bile ducts caused by cholecystectomy.
   Langenbecks Archiv fur Chirurgie , **373**, 345–54.
3. Larson, G.M., Vitale, G.C., Casey, J. *et al.* (1992).
   Multipractice analysis of laparoscopic cholecystectomy
   in 1983 patients. *American Journal of Surgery*, **163**,
   221–6.
4. Harvey, M.H., Cahill, J. and Wastell, C. (1992).
   Laparoscopic cholangiography: a simple inexpensive
   technique using readily available materials. *British
   Journal Surgery*, **79**, 1178–9.
5. Petelin, J.B. (1993). Clinical results of common bile
   duct exploration. *Endoscopic Surgery and Allied
   Technologies*, **1**, 125–9.
6. Pezet, D., Fondriuier, E., Rotman, N. *et al.* (1992)
   Parietal seeding of carcinoma of the gall bladder after
   laparoscopic cholecystectomy. *British Journal Surgery*,
   79, 230.
7. Cottier, D.J., McKay, C. and Anderson, J.R. (1991).
   Subtotal cholecystectomy. *British Journal Surgery*, **78**,
   1326–8.
8. Binnie, N.R., Nixon, S.J. and Palmer, K.R. (1992).
   Mirizzi syndrome managed by endoscopic stenting and
   laparoscopic cholecystectomy. *British Journal Surgery*,
   79, 647.
9. Perissat, J. (1993). Laparoscopic cholecystectomy: the
   European experience. *American Journal of Surgery*,
   165, 444–9.
10. Fitzgibbons, R.J., Annibali, R. and Litke, S. (1993).
    Gall bladder and gall stone removal, open versus closed
    laparoscopy and pneumoperitoneum. *American Journal
    of Surgery*, **165**, 497–504.
11. Lee, V.S., Chari, R.S. and Cucchiaro, G. (1993).
    Complications of laparoscopic cholecystectomy.
    American Journal of Surgery, **165**, 527–31.
12. McMillan, J. and Watt, I. (1993). Herniation at the site
    of cannula insertion after laparoscopic cholecystectomy.
    British Journal Surgery, **80**, 915.
13. Boyce, D.E., Wheeler, M.H. and Fligelstone, L.J.
    (1992). An unusual complication of laparoscopic chole-
    cystectomy. *Annals of the Royal College of Surgeons of
    England*, **74**, 254–5.

5

Laser versus electrocautery in laparoscopic cholecystectomy

Brock M. Bordelon and John G. Hunter

Introduction

Laparoscopic surgical techniques have gained wide acceptance in an exceedingly short period of time, and several authors have reported excellent results with laparoscopic cholecystectomy,[1,2,3,4] but controversies persist. That which has aroused most debate and discussion at meetings and in the literature is whether laser or electrosurgical dissection is the superior technique for dissecting the gallbladder from the liver bed.[5,6,7] The notable surplus of opinions regarding the superiority of laser or electrosurgical dissection during laparoscopic cholecystectomy is, unfortunately, matched only by a conspicuous lack of comparative data.

For many surgeons, the marriage of laser technology and laparoscopic surgery appears to be a perfect union of 'high tech' instrumentation and modern surgical techniques. In most cases, general surgeons were introduced to both technologies simultaneously during short laparoscopic cholecystectomy courses. These courses have been heavily influenced by the early work of two laparoscopic surgical teams in the United States: Reddick and Daniell in Nashville, Tennessee, and McKernan and Saye in Atlanta, Georgia. Each team included a gynaecologist proficient in laser laparoscopy and a general surgeon skilled at cholecystectomy. Thus, the union of laser and laparoscopic techniques for general surgeons was fashioned more by the experiences of gynaecologists with laser laparoscopy than by data supporting the superiority of laser over electrosurgery for gallbladder dissection.

Devastating complications resulted from surgeons applying recently learned laser laparoscopic cholecystectomy techniques without the benefit of extensive laser experience. For this reason, the safety of laser use in laparoscopic cholecystectomy has been questioned.[8,9] Advocates of laser dissection, however, contend that the lessons learned from complications encountered during the gynaecologic electrosurgery experience are being neglected.[10,11,12]

Laser and electrosurgical instruments are, in essence, two different devices that generate thermal energy. While thermal injury is their common end-product, laser and electrosurgical energy have fundamentally different characteristics that convey distinct tissue responses. A thorough understanding of the basic physics of laser and electrosurgical energy is necessary to address the debate surrounding their use.

Principles of monopolar electrosurgery

Electrosurgical generators produce electrical current at a frequency of 500,000–750,000 cycles/second. The current is conducted from the active electrode (cautery tip) through tissue back to an indifferent electrode (ground plate). The rapidly alternating current creates kinetic energy, and thereby tissue heat, by propelling ionized species adjacent to the active electrode to and fro within the electrical field.

Electrosurgical generators produce coagulating, cutting and blended waveforms. Coagulating current is characterized by rapid discharge of short bursts of high voltage energy, interrupted by short pauses that permit slower heating and better haemostasis. Electrosurgical cutting current is a continuous high frequency, low voltage sine wave discharge without intervening pauses, yielding rapid tissue heating and vaporization. Blended electrosurgical current is made up of short alternating discharges of high and low voltage electricity.

Effective coagulation requires deep and even tissue heating, and therefore deep and even penetration of electrical current. Electrosurgical tissue heating is related to current density, or the amount of current flowing through a particular cross-sectional area. Current density is directly proportional to applied power (voltage) and indirectly proportional to tissue resistance (impedance). Tissue resistance is high and current flow is low upon initial electrical contact, resulting only in superficial heating. Tissue heat increases with continued electrical current application, producing a fall in resistance and a proportional increase in current flow. As tissue heat increases, water evaporates and desiccation occurs. Desiccation increases tissue resistance, precipitating a fall in current density and cessation of cutting or coagulation. Increased tissue resistance can be overcome by increasing the power on the electrosurgical generator to a voltage high enough to propel current through the resistance.

With electrosurgical cutting, a high frequency (500 kHz), low voltage current rapidly heats tissue immediately adjacent to the electrode to >100°C. This generates tissue vaporization and produces a gap of steam between the electrode and the underlying tissue. Further electrical discharge results in current sparking across the steam gap. Electrosurgical cutting current swiftly vaporizes tissue in contact with the electrode, but does not penetrate deeply into adjacent tissue. This limits the lateral extent of thermal injury, but also prevents adequate coagulation.

Disadvantage of monopolar electrosurgical dissection

The introduction of laparoscopic surgical techniques allowed gynaecologists to perform minimally invasive tubal ligation, employing electrosurgical energy for fallopian tube vaporization. Unfortunately, intestinal injury remote to the site of surgery was occasionally seen with laparoscopic tubal ligation. This complication, with a reported frequency of 0.1–1.0%,[10,13] results from current leakage. Current leakage takes place because of inadequately insulated instruments, tissue conduction of electrical current, sparking of high voltage current, or capacitively coupled current.

The potential for intestinal injury from activation of a metal electrosurgical electrode with damaged or inadequate insulation is obvious. Frequently, however, the entire instrument is not in view during a laparoscopic procedure. Intestinal injury, which may be manifest only as tissue blanching, may go unrecognized in this situation. This problem can be avoided with careful inspection of electrosurgical instruments, especially heavily used instruments prone to damage during passage through trocar trumpet valves.

Tissue conduction occurs when electrical current passes from the tissue being coagulated to tissue in direct contact with it. One can readily appreciate the risk of conduction injury when electrosurgical energy is applied to an adhesion in contact with intestine. This injury may occur out of the laparoscopist's view, or the extent of tissue injury may be underestimated, leading to delayed identification and treatment. This complication can be easily prevented by close attention to the surgical field prior to application of electrosurgical current.

All surgeons are familiar with the phenomenon of sparking or arcing when high voltage electrosurgical current is used. In this situation, current arcs from an activated electrode to adjacent water-containing tissue. This is commonly seen with electrode activation prior to tissue contact. Alternatively, when electrode activation persists past the point of tissue desiccation, high voltage current may spark to adjacent viscera. The potential for this complication increases with increasing voltage, so FDA guidelines recommend a maximum peak-to-peak voltage of 1,200 volts for laparoscopic electrosurgical coagulation.

Capacitive coupling occurs when electrical current passes across *intact* insulation to tissue in contact with the instrument. This phenomenon was seen occasionally during early gynaecologic laparoscopic procedures, when operating telescopes were commonly employed. A considerable amount of the current going to an activated, ungrounded electrode placed through an operating telescope passes to the telescope. This capacitively coupled current must then discharge back to the ground plate. When the operating telescope is passed through a metal trocar, the current is discharged through the abdominal wall with insufficient power density to cause tissue injury. However, if the operating telescope is passed through a plastic trocar, the current is discharged to any grounded tissue in contact with the telescope, resulting in visceral injury.

Operating telescopes are rarely employed in current laparoscopic surgical procedures, but the potential for capacitively coupled electrical current injury persists. Any uninsulated instrument (such as a laparoscope) placed through a plastic trocar that contacts an activated, ungrounded electrode provides a vehicle for transmission of capacitively coupled current. A similar situation may arise when a metal trocar is used in conjunction with a plastic anchor; capacitively coupled current will flow from an activated, ungrounded electrode to the metal sleeve and from there to any contiguous viscera.

The risks of visceral injury with electrosurgical dissection during laparoscopic cholecystectomy can be minimized if the surgeon has a proper understanding of capacitive coupling and uses low voltage current. Conduction injuries of the common bile duct may result from current inadvertently applied to a surgical clip on the cystic duct, although this should be rare. A significant rate of bowel injury resulting from electrosurgical laparoscopic cholecystectomy, the most common concern expressed among proponents of laser dissection, has not materialized.

Principles of bipolar electrosurgery

The fundamental difference between monopolar and bipolar electrosurgery is the direction of current flow. In monopolar electrosurgery, current flows from the active electrode through tissue, mainly blood vessels, to the inactive electrode (ground plate). Bipolar electrosurgical instruments place the two electrodes in close proximity, so that current flows only through tissue in contact with both electrodes.

Disadvantages of bipolar electrosurgery

The requirement for dual electrodes in bipolar instruments creates some problems for the laparoscopic surgeon. A limited number of tip configurations are available. If the electrodes are placed in close proximity, current will bypass the tissue touching the instrument and travel to the inactive electrode along the path of least resistance. Both electrodes must be in contact with tissue in order for heating and coagulation to occur, a task that can be difficult to accomplish in some settings.

Power output can be increased with monopolar electrosurgical generators to overcome high tissue resistance in desiccated tissue. Until recently, this was impossible with bipolar generators, which had limited voltage and little ability to vaporize or cut tissue. Newer instruments designed specifically for laparoscopic applications appear to have surmounted this obstacle (BiLap, Everest Medical, St Paul, Minnesota), and are currently undergoing clinical trials.

Principles of laser

Laser is an acronym for *l*ight *a*mplification by *s*timulated *e*mission of *r*adiation. Lasers convert electrical energy to photons by directing electrical current into the lasing medium or into a bright lamp (flashlamp). When a photon from the flashlamp strikes an electron within the lasing medium, the electron is excited to a higher energy state by the absorption of energy. The electron rapidly returns to its resting state, releasing the absorbed energy as a photon characteristic of the lasing medium. This process is designated *spontaneous* emission. If this photon strikes an electron already excited to a higher energy state, return to the resting state is accompanied by the release of an identical photon of the same wavelength and with wavefronts synchronized (in phase) with each other. This process is designated *stimulated* emission. These two photons strike two more excited electrons, and the process multiplies exponentially as the photons are *amplified* between two mirrors.

Laser light is monochromatic (of a single wavelength) and that wavelength is determined by the lasing medium. It is termed coherent light, as all photons are in phase with each other across time and space. When two wave crests of laser light fall upon one another, a single wave crest is produced with twice the power and height of the original crests. The laser beam achieves its power from the energy of millions of these wave crests falling atop each other. While most lasers produce only a single wavelength (or colour) of light, some can be 'tuned' to emit light at several wavelengths of the electromagnetic spectrum.

Three lasers have been most commonly used for laparoscopic cholecystectomy. The neodymium-doped yttrium aluminum garnet (Nd:YAG) laser, $\lambda = 1,064$ nm, produces light in the near infrared portion of the spectrum. The potassium–titanyl–phosphate (KTP) laser, a frequency-doubled or wavelength-halved Nd:YAG laser, $\lambda = 532$ nm, emits green light. The argon laser, $\lambda = 488–514$ nm, produces blue light. In addition, a large amount of experience with pelviscopic use of the carbon dioxide laser, $\lambda = 10.6$ μm, has been reported in the gynaecologic literature.

The ability of laser light to heat tissue is dependent upon the laser wavelength, its power density, and the presence of tissue pigment. The most common tissue pigments, or chromophores, are water, melanin, and haemoglobin, each of which selectively absorbs light of different wavelengths. The extent of laser penetration into tissue, and therefore its effect, depends upon the quantity of each chromophore present and the extent of absorption of the wavelength in use by each chromophore. As a result, lasers of different wavelengths have different tissue effects, and their surgical applications vary dramatically.

CO₂ laser

Carbon dioxide laser energy ($\lambda = 10.6$ μm) is heavily absorbed by water. As a result, the CO_2 laser rapidly vaporizes tissue but penetrates only 50–100 μm, making it excellent for treatment of thin surface lesions.[14] Such shallow penetration, however, prevents the CO_2 laser from providing effective coagulation of vessels larger than 100–200 μm in diameter.

Additionally, CO_2 laser energy delivery requires a cumbersome set of mirrors in an articulating arm, making it difficult to use in laparoscopic surgery. Because it is heavily absorbed by any water-containing tissue, regardless of its pigmentation, the CO_2 laser should be used with a light backstop during laparoscopic procedures.

The CO_2 laser has been employed extensively in the laparoscopic treatment of endometriosis.[15,16] It has also been used as a cutting instrument in other pelviscopic procedures, such as oophorectomy, appendicectomy, hysterectomy, and adhesiolysis. However, the lack of a flexible fibre-optic fibre for CO_2 laser transmission and its inadequate coagulating abilities make this laser inappropriate for laparoscopic cholecystectomy.

Argon and KTP lasers

The argon ($\lambda = 488–514$ nm) and KTP ($\lambda = 532$ nm) lasers are poorly absorbed by water and heavily absorbed by haemoglobin. The majority of argon or KTP laser energy directed at vascularized tissue is rapidly absorbed, resulting in a uniform injury approximately 1 mm in depth.[17] Thus, these wavelengths provide excellent coagulation of superficial vascular lesions, such as colonic telangiectasias or deposits of endometriosis.[18] Such shallow penetration is inadequate for effective coagulation of larger vessels. Similarly, these lasers do not provide the deep tissue penetration and even heating necessary for coagulation of actively bleeding vessels. As a result, although heavily absorbed by haemoglobin, argon and KTP laser energy are relatively poor coagulators for laparoscopic surgery.

Nd:YAG laser

Free-beam Nd:YAG laser energy ($\lambda = 1,064$ nm) is poorly absorbed by haemoglobin and water, penetrating deeper to produce tissue injury 3–4 mm in depth.[17] Coagulation of the target tissue results, but vaporization, and hence cutting, does not occur, limiting the laparoscopic applications of free-beam Nd:YAG laser energy. Nd:YAG laser energy delivered with a contact tip, however, does vaporize tissue and produces a much shallower injury (< l mm), making it attractive for some laparoscopic procedures.[19]

Table 5.1. Contact Nd:YAG laser versus monopolar electrosurgery in 100 patients undergoing laparoscopic cholecystectomy

	Laser	*Electrocautery*	p
No. of patients	50	50	
Time to dissect gallbladder from liver (min, mean ± SD)	23.56 ± 9.56	19.24 ± 8.48	0.0187
Total no. of perforated gallbladders	15	8	NS
No. of liver injuries	18	14	NS
Estimated blood loss (graded 0–4, mean ± SD)	0.78 ± 0.85	0.34 ± 0.66	0.0052

NS = not significant.

Disadvantages of laser dissection

Photon energy of different wavelengths is selectively absorbed by different pigments, a phenomenon unique to lasers. This property is used to great advantage in the treatment of pigmented lesions, such as argon laser photocoagulation of endometriomas or vascular ectasias. This attribute similarly allows argon or KTP coagulation of small blood vessels during laparoscopic cholecystectomy dissection. However, laser energy of all wavelengths is heavily absorbed by black pigments. When eschar forms over a larger bleeding vessel, photocoagulation cannot proceed unless the eschar is removed. In contrast, electrical current is colour blind, and high peak voltage coagulation current will readily arc across thin eschar to coagulate the underlying vessel. Additionally, most monopolar electrical current passes back to the ground plate through the circulatory system. This produces the highest current density, and thus heating, in blood vessels. As a result, laser dissection during laparoscopic cholecystectomy, even with the Nd:YAG laser, can be expected to be bloodier than electrosurgical dissection.

A few obstacles are encountered when free-beam laser fibres are used laparoscopically. Dissection with a free laser beam provides no tactile feedback to the surgeon, and accurate targeting may prove difficult. Past-pointing injuries of nearby viscera may result. Contact tip fibres, while more expensive, do provide tactile feedback and allow the surgeon to cut tissue with the side of the fibre. Fine-pointed contact tips heat so rapidly that all of the thermal energy is quickly transmitted to tissue, resulting in tissue vaporization. Large orbed contact tips heat much more slowly, generating a slower increase in tissue temperature and producing tissue coagulation. However, contact laser fibre tips remain hot for 5–10 seconds following cessation of activation, and may cause inadvertent visceral injury.

Comparative data

To date, two reports comparing laser dissection with electrosurgical dissection during laparoscopic cholecystectomy have been published. The first report, a retrospective evaluation of 50 patients undergoing laparoscopic cholecystectomy, found free-beam KTP laser dissection to average 20 minutes longer and cost $500 more than electrosurgical dissection.[5] A study bias in favour of electrosurgical dissection exists in this review, however, as the laser-dissected patients underwent cholecystectomy earlier in the author's experience than electrosurgically dissected patients. Another author reported a prospective study of 300 patients undergoing laparoscopic cholecystectomy with contact Nd:YAG laser, free-beam KTP laser, or electrosurgical dissection.[6] Although concluding that electrosurgical dissection was cheaper, less bloody, and faster than laser dissection, no numerical data were provided in this report.

We undertook a prospective, randomized trial comparing laser and electrosurgical dissection during laparoscopic cholecystectomy. For the reasons outlined earlier, a contact Nd:YAG laser system using 1,200 μm orb-tipped fibres was chosen. With laser set-up and calibration time excluded, we found laser dissection of the gallbladder from the liver bed averaged 4 minutes longer than electrosurgical dissection $(p < 0.05)$[20] (see Table 5.1). This finding was influenced by significantly greater blood loss accompanying laser dissection $(p < 0.05)$. Dissection time was additionally prolonged by laser malfunction or fibre breakage in 6 of 50 patients in the laser group. No complications attributable to dissection with either instrument were noted.

Conclusions

The evidence gathered to date clearly does not support the contention that laser dissection in laparoscopic cholecystectomy is safer and superior to electrosurgical dissection. On the contrary, electrosurgical devices provide better coagulation and faster dissection than lasers. Certainly, there is no reason for the experienced laser laparoscopist to abandon laser use. However, undertaking the significant training and start-up costs associated with lasers does not appear justified for the average laparoscopic surgeon.

References

1. Peters, J.H., Ellison, E.C., Innes, J.T. *et al.* (1991). Safety and efficacy of laparoscopic cholecystectomy. *Annals of Surgery*, **213**, 3–12.
2. The Southern Surgeons Club (1991). A prospective analysis of 1518 laparoscopic cholecystectomies. *New England Journal of Medicine*, **324**, 1073–8.
3. Goodman, G.R. and Hunter, J.G. (1990). Results of laparoscopic cholecystectomy in a university hospital. *American Journal of Surgery*, **162**, 576–9.
4. Bailey, R.W., Zucker, K.A., Flowers, J.L. *et al.* (1991). Laparoscopic cholecystectomy: experience with 375 consecutive patients. *Annals of Surgery*, **214**, 531–41.
5. Voyles, C.R., Petro, A.B., Meena, A.L. *et al.* (1991). A practical approach to laparoscopic cholecystectomy. *American Journal of Surgery*, **161**, 365–70.
6. Corbitt, J.D. (1991). Laparoscopic cholecystectomy: laser versus electrosurgery. *Surgical Laparoscopy and Endoscopy*, **1**, 85–8.
7. Hunter, J.G. (1991). Laser or electrocautery for laparoscopic cholecystectomy? *American Journal of Surgery*, **161**, 345–9.
8. Easter, D.W. and Moosa, A.R. (1991). Laser and laparoscopic cholecystectomy: a hazardous union? *Archives of Surgery*, **126**, 423.
9. Voyles, C.R., Meena, A.L., Petro, A.B. *et al.* (1990). Electrocautery is superior to laser for laparoscopic cholecystectomy. *American Journal of Surgery*, **160**, 457.
10. Thompson, B.H. and Wheeless, C.R. (1973). Gastrointestinal complications of laparoscopy sterilization. *Obstetrics Gynecology*, **41**, 669–76.
11. Valez, M., Reddick, E. and Kaivc, M. (1991). Should electrosurgery be used laparoscopically? *The Halsted Health Harbinger*, March, 1–4.
12. American Health Consultants (1991). Are general surgeons ignoring lessons of gynecology? *Clinical Laser Monthly*, **9**, 1–4.
13. Phillips, J.M. (1975). Survey of gynecologic laparoscopy for 1974. *Journal of Reproductive Medicine*, **15**, 45–50.
14. Dixon, J.A. (1988). Current laser applications in general surgery. *Annals of Surgery*, **207**, 355–72.
15. Martin, D.C. (1986). CO_2 laser laparoscopy for endometriosis associated with infertility. *Journal of Reproductive Medicine*, **31**, 1089–94.
16. Adamson, G.D., Lu, J. and Subak, L.L. (1988) Laparoscopic CO_2 laser vaporization of endometriosis compared with traditional treatments. *Fertility and Sterility*, **50**, 704–10.
17. Hunter, J.G., Burt, R.W., Becker, J.M. *et al.* (1989). Quantitation of colonic injury from argon laser, neodymium : YAG laser and monopolar electrocautery applied to flat mucosa and small sessile polyps of the canine colon. *Gastrointestinal Endoscopy*, **35**, 16–21.
18. Keye, W.R. (1989). Laparoscopic treatment of endometriosis. *Obstetrics Gynecology Clinics of North America*, **16**, 157–66.
19. Corson, S.L., Woodland, M., Frishman, G., *et al.* (1989). Treatment of endometriosis with a Nd:YAG tissue contact laser probe via laparoscopy. *International Journal of Fertility*, **34**, 284–8.
20. Bordelon, B.M., Hobday, K.A. and Hunter, J.G. (1993) Laser versus electrosurgery during laparoscopic cholecystectomy: a prospective, randomized trial. *Archives of Surgery*, **128**, 233–6.

6

The results of laparoscopic cholecystectomy

R.G. Wilson

Introduction

The first successful laparoscopic cholecystectomy was performed by Mouret in Lyons, France, in 1987. Although Mouret has never published an account of this, the operation was rapidly adopted by Dubois and co-workers in Paris[1] and the technique spread rapidly through France[2] and Germany.[3] Almost simultaneously in the United States several centres were also developing a similar laparoscopic approach to cholecystectomy. This was first reported in print by Reddick and Olsen[4] with the major difference to the French approach being the use of and emphasis on the laser. Since then the operation has become well established throughout the Western world and is already being referred to as the gold standard procedure for symptomatic gallstones.

Review of the literature shows that there are some immediately apparent benefits to the patient when it is compared to open cholecystectomy. The rapid introduction of this technique has, however, not been without controversy.[5,6,7] There are perceived weaknesses of the procedure such as an increased incidence of common bile duct injury which will probably diminish as surgeons gain more experience with this technique.

Success of laparoscopic cholecystectomy

The early proponents of laparoscopic cholecystectomy in Europe wisely counselled a lengthy list of contraindications to attempting the procedure.[8] In Cuschieri's survey of 20 different surgeons there was 100% consensus that severe acute cholecystitis or empyema should be considered as contraindications as should jaundice, portal hypertension and pregnancy. Most also agreed that ductal calculi, acute pancreatitis and previous surgery were relative contraindications. Many of these contraindications were accepted and applied in the early reported series of cholecystectomy, but sadly few authors have given a clear indication of how many patients were excluded. Given that laparoscopic cholecystectomy in most series includes a degree of patient selection, the applicability of the technique should be interpreted with respect to the reported rates of conversion to open operation as this is one important yardstick of success. Conversion, during the learning phase in particular, should not be regarded as failure.

The conversion rate in published series is shown in Table 6.1. Although some have reported conversion rates as high as 13%, without a selective approach,[9] a commonly quoted figure for conversion is 5% and many of the early series were remarkably consistent in this regard. However, as surgical experience and confidence with the procedure grow it is likely that this figure will fall progressively. The first 400 laparoscopic cholecystectomies performed at the Western General Hospital, Edinburgh, were audited on a prospective basis with no patients presenting for cholecystectomy being excluded. The conversion rate was 2%. This has been bettered by Reddick and Spaw, pioneers of laser laparoscopic

Table 6.1 Conversion rates in published series

Series	n	Conversions	Forced	Elective
Grace[9]	100	14 (14%)	4	10
Schirmer[10]	152	13 (8.5%)	6	7
Graves[11]*	304	21 (6.9%)	2	19
Wilson[12]	180	10 (6.0%)	5	5
Dubois[13]*	690	40 (5.8%)	4	36
Zucker[14]*	100	5 (5.0%)	2	3
Berci[15]*	418	22 (5.0%)	not stated	
Voyles[16]*	453	24 (5.0%)	0	24
Southern Surgeons[17]*	1,518	72 (4.7%)	16	56
Gadacz[18]*	60	3 (4.4%)	2	1
Davis[19]*	622	26 (4.2%)	10	16
Peters[20]*	100	4 (4.0%)	1	3
European Multicentre[8]*	1236	45 (3.6%)	12	33
Perissat[2]	104	3 (2.9%)	2	1
Soper[21]	618	18 (2.9%)	1	17
Ferzli[22]	111	3 (2.0%)	2†	1
McKernan[23]	50	1 (2.0%)	1	
Spaw[24]	500	9 (1.8%)	3	6
Total	7,316	333 (4.5%)		

*Denotes series which state if patients were selected for operation.
†Includes one major vascular injury

cholecystectomy, who achieved a conversion rate of 1.8% in their first 500 patients.[24]

Some smaller series have reported conversion rates of zero.[25,26] A conversion rate of no more than 2% or less should be feasible even in unselected groups of patients who have had previous abdominal surgery. In our own series of 400 patients 54% had had some form of previous abdominal procedure. This includes patients with partial gastrectomy and patients with previous major colorectal resections.

The proportion of conversions which were due to an elective decision or were forced by an adverse event are also listed in Table 6.1. In the majority of cases this was due to an inability to proceed with the operation either because of abdominal adhesions or the surgeon perceiving there to be adverse inflammatory reaction around the gallbladder making dissection difficult. A smaller proportion of conversions are due to the surgeon's hand being 'forced'. A common reason cited in several series is bleeding from the cystic artery. This appears to be a more common event in those series where a blunt dissection technique is used as opposed to a diathermy dissection technique. In our own experience in Edinburgh, no patients have required conversion to open procedure due to haemorrhage

from the cystic artery. It is likely that this particular complication is related to dissection technique and should be less frequently reported as an indication for conversion as surgical expertise increases.

Another common procedure-related indication for forced conversion is common bile duct injury. This was cited as the reason for two enforced conversions in a large European study of 1,236 procedures. It also accounted for conversions in several of the early series reported in the United States.[14,15,20] In the large Southern Surgeons series,[17] seven injuries to major bile ducts occurred during operation for a rate of 0.5%. Four of these injuries, described as simple lacerations, were recognized and were repaired during the initial surgery.

Laparoscopic procedures have a small but well-documented incidence of both visceral and vascular injury estimated at between 0.3 and 2%.[27] It is inevitable that such complications will occur during laparoscopic cholecystectomy. In the Southern Surgeons review 0.3% of patients (4 out of 1518) required conversion to an open procedure for bowel injury and others have reported isolated cases.[12,22,24]

Ferzli and Kloss[22] have reported a single case of major vascular injury during laparoscopic cholecystectomy.

Table 6.2   Post-operative complications (excludes retained CBD stones)

Series	n	Total	Major		Minor	
			Biloma	Other	Wound	Other
Grace[9]	100	12 (12.0%)	2	2	1	7
Peters[20]	100	11 (11.0%)	2	–	2	7
Schirmer[10]	152	16 (10.5%)	–	5	5	6
Wilson[12]	180	12 (6.7%)	1	2	2	7
Southern Surgeons[17]	1,518	59 (3.9%)	6	5	16	32
Davis[19]	622	23 (3.4%)	3	6	8	6
Spaw[24]	500	13 (2.6%)	1	4	0	8
Perissat[2]	114	3 (2.6%)	3	0	0	0
Soper[21]	618	16 (2.3%)	1	3	4	6
McKernan[23]	50	1 (2.0%)	1	0	0	0
Graves[11]	304	6 (2.0%)	0	0	0	6
Nottle[35]	50	1 (2.0%)	1	0	0	0
European Multicentre[8]	1,236	18 (1.5%)	2	5	5	6
Dubois[13]	690	7 (1.1%)	4	3	–	–
Voyles[16]	453	5 (1.1%)	1	2	–	–
Zucker[14]	100	1 (1.0)	–	–	1	0
Berci[15]	418	1 (0.2%)	0	1	0	0
Ferzli[22]111	0	0	0	0	0	0
Total	7,316	205 (2.8%)				

With improved techniques of laparoscopic suturing it is likely that in the future visceral injury if recognized will be dealt with laparoscopically. Major vascular injury should be a preventable complication of laparoscopy if correct procedures are adhered to but is one reason why a completely open technique for initiation of laparoscopy has been advocated by some.[23]

Finally, equipment failure has on occasion been reported as a reason for conversion.[8,9] With the increasing use of laparoscopic surgery it is likely that equipment failure will be obviated as a cause of conversion once equipment back-up becomes widely available.

Mortality

The reported mortality of open cholecystectomy in recent series ranges from 0.15 to 1.8%.[15,28,29,30] In Lothian the mortality following 6,700 open cholecystectomies between 1980 and 1988 was 0.6% for cholecystectomy alone rising to 0.9% when explorations of the common bile duct were included. This mortality was virtually confined to the over 60 age group.[31] Mortality following laparoscopic cholecystectomy has been low in reported series with no deaths in the largest European

study to date.[8] The only death in the Southern Surgeons series was the result of misdiagnosis (the patient dying from an undiagnosed leaking abdominal aortic aneurysm). In Dubois' series the only death in 690 cases was from a presumed pulmonary embolus.[13] Several large individual series have been reported with no deaths.[19,21,32] The Royal College of Surgeons of England confidential audit reported a mortality of 0.12% in 1,600 patients which was four times less than that following open cholecystectomy in the same period.[33]

It is reasonable to conclude therefore that laparoscopic cholecystectomy has a lower mortality rate than the open procedure.

Morbidity

One of the major sources of complications in conventional open cholecystectomy is the abdominal incision.[34] It might be expected that overall complications will therefore be lower with the laparoscopic procedure. The incidence of general complications in major series of laparoscopic cholecystectomy are summarized in Table 6.2. Overall the incidence of general complications is lower than for open cholecystectomy. Of the common complications of cholecystectomy, wound infection has

Table 6.3 Percentage bile duct injuries in laparoscopic cholecystectomy series

Series	n	% Bile duct injury	% Operative cholangiography
McKernan[23]	50	2.0	0.0
Zucker[14]	100	2.0	31.0
Neugebauer[3]	100	1.0	–
Peters[20]	100	1.0	8.0
Goodman[38]	100	1.0	76.0
Wilson[12]	180	0.6	0.0
Schirmer[10]	152	0.6	66.0
Southern Surgeons[17]	1,518	0.5	29.2
Berci[15]	418	0.5	90.0
European Multicentre[8]	1,236	0.34	–
Soper[21]	618	0.2	–
Graves[11]	304	0.3	34.0
Davis[19]	622	0.14	14.7
Graffis[32]	900	0.02	–
Voyles[16]	453	0	9.3
WGH*	500	0.0	6.0
Grace[9]	100	0.0	0.0
Spaw[24]	500	0.0	79.0
Perissat[2]	104	0.0	0.0
Ferzli[22]	111	0.0	21.0
Dubois[13]	690	0.0	0.0
Total	9,456	0.48%	

*Western General Hospital, Edinburgh.

a lower incidence with the laparoscopic technique while chest infections, deep venous thrombosis and pulmonary embolism have seldom been reported, although, as noted above, pulmonary embolus was thought to be the cause of death in a single case in Dubois' personal series.

Two sources of post-operative morbidity have, however, been highlighted in laparoscopic cholecystectomy in particular. These are firstly injury to the bile duct and secondly post-operative biliary leakage. Injury to the bile duct is the most serious morbidity associated with the operation and has an incidence of between 0.1 and 0.4% in recent series of open cholecystectomy.[28,30,36] Even following open cholecystectomy it is difficult to estimate a precise incidence due to under-reporting and because it is an uncommon complication. Perhaps the most accurate figures are those from Sweden where Andren-Sandberg *et al.*[27] recorded an incidence of 0.05% in the mid-1980s. The numbers of bile duct injuries in reported series of laparoscopic cholecystectomy are shown in Table 6.3. Most of these series do not identify the reasons for bile duct injury but several do report lacerations of the

common bile duct which they attribute to excessive traction on the cystic duct. Easter and Moosa have described six bile duct injuries following laparoscopic cholecystectomy, five of which were associated with the use of a laser.[39] There have also been anecdotal reports which suggest that the incidence of bile duct injury may be higher than in reported series.[40,41] Hunter suggests that bile duct injury can be avoided by routine use of a 30° laparoscope, maintaining firm cephalic traction on the fundus of the gallbladder, lateral traction on the infundibulum of the gallbladder to place the cystic duct as perpendicular to the bile duct as possible, and routine operative cholangiography.[42]

The use of routine operative cholangiography to clarify duct anatomy remains controversial. Sackier *et al.*,[43] who strongly advocate cholangiography, converted 12 of 464 cases because of findings on cholangiography. Eight had common bile duct stones. In two cases conversion was required for bile duct injuries which occurred during or after cholangiography and a further 2 patients were unnecessarily converted because of failure to visualize the proximal bile ducts which were subsequently found to be intact. Operative cholangiography may be performed too late to avoid biliary injury. Dubois, who does not perform routine operative cholangiography, has had no major bile duct injury in 640 patients and in our own hospital series where a policy of selective cholangiography has been used there has been no major bile duct injury in more than 550 patients.

Andren-Sandberg *et al.*[37] found that most bile duct injuries were caused by trainee surgeons who had previously performed between 25 and 100 cholecystectomies. It seems likely that the incidence of bile duct injury will decrease during laparoscopic surgery as surgeons gain experience with the technique. The increased incidence of this major complication in early series underlines the need for adequate training in this procedure. Blumgart's conclusion is just as relevant to laparoscopic as it was to open cholecystectomy. He suggested that bile duct strictures are inflicted as a result of imprecise dissection and poor visualization of anatomical structures.[44]

Post-operative biliary fistulae and bile collections have also been reported in several series of laparoscopic cholecystectomy. Some have been due to failure of the clips used to secure the cystic duct.[13,18] Others have been due to leaks from the hepatic duct as in Dubois' series[13] where 2 patients presented late with small fistulae thought to be secondary to diathermy injury. A third reported source of bile leak following laparoscopic cholecystectomy is leakage from accessory ducts of Lushka.[12,20,23,35] While some have advocated laparotomy for these complications[12,20] other have dealt with them by endoscopic biliary drainage and percutaneous abdominal drainage.[20] A third approach which we have favoured in our own patients is relaparoscopy for peritoneal toilet and placement of a subhepatic drain. We have successfully employed this technique in 3 patients who developed post-operative biliary peritonitis, in two cases due to drainage from an accessory bile duct and in one case due to failure of the cystic duct clip.

The majority of centres reporting laparoscopic cholecystectomy have attempted to identify and treat choledocholithiasis pre-operatively with ERC. Although this may change as laparoscopic techniques to explore the common bile duct are perfected there is little evidence to suggest that laparoscopic

Table 6.4 Reported incidence of retained common duct stones following laparoscopic cholecystectomy

Series	n	%	Operative cholangiography
WGH*	400	2	Selective
Wilson[12]	180	1.6	No
Grace[9]	100	1	No
Zucker[14]	100	1	Routine
Peters[20]	100	1	Selective
Voyles[16]	423	0.5	Selective
Southern Surgeons[17]	1,518	0.4	Selective
Soper[21]	618	0.3	Selective
Davis[19]	622	0.16	Selective
Spaw[24]	500	0.0	Routine
Graffis[32]	900	0.0	Selective

*Western General Hospital, Edinburgh.
Minimum follow-up of 6/12 as of April 1992, in other series follow-up limited to a few weeks to months.

Table 6.5 Mean post-operative hospital stay

Series	n	Days
Spaw[24]	500	0.98
Berci[15]	418	1.0
Peters[20]	100	1.1
Schirmer[10]	139	1.2
Southern Surgeons[17]	1,518	1.2
Ferzli[22]	111	1.4
Davis[19]	622	1.8
WGH*	400	1.8
Nathanson[49]	60	2.9
European study[8]	1,236	3.0
Neugebauer[3]	100	3.0
Grace[9]	100	4.1

*Western General Hospital, Edinburgh.

cholecystectomy results in increased numbers of patients presenting with symptomatic choledocholithiasis following cholecystectomy (Table 6.4). To date those that have been reported have all been dealt with successfully by endoscopy with one exception: Graffis[32] describes a single case of open choledochotomy following a previous laparoscopic cholecystectomy.

Some series have reported morbidity which is peculiar to the laparoscopic approach. The most common is readmission after discharge with unexplained upper abdominal pain. In these patients investigations are normal and symptoms resolve spontaneously.[10,12,17,20] Wilson *et al.* have also reported delayed recognition of

Table 6.6 Return to full-time work

	n	*Return to full-time work*	
Southern Surgeons[17]	139	79% within 10	
Spaw[24]	500	Mean	5.2
Wilson[12]	180	Median	12
Peters[20]	100	Median	12.8
European Multicentre[8]	1,236	Median	11
Zucker[14]	100	94% within 1 week	
Nottle[35]	50	Mean	11
Graves[11]	304	Mean	7.2
Grace[9]	100	Mean	13.7
WGH*	400	Mean	12.0

*Western General Hospital, Edinburgh.

visceral injury[20] which presented as an enteral fistula through a cannula site and settled with conservative management.

Post-operative stay

The major benefit for the patient which is most readily measured following laparoscopic chole-cystectomy is reduced hospital stay. Mean hospital stay in major published series is shown in Table 6.5. In the United States this averages about 1 day with the 23 hour admission being particularly popular, although Reddick and Olsen have in particular emphasized that laparoscopic cholecystectomy is feasible as a day case procedure.[45] In Europe the stay has been longer averaging either 2 or 3 days. It is likely that this figure will reduce as surgeons appreciate that it is rarely necessary for the patient to have a bladder catheter, an IV infusion, or opiate analgesia. This is underlined by our own experience in which the mean post-operative stay in hospital for our first 100 patients was 2.4 days whereas for the fourth 100 patients it was 1.2 days. The average post-operative stay in the United States following open cholecystectomy is 6.2 days.[46] This figure is identical to a recent audit of open cholecystectomy in Lothian. Short stay admissions for standard open cholecystectomy has long been an accepted practice[47,48] but has not been widely practised, perhaps because of the need for skilled back-up once the patient is discharged into the community. The principal advantage of laparoscopic cholecystectomy is that patients can be discharged without special provision after a short hospital stay.

An additional benefit of laparoscopic cholecystectomy is that patients return to work earlier than following the open procedure. The time to return to work in major published series is shown in Table 6.6. Return to work has tended to be faster in the United States than in Europe, a trend which was highlighted by the comparative study of Vitale *et al.*[50] In Spaw's series[24] the mean time to return to work is 5.2 days and in that of the Southern Surgeons 79% of patients returned to work within 10 days.[17] In the European Multicentre study reported by Cuschieri the median was 11 days,[8] in the study of Wilson *et al.* 12 days[12] and in our own Edinburgh experience 14 days, which is identical to that of an Irish study.[9] This in part is a reflection of advice given by surgeons which presumably tended to be conservative until more experience was gained. It may also reflect the unwillingness of general practitioners to allow patients to return to work early after cholecystectomy.

Symptomatic outcome

While it has been postulated[51] that the absence of an abdominal wound will result in an increased number of patients who remain asymptomatic after removal of the gallbladder there is little data on the long-term outcome after laparoscopic cholecystectomy. Peters *et al.*[20] reported a 3 month follow-up in 52 cases of laparoscopic cholecystectomy of whom 77% considered their symptoms improved.

We have recently completed a survey of the symptomatic outcome in a cohort of 115

Table 6.7. Symptomatic outcome a minimum of one year after surgery

	Percentage of patients (95% confidence interval) having symptoms every day or most days		
	Laparoscopic cholecystectomy n = 100	*Open cholecystectomy* n = 167	*Inguinal hernia repair* n = 163
Abdominal pain	6 (2.2 12.6)	6.6 (3.3 11.5)	6.1 (3.0 11.0)
Nausea/vomiting	10 (4.9 17.6)	3.6 (1.3 7.7)	4.9 (2.1 9.4)
Heartburn	14 (7.9 22.4)	9.6 (5.6 15.1)	10.4 (5.7 15.1)
Bloating	12 (6.4 20.0)	14.4 (9.1 19.7)	4.9 (2.1 9.4)
Flatulence	17 (10.2 25.8)	20.4 (14.3 26.5)	14.1 (8.8 19.5)
Antacids	23 (15.2 32.5)	12.0 (7.1 16.9)	15.3 (9.8 20.9)
Diarrhoea	6 (2.2 12.6)	4.2 (1.7 8.4)	1.2 (0.2 4.4)

patients who had a laparoscopic cholecystectomy at least 1 year previously. For controls the same questionnaire was sent to 200 patients after open cholecystectomy and as a control group 200 patients who had inguinal hernia repair. Return of questionnaires was highest following laparoscopic cholecystectomy (100/115, 87.7%) than after open cholecystectomy (167/200, 83.5%) or inguinal hernia repair (163/200, 81.5%). In each case patients were asked to indicate whether in the previous 6 months they had experienced the listed symptoms every day, most days, occasionally or never. Patients were asked about their appetite, enjoyment of food and specific food intolerance. They were also asked if they consulted their GP about stomach pains since the operation and if so to give the reasons. Details about pre-operative symptoms and indications for the operation had been recorded prospectively for patients having laparoscopic cholecystectomy.

There was no difference in the number of patients who considered the operation to have cured or improved their pre-operative symptoms after laparoscopic cholecystectomy (94%), open cholecystectomy (94%) or inguinal hernia (94.5%). Similarly, equal numbers in each group considered their operation to have been a success (LC 94%, OC 95.2% and IH 94.5%).

The proportion of patients having symptoms every day or most days following each of the operations is shown in Table 6.7. There were no differences between the laparoscopic and open cholecystectomy groups for any of the symptoms. Antacid consumption was signifi-

cantly higher following laparoscopic cholecystectomy than open cholecystectomy as was the presence of diarrhoea but this did not reach statistical significance.

Of the laparoscopic cholecystectomy group (95% confidence limit 80–93.6%) 98% enjoyed a good appetite as did 88% of those who had an open procedure (95% confidence limit 83.1–92.9%). Enjoyment of food was similar in both groups (LC 89%, OC 95%) as was the incidence of intolerance to certain food stuffs (42% versus 47%). The majority of patients who undergo laparoscopic cholecystectomy in our Institution had presented in both the open and laparoscopic groups with acute cholecystitis or with acute symptomatic biliary pain. In our study we have found a higher incidence of satisfaction with the operation than in previous studies which only looked at open cholecystectomy. Thus Ros and Zambon evaluated 93 patients before and 2 years after open cholecystectomy at which time they found that only 53% were completely symptom free.[52] In most of these patients, however, the indication for the operation had been flatulent dyspepsia. In our own study only 17% of patients after laparoscopic cholecystectomy and 20.3% after open cholecystectomy complained of flatulence every day or most days. The antacid consumption noted particularly in the laparoscopic cholecystectomy group is presumably an attempt to treat this and the heartburn, which in our series was present in 14% of patients every day or most days after laparoscopic cholecystectomy.

A similar prevalence of these other symptoms such as stomach pain in the control group when compared to cholecystectomy patients is in keeping with previous observations on hernia operations and the general population.[53,54] It is therefore not unusual for these symptoms to have been present in patients following a cholecystectomy.

Previous studies have concluded that chronic pain in the abdominal wound was the major source of pain following open cholecystectomy in 24%[55] to 27%[52] of patients. Although we did not ask patients to specify if their abdominal pain was wound related the similar incidence of pain in the open cholecystectomy group compared to the laparoscopic cholecystectomy group does suggest that wound-related problems are not a major factor in our patients' outcome.

The high proportion of patients presenting with acute symptoms in our series may be an additional factor to explain the superior symptomatic outcome in our patients.

Perhaps the single most important question in a survey such as this is whether the operation was a success or the symptoms cured or improved as judged by the patient. Of our patients 93% considered the laparoscopic cholecystectomy to have been a success while 94% felt that their initial problems had been cured or improved. Postulated long-term benefits of laparoscopic over open cholecystectomy due to reduced wound-related symptoms have not been borne out by our study. What can certainly be concluded is that laparoscopic cholecystectomy will achieve the same rate of patient satisfaction as open cholecystectomy and none of the specific symptoms we enquired about were different a minimum of 1 year after the two types of operation.

Laparoscopic cholecystectomy for acute cholecystitis

Much of the above literature review pertains to elective cholecystectomy as cases with acute cholecystitis, severe inflammatory cholecystitis and epyema in particular were generally considered to be contraindications by the first surgeons to perform laparoscopic cholecystectomy.[8] Several centres have reported a high conversion rate when attempting laparoscopic cholecystectomy in the presence of severe acute cholecystitis and conclude that this should still be regarded as a contraindica-

tion.[9,10,12] In most major series the majority of conversions are elective at the discretion of the surgeon and in most of these series one of the prime factors prompting conversion to an open procedure was severe inflammation in the gallbladder. Despite this, laparoscopic cholecystectomy for severe acute cholecystitis has been reported with a varied degree of technical success in limited numbers of patients.[56-58] Cooperman[56] successfully performed laparoscopic cholecystectomy in 11 out of 12 patients with empyema while Flowers *et al.*[57] were more cautious in their enthusiasm for the technique and were only able to complete 10 out of 15 attempted cases laparoscopically. Unger *et al.*[58] have reported laparoscopic cholecystectomy in 55 patients with varied degrees of acute cholecystitis. This series includes five cases of empyema and 4 patients with frankly necrotic gallbladders. The remainder of their patients had a combination of acute/chronic inflammation and in 2 patients carcinoma of the gallbladder. Four of these patients required conversion to an open procedure.

In all of the above series the patients required a slightly longer post-operative stay than in cold elective cases. Our own experience of laparoscopic cholecystectomy for acutely diseased gallbladders is similar to that of Cooperman but more extensive.[59] Thirty-two patients have presented with severe complicated acute gallbladder disease which required emergency surgery within 72 hours of presentation despite intensive conservative management. Twenty-one had an empyema which had perforated in four cases and the remaining 10 patients had severe cholecystitis with transmural inflammation and a subhepatic inflammatory mass or gangrene. Only two of these cases required conversion to an open procedure. The first was a patient who had had a partial gastrectomy and who was operated on by a visiting pioneer of laparoscopic techniques, Dr E.J. Reddick. Despite his considerable experience he was forced to retreat when faced with extensive intra-abdominal adhesions. The second patient was converted because the surgeon was unable to identify with safety the cystic pedicle. There was no operative mortality and morbidity was minimal. One of the patients converted to open operation developed urinary retention and there were two complications in the laparoscopic cholecystectomy group. One of

Table 6.8. Comparison of elective and emergency laparoscopic cholecystectomy : WGH* experience

	Elective 368	Emergency 32
Conversion	6 (1.6%)	2 (6.0%)
Operation time (min)	95 (25–300)	106 (60–185)
Post-operative stay	1.4 (0–21)	2.0 (1–60)
IV Fluids	22	32
IV Antibiotics	20	27

*Western General Hospital, Edinburgh.

those was a minor wound infection and the second complication was a common bile duct stone which presented 6 weeks post-operatively and was successfully dealt with by ERCP and papillotomy.

The results experienced by these patients compared to those undergoing elective surgery during the same period are compared in Table 6.8. The median post-operative stay required was 2 days and the majority of the emergency patients required intravenous fluids and antibiotics for a 24 hour period. In many cases, presumably due to the relief of severe pain, they recovered faster than some elective patients. We have concluded that emergency laparoscopic cholecystectomy is a safe and effective treatment even for the most severe complicated acute cholecystitis. It has a low morbidity, takes no longer than elective laparoscopic surgery and confers similar benefits to the patient.

Summary

Laparoscopic cholecystectomy must now be regarded as the gold standard treatment for patients with symptomatic gallstones. Although the initial reports of this procedure appeared to show an increased risk of bile duct injury, analysis of later, larger series shows that the trend is decreasing and it seems reasonable to predict that the complication of bile duct injury has been simply a representation of the general surgical community's learning curve with a new procedure. It is now already established that the procedure has a lower mortality rate than open cholecystomy and in addition to a decreased morbidity rate the morbidity tends to be less severe.

Conversion rates for all cholecystectomies can reasonably be expected to fall to less than 2%. It seems reasonable now to consider the procedure for all comers. The contraindications suggested by Udwadia remain the most appropriate:[60] where the patient is unfit for general anaesthesia, although successful laparoscopic cholecystectomy has been reported under epidural anaesthesia;[61] acute pancreatitis when laparoscopic cholecystectomy alone will not improve the patient's clinical course; cholecystoenteric fistula; doubts about gallbladder malignancy; and finally pregnancy, although again successful cases have been reported.[62]

For patients who present with gallbladder stones the operation can now be recommended in a number which is nudging very close to 100%.

From this review of the literature it can be concluded that laparoscopic cholecystectomy is the treatment of choice for patients with symptomatic gallbladder stones. The patient can anticipate a post-operative hospital stay of less than 2 days without the need for an intravenous infusion and without opiate analgesia.

Operative cholangiography policy remains controversial but there is little evidence to support the view that routine cholangiography will prevent major bile duct injury. Given that laparoscopic methods to explore the bile duct are being increasingly reported it seems likely that most surgeons will adopt a selective cholangiography policy.

Laparoscopic cholecystectomy is undoubtedly here to stay despite the absence of a controlled clinical trial and the last remaining doubts about the efficacy of this procedure will be laid to rest as further well-audited prospective series are reported.

References

1. Dubois, F. Icard, P., Bertholet, G. and Levard, H. (1990). Coelioscopic cholecystectomy: preliminary report of 36 cases. *Annals of Surgery*, **211**, 60–2.
2. Perissat, J., Collet, D., Vitale, G., Belliard, R. and Sosso, M. (1991). Laparoscopic cholecystectomy using intracorporeal lithotripsy. *American Journal of Surgery*, **161**, 371–6.
3. Neugebauer, E., Troidl, H., Spangenberger, W., Dietrich, A. and Lefering, R. (1991). The Cholecystectomy Study Group. Conventional verus laparoscopic cholecystectomy and the randomized controlled trial. *British Journal of Surgery*, **78**, 150–4.

4. Reddick, E.J., Olsen, D.O., Daniell, J.F., Saye, W.B., McKernan, J.B., Miller, W. and Hoback, M. (1989). Laparoscopic laser cholecystectomy. *Laser Medicine and Surgery News and Advances*, February, 38–40.

5. Stoney, W.S. (1991). Laparoscopic cholecystectomy. Problems of rapid growth (editorial). *The Southern Medical Journal*, **84**, 681–3.

6. Baxter, J.N. and O'Dwyer, P.J. (1992). Laparoscopic or minilaparotomy cholecystectomy: for debate. *British Medical Journal*, **304**, 559–60.

7. Smith, R. (1991). Laparoscopic cholecystectomy (letter). *British Medical Journal*, **302**, 593.

8. Cuschieri, A., Dubois, F., Mouiel, J., Mouret, P., Becker, H., Buess, G., Trede, M., Troidl, H. (1991). The European experience with laparoscopic cholecystectomy. *American Journal of Surgery*, **161**, 385–7.

9. Grace, P., Quereshi, A., Darzi, A. *et al.* (1991). Laparoscopic cholecystectomy; a hundred consecutive cases. *Irish Medical Journal*, **84**, 12–14.

10. Schirmer, B.D., Edge, S.B., Dix, J., Hyster, M.J., Hanks, J.B. and Jones, R.S. (1991). Laparoscopic cholecystectomy. *Annals of Surgery*, *213*, 665–76.

11. Graves, H.A., Ballinger, J.F. and Anderson, W.J. (1991). Appraisal of laparoscopic cholecystectomy. *Annals of Surgery*, **213**, 655–64.

12. Wilson, P., Leese, T., Morgan, W.P., Kelly, J.F. and Brigg, J.K. (1991). Elective laparoscopic cholecystectomy for 'all-comers'. *Lancet*, **338**, 795–7.

13. Dubois, F., Berthelot, G. and Levard, H. (1991). Laparoscopic cholecystectomy: historic perspective and personal experience. *Surgical Laparoscopy and Endoscopy*, **1**, 52–7.

14. Zucker, K.A., Bailey, R.W., Gadecz, T.R. and Imbembo, A.L. (1991). Laparoscopic guided cholecystectomy. *American Journal of Surgery*, **161**, 36–44.

15. Berci, G. and Sackier, J.M. (1991). The Los Angeles experience with laparoscopic cholecystectomy. *American Journal of Surgery*, **161**, 382–4.

16. Voyles, C.R., Petro, A.B., Meena, A.L., Baick, A.J. and Koury, A.M. (1991). A practical approach to laparoscopic cholecystectomy. *American Journal of Surgery*, **161**, 365–70.

17. The Southern Surgeons Club (1991). A prospective analysis of 1518 laparoscopic cholecystectomies. *New England Journal of Medicine*, **324**, 1073–8.

18. Gadacz, T.R., Talamini, M.A., Lilliemoe, K.D. and Yeo, C.J. (1990). Laparoscopic cholecystectomy. *Surgical Clinics of North America*, **70**, 1249–62.

19. Davis, C., Arregui, M., Nagan, R.F. and Shaar, C. (1992). Laparoscopic cholecystectomy: the St. Vincent experience. *Surgical Laparoscopy and Endoscopy*, **2**, 64–9.

20. Peters, J.H., Ellison, E.C., Innes, J.T. *et al.* (1991). Safety and efficacy of laparoscopic cholecystectomy. A prospective analysis of 100 initial patients. *Annals of Surgery*, **213**, 3–12.

21. Soper, N.J., Barteau, J.A., Clayman, R.V., Ashley, S.W. and Dunnegan, D.L. (1992). Laparoscopic v standard open cholecystectomy: comparison of early

results. *Surgery, Gynecology and Obstetrics*, **174**, 114–8.

22. Ferzli, G. and Koss, D.A. (1991). Laparoscopic cholecystectomy: 111 consecutive cases. *American Journal of Gastroenterology*, **86**, 1176–8.

23. McKernan, J.B. (1991). Laparoscopic cholecystectomy. American Surgeon, **57**, 311–12.

24. Spaw, A.T., Reddick, E.J. and Olsen, D.O. (1991). Laparoscopic laser cholecystectomy: analysis of 500 procedures. *Surgical Laparoscopy and Endoscopy*, **1**, 2–7.

25. Dion, Y.M. and Moin, M. (1990). Laparoscopic cholecystectomy: a report of 60 cases. *Canadian Journal of Surgery*, **53**, 483–6.

26. Espiner, H.J., Eltringham, W.K., Rowe, A. and Miller, R. (1991) Laparoscopic cholecystectomy (letter). *British Medical Journal*, **302**, 847.

27. Chamberlain, G. and Brown, J.C. (1978). Gynaecological laparoscopy. The report of the working party of the confidential enquiry into gynaecological laparoscopy. *Royal College of Obstetrics and Gynaecology of London*, April, 105–53.

28. Habib, N.A., Foo, C.F., Cox, S. *et al.* (1990). Complications of cholecystectomy in district general hospitals. *British Journal of Clinical Practice*, **66**, 189–92.

29. McSherry, C.K. and Glenn, F. (1990). The incidence and causes of death following surgery for non malignant biliary tract disease. *Annals of Surgery*, **191**, 271–5.

30. Morgernstern, L., Wong, L. and Berci, G. (1992). Twelve hundred consecutive cholecystectomies before the laparoscopic era. *Archives of Surgery*, **127**, 401–3.

31. Garden, O.J. (1988). Cholelithiasis. Lothian Surgical Audit Annual Report.

32. Graffis, R. (1992). Laparoscopic cholecystectomy: the methodist hospital experience. *Surgical Laparoscopy and Endoscopy*, **2**, 69–74.

33. Dunn, D.C. (1991). Voluntary confidential audit of outcome of surgery. *British Medical Journal*, **303**, 1272.

34. Merrill, J.R. (1988). Minimal trauma cholecystectomy. *American Surgeon*, **54**, 256–61.

35. Nottle, P.D., Wale, R.J. and Johnson, W.R. (1991). Percutaneous laparoscopic cholecystectomy: the first fifty. *Australian and New Zealand Journal of Surgery*, **61**, 254–60.

36. Raute, M. and Schaupp, W. (1988). Iatrogenic damage of the bile ducts caused by cholecystectomy. *Langenbecks Archives of Chirurgie*, **373**, 345–54.

37. Andren-Sandberg, A., Alinder, G. and Bengmark, S. (1985). Accidental lesions of the common bile duct at cholecystectomy. *Annals of Surgery*, **201**, 328–32.

38. Goodman, G.R. and Hunter, J.G. (1991). Results of laparoscopic cholecystectomy in a university teaching hospital. *American Journal of Surgery*, **162**, 576–80.

39. Easter, D.W. and Moosa, A.R. (1991). Laser and laparoscopic cholecystectomy. A hazardous union? *Archives of Surgery*, **126**, 423.

40. Shanahan, D. and Knight, M. (1992). Laparoscopic cholecystectomy (letter). *British Medical Journal*, **304**, 777.

41. Cheslyn-Curtis, S., Emberton, M., Ahmed, H., Williamson, R.C.N. and Habib, N.A. (1992). Bile duct injury following laparoscopic cholecystectomy. *British Journal of Surgery*, **79**, 231–2.

42. Hunter, J.G. (1991). Avoidance of bile duct injury during laparoscopic cholecystectomy. *American Journal of Surgery*, **162**, 71–6.

43. Sackier, J.M., Berci, G., Phillips, E., Carroll, B., Shapiro, S. and Paz-partlow, M. (1991). The role of cholangiography in laparoscopic cholecystectomy. *Archives of Surgery*, **126**, 1021–6.

44. Blumgart, L.H., Kelly, C.J. and Benjamin, I.S. (1987). Benign bile duct stricture following cholecystectomy: critical factors in management. *British Journal of Surgery*, **71**, 836–43.

45. Reddick, E.J. and Olsen, D.O. (1991). Outpatient laparoscopic laser cholecystectomy. *American Journal of Surgery*, **160**, 485–7.

46. National Inpatient Profile. Healthcare Knowledge Systems. Ann. Arbor. Michigan. 1989; 360.

47. Hall, R.C. (1987). Short surgical stay: two hospital days for cholecystectomy. *American Journal of Surgery*, **154**, 510–14.

48. Moss, G. (1986). Discharge within 24 hours of elective cholecystectomy. *Archives of Surgery*, **121**, 1159–61.

49. Nathanson, L.K., Shimi, S. and Cuschieri, A. (1991). Laparoscopic cholelcystectomy: the Dundee technique. *British Journal of Surgery*, **78**, 155–9.

50. Vitale, G.C., Collet, D., Larson, G.M., Cheadle, W.G., Miller, F.B. and Perissat, J. (1991). Interruption of professional and home activity after laparoscopic cholecystectomy among French and American patients. *American Journal of Surgery*, **161**, 396–8.

51. Brookes, D.C., Becker, J.M. and Carr-Locke, D.L. (1991). Laparoscopic cholecystectomy. *Baillieres Clinics in Gastroenterology*, **5**, 225–38.

52. Ros, E. and Zambon, D. (1987) Post cholecystectomy symptoms. A prospective study of gall stone patients before and two years after surgery. *Gut*, **28**, 1500–4.

53. Hannay, D.R. (1978). Symptom prevalence in the community. *Journal of the Royal College of General Practitioners*, **28**, 492–9.

54. Salaman, J.R., Harvey, J. and Duthie, H.L. (1981). Importance of symptoms after highly selective vagotomy. *British Medical Journal*, **283**, 1438.

55. Bates, T., Ebbs, S.R., Harrison, M. and A'Hern, R.P. (1991). Influence of cholecystectomy on symptoms. *British Journal Surgery*, **78**, 964–7.

56. Cooperman, A.M. (1990). Laparoscopic cholecystectomy for severe acute, embedded and gangrenous cholecystitis. *Journal of Laparoscopic Surgery*, **1**, 37–40.

57. Flowers, J.L., Bailey, R.W., Scovill, W.A. and Zucker, K.A. (1991). The Baltimore experience with laparoscopic management of acute cholecystitis. *American Journal of Surgery*, **161**, 388–92.

58. Unger, S.W., Edelman, D.S., Scott, J.S. and Unger, H.M. (1991) Laparoscopic treatment of acute cholecystitis. *Surgical Endoscopy*, **1**, 14–16.

59. Wilson, R.G., Macintyre, I.M.C., Nixon, S.J., Saunders, J.H. and Varma, J.S. (1992). Laparoscopic cholecystectomy: a safe and effective treatment for complicated acute cholecystitis. *British Medical Journal*, **305**, 394–6.

60. Udwadia, T.E. (1991). *Laparoscopic Cholecystectomy*. Oxford University Press, India.

61. Edelman, D.S. (1991). Laparoscopic cholecystectomy under continuous epidural anaesthesia in patients with cystic fibrosis. *American Journal of Diseases in Children*, **145**, 723–4.

62. Pucci, R.D. and Seed, R.W. (1991). Case report of laparoscopic cholecystectomy in the third trimester of pregnancy. *American Journal of Obstetrics and Gynecology*, **165**, 401–2.

7

Alternatives to laparoscopic cholecystectomy

Sarah Cheslyn-Curtis and R.C.G. Russell

Introduction

Those interested in laparoscopic surgery have grown complacement and consider that the only technique suitable for patients with gallstones is laparoscopic surgery. A keystone of good laparoscopic technique is an awareness both pre-operatively and per-operatively when the laparoscopic approach is inappropriate. Further, there are some patients who prefer to have their gallbladder preserved; these patients are usually younger people who have had only a few episodes of biliary colic and feel that they wish to preserve their gallbladder for fear of developing symptoms after the cholecystectomy and due to the absence of the gallbladder. Finally, there is a group of patients who are temporarily, such as after major surgery, or long term, unfit for laparoscopic surgery due to general medical problems, and should be treated by a non-invasive approach which does not involve general anaesthesia.

At present, the strict parameters of laparoscopic cholecystectomy have not been defined and many of the most experienced laparoscopic surgeons find that they are unable to attempt all cholecystectomies by the laparoscopic technique. Nevertheless, the beginner must be very aware of the difficulties that may be encountered during laparoscopic cholecystectomy especially in the patient with a fibrous small gallbladder in which there is much fibrosis around the triangle of Calot, or the patient who has evidence of recent acute inflamma-

tion, for here the bleeding associated with the acute inflammation can make accurate anatomical dissection difficult leading to errors in judgement. Despite good imaging it is not always possible to select such patients pre-operatively and hence even at laparoscopy the surgeon must be prepared to adopt alternative techniques. These alternative techniques can be either to perform a drainage procedure such as a percutaneous cholecystolithotomy under laparoscopic vision or to convert the procedure to a minilaparotomy. The safety of the patient remains paramount and there must be no shame to consider that alternative treatments are better for a particular patient.

Much emphasis has been laid on determining whether a laparoscopic cholecystectomy has a better outcome or greater advantages for the patient than some of the alternatives. Such debate is perhaps inappropriate and certainly the idea of establishing a controlled trial to determine which procedure is preferable is unlikely to yield a result as certain techniques have advantages for particular patients. The consensus view among patients is that the laparoscopic technique provides a better outcome and less pain than the other techniques; most surgeons have little difficulty agreeing with this concept. However, the surgeon must determine that for him the laparoscopic technique is the ideal for a particular patient and if it is not the ideal then he must be prepared to offer one of the alternative treatments. It is our contention that a service offering laparoscopic cholecystectomy

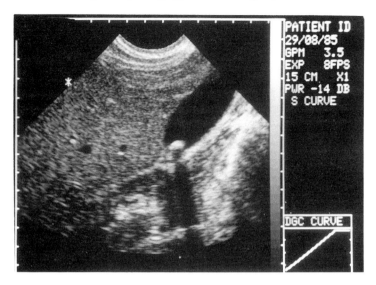

Fig. 7.1 Ultrasound of gallbladder showing a solitary stone with its acoustic shadow in a thin-walled uninflamed gallbladder.

should also be able to offer or have access to a number of the alternative techniques such as percutaneous cholecystolithotomy, endoscopic sphincterotomy and minicholecystectomy as a minimum. Thus, once the surgeon has made the decision that treatment for gallstones is appropriate, the surgeon should be able to discuss, without prejudice, the alternative treatments open to the patient. He must determine the suitability of the patient for a particular therapy on the basis of a well-defined assessment plan.

Assessment of patients for alternative treatments

The selection of the patient begins with a clinical history which determines the fitness of the patient for operative intervention. A detailed ultrasound assessment is then undertaken. It has been found useful to agree with the ultrasonographer a defined protocol. The ultrasonographer should determine the presence or absence of stones in the gallbladder, the stone size and their number (Figure 7.1). It is useful to establish the position of the gallbladder and in particular whether it is accessible for imaging or percutaneous access. For instance, a gallbladder that is difficult to image is unsuitable for most lithotripsy techniques. Similarly, a gallbladder that is largely intrahepatic can present particular problems for the inexperi-

enced laparoscopist. It is useful to determine the thickness of the wall of the gallbladder as this gives some indication of the degree of fibrosis around the gallbladder. Finally, by means of a fatty meal the contractability of the gallbladder should be assessed. The gallbladder emptying can be determined by measuring a change in the fasting gallbladder volume. Using the ellipsoid method,[1] long-axis and transverse images of the gallbladder (Figure 7.2a and b) are obtained and the volume calculated from the following formula:

$$\text{Gallbladder volume (ml)} = \frac{p.\text{length.width.height}}{6}$$

A reduction in volume of 30% or more is regarded as adequate gallbladder emptying. The ultrasonographer should then be asked to determine the size of the bile duct (Figure 7.3). It is useful to determine the size of the common hepatic duct, the common bile duct both above the duodenum and retroduodenally. A bile duct which has a size of less than 6 mm throughout its length is unlikely to contain a stone.

If a patient is being considered for dissolution therapy or extracorporeal shockwave lithotripsy, computed tomography is much more sensitive than conventional radiography in assessing calcification and can distinguish most pigment stones which are less appropriate for these techniques from cholesterol

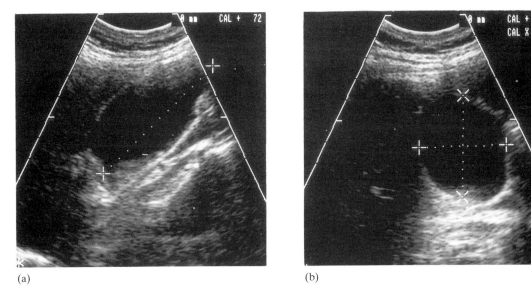

Fig. 7.2 Calculation of the gallbladder volume by measuring the longitudinal (a) and transverse (b) images of the gallbladder and applying the ellipsoid formula.

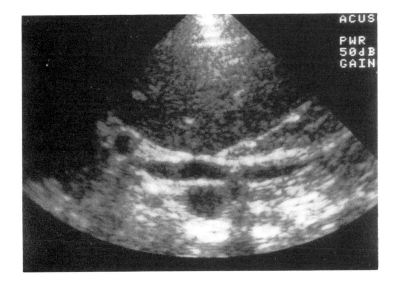

Fig. 7.3 Ultrasound of the bile duct showing a stone with a typical acoustic shadow.

stones (Figure 7.4). In a study of 28 patients with gallbladder or bile duct stones, the stone density was measured before cholecystectomy or endoscopic removal and compared with stone composition.[2] The range of attenuation values (Hounsfield units) for cholesterol stones (28–98 HU) was significantly different from the range of pigment stones.

If there is doubt about the size of the common bile duct or the anatomy of the biliary tree or the presence or absence of stones, it is appropriate to undertake further imaging. Intravenous cholangiography has gained in popularity, particularly among French surgeons, as a means of obtaining accurate information about the bile duct, its anatomy and contents, pre-operatively. With modern contrast medium this is undoubtedly done rapidly and quickly. Safety, which has always been in doubt, with this technique is

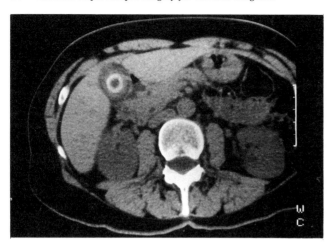

Fig. 7.4 CT scan showing a heavily calcified stone in the gallbladder. Such a stone would be unsuitable for dissolution or lithotripsy.

now less of a problem with the newer contrast agents, and reactions are now rarely recorded. If there is any doubt about the common bile duct either on account of unusual anatomy or the presence of stones then a pre-operative endoscopic cholangiogram is appropriate with provision for an endoscopic sphincterotomy and duct clearance to be performed at the time of the procedure.

Non-invasive techniques

Oral dissolution therapy

Background

Several agents for gallstone dissolution have been described for oral administration or for direct instillation into the gallbladder.[3] Dissolution therapy with bile acids was first used in 1970.[4] Two bile acids, chenodeoxycholic acid and its 7b-epimer, ursodeoxycholic acid, correct the hepatic metabolic defect that results in hypersecretion of cholesterol in bile. Ursodeoxycholic acid is more effective than chenodeoxycholic acid as it desaturates the bile to a greater extent and eliminates cholesterol as stable liquid crystalline dispersions. These acids have been shown to be effective in dissolving cholesterol gallstones at doses of about $15 \, mg \, kg^{-1} \, day^{-1}$ for chenodeoxycholic acid and $8–13 \, mg \, kg^{-1} \, day^{-1}$ for ursodeoxycholic acid.[5] Chenodeoxycholic acid has side effects, particularly diarrhoea, which lead to poor patient compliance. Other side effects are skin rash, changes in liver function tests, an increase in low density lipoprotein cholesterol and hepatotoxicity. Ursodeoxycholic acid is virtually free from side effects but is expensive. For these reasons, a combination of the two agents is commonly used and this is at least as effective as either agent alone.[6]

Selection

The ideal patient should have radiolucent stones measuring less than 15 mm in diameter (preferably < 10 mm) to give the best surface area:volume ratio, and should have a functioning gallbladder. Using these selection criteria, less than 30% of patients are suitable for oral dissolution therapy, but if account is taken of patient compliance, obesity and the presence of radiolucent insoluble pigment stones, this figure may be as low as 10%. Improved selection can be obtained by computed tomography. The effect of selecting patients by computed tomography on the results of bile acid therapy has yet to be determined but in a small study of 24 patients selected by computed tomography and treated with bile acid therapy, 64% were stone free by 18 months compared with 20% selected without computed tomography.[7]

Results

The overall efficacy of dissolution therapy is disappointingly low at about 38%, and the treatment is prolonged (6–24 months).[8] The finding on oral cholecystography of floating stones (consistent with a high cholesterol content) is associated with successful dissolution in 80–90% of cases and is the best indication for this form of therapy.[9,10] When the stones are small in number (< 1 cm in diameter within a well-functioning gallbladder) and the patient complies with the treatment, the chance of success is about 60%. Patients with larger stones which occupy most of the gallbladder volume are less likely to respond to bile acid therapy because of the greater stone burden and reduced surface area:volume ratio.

Complications occasionally develop during treatment but whether they occur with greater frequency than would happen spontaneously is unknown. Gleeson *et al.*[11] have reported cystic duct obstruction in 20% of patients after 4 years of treatment with ursodeoxycholic acid and other complications, such as recurrent biliary colic, pancreatitis and cholecystitis, in 16.8% of patients after 18 months of treatment, necessitating referral for cholecystectomy.

Recurrence

Recurrent stone formation is expected once treatment is stopped but to assume that all patients will develop stone recurrence is incorrect.[12] In the British–Belgian Gallstone Study Group's trial,[13] 83 of the original 93 patients with complete dissolution of their gallstones were followed up for 3.5–5 years. At the end of 5 years, less than 50% of the patients had developed stone recurrence and only two of 21 patients were symptomatic. The highest recurrence rate was noted in those patients with the most recent dissolution of their gallstones which indicates the stone clearance may have been incomplete. The rate was lower in patients who had remained stone free for at least 9 months, and after 2.5 years there were no further recurrences to the end of the trial. O'Donnell and Heaton[14] reported on 40 patients with complete dissolution of their gallstones of whom 27 had been followed up for over 4 years (range 0.5–11 years). The recurrence rate was approximately 10% per year for the first 5 years and then reached a plateau without additional recurrences in the subsequent 6 years. In another study[15] with a 12 year follow-up period, there were 96 complete dissolutions in 86 patients (some patients being treated for recurrent stones).

The overall recurrence rate was 12.5% in the first year rising to 61% in the eleventh year. In the early part of this study stone clearance was assessed by oral cholecystography rather than ultrasonography and so dissolution may have been overestimated leading to a higher recurrence rate. Only 10% of patients who were treated for solitary stones developed a recurrence by the sixth year, suggesting that the majority of these patients are unlikely to reform stones in the future. Similarly in the British-Belgian Gallstone Study Group's trial[16] only 15% of patients treated for solitary stones developed recurrence after 4 years. In both studies the rate of recurrence was significantly higher in patients treated for multiple stones. Such patients may have a greater degree of nucleating defects or more seeding factors increasing their propensity to reform gallstones.

The efficacy of post-dissolution therapy is uncertain and while its long-term administration has been shown significantly to reduce the overall recurrence rate, this is mainly due to an effect on patients under 50 years of age.[15] In the British–Belgian Gallstone Study Group's trial, post-dissolution therapy (3 mg ursodeoxycholic acid kg^{-1} day^{-1}) was given to one-third of patients.[13] This group contained a larger number of patients with recent stone dissolution and these patients may have been at greater risk of recurrence. However, the ursodeoxycholic acid-treated group showed a 50% decrease in recurrence compared with projected rates. Continuing oral dissolution therapy indefinitely after stone clearance is usually inappropriate because approximately 40% of patients will remain stone free for at least 12 years. There has been recent interest in altering cholesterol nucleation with non-steroidal anti-inflammatory agents. A significantly lower incidence of post-dissolution recurrence has been noted in patients on therapeutic doses of non-steroidal anti-inflammatory drugs for rheumatic complaints.[17] Also the rate of gallstone formation, in obese patients undergoing rapid weight loss, has been significantly reduced with ursodeoxycholic acid and to a lesser extent with aspirin (1,300 mg day^{-1})[18] However, aspirin (1,000 mg day^{-1}) has not been shown to reduce the risk of hospitalization for gallstone disease when given as part of a large (4,524 patient), double-blind, randomized, controlled trial of aspirin or placebo for the prevention of cardiovascular events.[19] If stones reform, immediate treatment may not be indicated, especially if they are not symptomatic.

Summary

Provided patients are carefully selected, which may mean that as few as 10% are suitable for treatment, oral dissolution therapy is moderately effective and will completely dissolve stones in 40–60% of treated patients. The treatment takes up to 2 years for complete stone dissolution and is expensive. Stone recurrence will occur in approximately 50% of patients within 5 years.

Extracorporeal shockwave lithotripsy

History

Extracorporeal shockwave lithotripsy was pioneered in Munich and first used for the treatment of kidney stones in 1980.[20] Experimental work was performed on human gallstones implanted in the gallbladders of dogs[21] and in 1986 Sauerbruch *et al.*[22] reported the successful fragmentation of gallstones in 9 patients.

Shockwaves

A shockwave is a highly distorted sinusoidal wave with a very rapid increase in amplitude and slower decline, it is created when the velocity of a pressure front exceeds the speed of sound.[23] In extracorporeal shockwave lithotripsy, the shockwaves are generated, focused and transmitted to the body through a liquid medium, usually water, which has a similar acoustic impedance to body tissues. The shockwaves spread through the body with little energy loss and therefore minimal tissue damage. Accurate positioning of the stone at the focal point of the wave is necessary for release of the high energy on impact which creates mechanical stresses and leads to fragmentation of the stone.

Lithotripsy machines

All extracorporeal lithotripters incorporate underwater shockwave generation, a focusing system, a liquid medium to transmit shock-waves from the machine to the body and an imaging system to target the shockwaves accurately on the stone. The original first generation Dornier (Germering, Germany) machine used the spark-gap principle to generate shockwaves which were focused on the stone with a fluoroscopic guidance system. The treatment involved the patient being partially immersed in a water bath under general anaesthesia. Several second generation machines are on the market using three different systems to generate shockwaves: underwater spark discharge, piezoelectric elements and electromagnetic deflection of a metal membrane. Focusing of the shockwaves is achieved by an elliptical reflector, by arraying the piezoceramic elements on a hemispherical dish or by an acoustic lens. Most manufacturers have replaced the water bath with a compressible water bag and have both ultrasound and radiographic targeting systems.

Intravenous sedoanalgesia is still necessary when using the spark-gap system. The advantage of the piezoelectric system is that it causes minimal trauma and is almost painless; treatment can be performed on an outpatient basis without anaesthesia or analgesia.[24] The disadvantage of the piezoelectric system is that a much higher proportion of patients require multiple treatment sessions to produce stone fragmentation. The more powerful shock-waves produced by the newer machines may overcome this difficulty.

Adjuvant therapy

Following stone fragmentation by lithotripsy the spontaneous discharge of stone fragments is unlikely to be complete. These fragments must negotiate the cystic duct with its valves of Heister, the common bile duct which has no peristalsis, and the sphincter of Oddi to reach the duodenum. Emptying of the normal gallbladder is a slow and incomplete process and in patients with gallstones is significantly impaired.[25,26] This impairment may be due to the physical presence of the stones, to chronic inflammation of the gallbladder wall or it may be related to the aetiology of stone formation. For these reasons adjuvant therapy is given, usually in the form of oral bile acids, but such treatment also impairs gallbladder emptying.[25] Although adjuvant therapy is thought to be necessary, studies to determine whether extracorporeal shockwave lithotripsy is effective without it have been conducted in the UK, the USA and Canada. Other adjuvant therapies that can be used are contact dissolution therapy or percutaneous cholecystolithotomy.

Selection

Patients are usually selected for extracorporeal shockwave lithotripsy according to criteria laid down in the Munich study.[27] These criteria are based on the assumption that dissolution therapy is necessary to achieve complete clearance of stone fragments which means that only cholesterol stones are suitable for treatment. Stones should be radiolucent, less than 3 cm in diameter and number not more than three. The gallbladder must function to allow bile acids to reach the stones and for the spontaneous passage of stone fragments. In the original Munich study[27] 28% of patients with gallstones were accepted for treatment but in the recent updated report,[28] 711 patients were treated over 5 years representing 19% of those referred. Examination of the number and size of gallstones in gallbladders removed at cholecystectomy suggests that only 15% of patients are suitable for lithotripsy.[29] Darzi *et al.*[30] have questioned the validity of current selection criteria and in their study of 108 patients, treated by lithotripsy combined with adjuvant bile acid and terpene administration, only one-third of patients would have been selected using the Munich criteria. The remaining patients had stones that were more than 3 cm in diameter, more than three in number, or radio-opaque. Although the initial stone clearance was slower, overall clearance at 12–18 months was 78%. Greiner *et al.*[31] examined some fragments in the faeces of 21 patients after extracorporeal shockwave lithotripsy and found that most fragments were from mixed stones and concluded that lithotripsy does not seem to be limited to pure cholesterol stones. In a study of 38 patients with calcified stones treated by lithotripsy,[32] only 3 of 19 patients followed up for a mean 18 weeks were free of residual fragments. When compared with non-calcified stones, calcified stones required 50% more shockwaves for successful fragmentation, the clearance of fragments from the gallbladder was slower and there was a higher incidence of complications. These studies indicate that some patients, who were previously regarded as unsuitable for extracorporeal shockwave lithotripsy, may be successfully treated. However, the results of treating patients with calcified stones are disappointing.

Results – stone fragmentation

Sackmann *et al.*[27] reported the Munich experience of the first 175 patients treated between 1985 and 1987 on the Dornier prototype spark-gap machine with adjuvant bile acid therapy. Eighty-three per cent of patients had solitary stones. Stone fragmentation occurred in all but 1 patient and 78% of stones were reduced to fragments of less than 3 mm in diameter, with a retreatment rate of only 5%. A total of 711 patients have now been treated, latterly using the second generation MPL9000 Dornier machine.[28] Eighty per cent had solitary stones. Complete stone fragmentation was achieved for 83% of solitary stones with diameters of up to 20 mm, for 64% of larger solitary stones and for only 32% of patients with two or three stones. In another study,[33] 38 patients were treated by piezoelectric lithotripsy and stone fragmentation was achieved in 34 patients (89%) but 25 required multiple treatment sessions (range 1–5). Other centres have achieved fragmentation rates of 75–95% with a variety of machines but with higher retreatment rates and larger fragment size than the Munich study.[34,35,36,37] Stone fragmentation has been most successful with solitary stones of less than 20 mm in diameter.[28,35,37] The poorer fragmentation rate with multiple stones and larger solitary stones may be due to the greater stone burden and the difficulties encountered in focusing shockwaves on a stone in the presence of multiple stones and fragments.

Stone clearance

In the Munich study of the first 175 patients,[27] complete stone clearance was achieved in 63% of patients at 4–8 months, in 78% of patients at 8–12 months, and in 91% of patients at 12–18 months. In patients with solitary stones of up to 20 mm in diameter the corresponding values were higher, 78, 86 and 95% respectively. Relatively poor clearance rates were observed for multiple stones, 29, 40 and 67% respectively. Similar results were obtained with the Dornier MPL9000 machine.[28] The early results of the USA Cooperative Study in which 223 patients were treated by extracorporeal shockwave lithotripsy and adjuvant ursodeoxycholic acid therapy show that 90% of patients with solitary stones of less than 20 mm in diameter and 36% overall were stone free 6 months after lithotripsy. Approximately 1,500 patients have been treated on the Wolf (Knittlingen, Germany) piezoelectric machine with a stone-free rate at 1 year of 73% for solitary stones and of 51% for multiple stones (European piezolith user meeting, unpublished results). Therefore, it seems that extracorporeal shockwave lithotripsy gives good results for solitary stones of up to 20 mm in diameter but that its value for the treatment of multiple stones is less certain.

The need for adjuvant bile acid therapy has been questioned. Fache et al.[38] treated 136 symptomatic gallstone patients with extracorporeal lithotripsy without oral dissolution therapy and obtained complete stone clearance in 61% of patients followed up for 12 months. They concluded that the results of treatment with lithotripsy alone were comparable to those with combined lithotripsy and dissolution therapy. However, a small study of 35 patients randomized to lithotripsy alone, dissolution therapy alone or combined lithotripsy and dissolution therapy showed that gallstone clearance following lithotripsy appears to be dependent upon dissolution therapy.[39] A multi-centre trial of 600 symptomatic patients with gallstones, randomized to receive ursodeoxycholic acid or placebo for 6 months, has since shown that adjuvant bile acid therapy doubled the stone-free rate (21% versus 9% respectively).[40] In this trial, successful fragmentation was achieved in 47% of patients compared with 78% in the Munich study. The stone-free rate at 6 months was also less at 21%. Maher et al.,[41] participating in this study, continued to follow their 133 patients but the patients receiving placebo were crossed over to receive bile acid therapy and by 12 months the significant advantage of patients treated with bile acid therapy over placebo had disappeared. Therefore, oral dissolution therapy appears to be an important adjunct to successful extracorporeal shockwave lithotripsy.

Complications and soft-tissue effects

Complications following lithotripsy are common but are usually minor and include transient biliary pain (36%), pancreatitis (2%), cholestasis (1%), skin petechiae (8%) and transient haematuria (4%).[28] Extracorporeal shockwave lithotripsy has the potential for causing significant soft tissue damage in the high pressure area around the focus of the shockwave.[21,42,43] Oedema of the gallbladder wall with vascular dilatation, petechial haemorrhages and variable mucosal denudation have been observed, but these changes, apart from mucosal denudation, were absent from gallbladders excised 24–48 hours and 5 days after lithotripsy.[44] The changes that occur seem to be rapidly reversible. Pulmonary damage reported in dogs has not been observed in patients.[38]

Recurrence

Only very limited data on gallstone recurrence following stone clearance by extracorporeal shockwave lithotripsy and adjuvant dissolution therapy are available because of the short follow-up period, but recurrence rates are expected to be similar to those following bile acid therapy. Sackmann et al.[45] followed up 58 of the first 60 patients to become stone free after lithotripsy for a mean period of 18 months (range 12–37 months) after discontinuation of adjuvant bile acid therapy. The rate of gallstone recurrence was 9% in the first year. The probability of stone recurrence was 11% at 18 months but no further increase was observed up to 3 years. Darzi et al.[46] have reported stone recurrence in 4 of 49 patients who had complete stone clearance for a mean 8 months (range 1–20 months) after discontinuation of dissolution therapy. In both studies the recurrent stones were small and multiple in all patients. Multiple, tiny, residual stone fragments undetected by ultrasonography may provide the nidus for recurrent stone formation.

Summary

Extracorporeal shockwave lithotripsy using second generation machines is usually painless and can be performed without anaesthesia on an outpatient basis. However, only 10–20% of patients with gallstones are suitable for treatment. The results of lithotripsy are promising with fragmentation rates of 75–90% being achieved, followed by complete stone clearance in up to 90% of patients at 12–18 months. The best results are obtained with solitary stones which occur in 5% of patients; the value of lithotripsy for treating multiple stones is less certain.

Percutaneous gallbladder procedures

The ability to puncture the gallbladder percutaneously under radiological control or laparoscopically under direct vision has opened new avenues for the non-operative management of biliary disease.

Diagnostic techniques

Transhepatic puncture of the gallbladder can be used to obtain a choolecystogram and a cholangiogram which is of use when percutaneous transhepatic cholangiography has failed. It is also useful for aspiration of bile or pus for culture in suspected cases of acute cholecystitis or empyema, and for biopsy of lesions within the gallbladder.

Therapeutic techniques

The ability to access the gallbladder percutaneously has resulted in the development of new therapeutic techniques, including percutaneous cholecystostomy, contact dissolution of gallstones and percutaneous cholecystolithotomy.

Percutaneous cholecystostomy

The transhepatic introduction of a 7–10Fr drainage catheter into the gallbladder under ultrasound control with local anaesthesia is being increasingly used to treat the acute complications of gallstone disease (Figure 7.5). Percutaneous drainage of the gallbladder under these conditions, as with any infected collection or obstructed ductal system, produces immediate relief of symptoms with resolution of pyrexia and raised white cell count. It is a very effective and safe method of managing the elderly and high risk patient with acute cholecystitis, an empyema or gangrenous perforation of the gallbladder associated with localized abscess formation. Urgent or emergency cholecystectomy in this group of patients carries a mortality of 10–14% and even the lesser procedure of

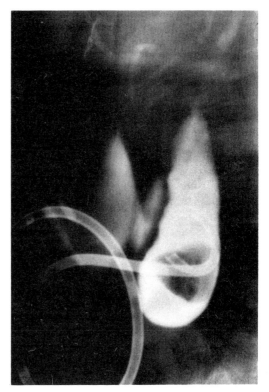

Fig. 7.5 A catheter placed in the gallbladder – contrast is seen adjacent to the gallbladder indicating a leak occurring at the time of the puncture. Such collections resolve rapidly.

operative cholecystostomy has a mortality rate of 5%.

After resolution of the acute phase of recovery of the patient, the gallbladder and any bile duct stones can be removed by percutaneous or endoscopic techniques without the need for interval cholecystectomy.

Contact dissolution therapy

Background

The Mayo Clinic introduced contact dissolution therapy with methyl tert-butyl ether (MTBE) in 1985.[47] MTBE is the most potent solvent for cholesterol stones and at present is preferred for the dissolution of gallbladder stones. Mono-octanoin and d-limonene dissolve cholesterol more slowly and are used for bile duct stones. MTBE is an alkyl ether similar to the anaesthetic agent diethyl ether, but it is liquid at body temperature, boiling at 55°C. It is capable of dissolving more than twice its own volume of cholesterol. Solitary stones have been dissolved *in vitro* in 60–100 minutes and when multiple stones have been placed in dogs' gallbladders dissolution has occurred within 4–16 hours.[48] As with bile acid therapy, MTBE is ineffective against pigment or calcified stones, but it can dissolve the cholesterol in mixed stones, leaving a residue of mud or gravel.

Technique

MTBE is administered via a 5Fr percutaneous transhepatic catheter placed in the gallbladder under intravenous sedation and local anaesthesia.[49] Before the MTBE is administered, contrast medium is injected into the gallbladder to estimate the volume needed to produce overflow into the cystic duct. Thistle *et al.*[49] continuously infuse and aspirate MTBE 4–6 times a minute by hand, for an average of 5 hours per day, for 2–3 days. At the end of the procedure, a catheter is either left in the gallbladder or can be removed with the use of ceruletide which stimulates gallbladder contraction preventing bile leakage.[50] The solvent needs to be continuously agitated and stirred as the rate of dissolution is dependent on its flow over the stone surface. *In vitro* studies have shown that the speed of dissolution may be increased by several methods: a microprocessor-assisted solvent transfer system,[51] flotation in contrast medium,[52] transcutaneous ultrasound energy[53] and stone fragmentation with a tunable dye laser[54] or ESWL prior to MTBE instillation. The microprocessor-assisted solvent transfer system simultaneously infuses and aspirates MTBE into and from the gallbladder at a high flow rate and regulates intragallbladder pressure to prevent solvent escape into the duodenum.

Selection

Only patients with cholesterol stones are suitable for treatment as MTBE is ineffective against pigment or calcified stones. Leuschner *et al.* carefully selected 120 patients from a group of 612 patients (20%) for MTBE therapy.[53]

Results

Thistle *et al.*[49] reported that MTBE resulted in complete or more than 95% dissolution of stones in 72 of 75 patients (96%). However, only 21 were completely stone free, the other 51 had residual debris in their gallbladders which would be expected to act as a nidus for recurrent stone formation. The overall 1 year stone recurrence rate for MTBE dissolution was 29%.[56]

Leuschner *et al.*[55] were successful in puncturing the gallbladder in 117 of 120 patients (98%) and achieved stone dissolution in 113 (97%). Other studies report dissolution rates of 50%[57] and over 80%.[58] The mean dissolution time for solitary stones was 3 hours and for multiple stones 10 hours.[54] After treatment 34% had some residue in the gallbladder and two of these patients developed recurrent stones. McNulty *et al.*[59] found that 4 of 18 patients (22%) developed recurrent stones within 6–18 months following complete dissolution with MTBE.

There have been several problems with this technique, not least the side effects, which include severe burning pain due to intraperitoneal leakage, transient sedation due to systemic absorption, intravascular haemolysis, nausea, vomiting, duodenal erosions, haematobilia, abnormalities in liver function tests, renal failure and destruction of certain catheter materials. MTBE does not appear to damage the gallbladder mucosa apart from producing mild inflammation and oedema.[60]

The treatment is very labour intensive requiring considerable care and skill and, because of the potential for complications, is only suited to a few specialist centres. The early stone recurrence rate appears to be higher than other gallbladder preserving treatments and is of concern.

Combined contact dissolution therapy and extracorporeal shockwave lithotripsy

Oral dissolution therapy as an adjunct to extracorporeal lithotripsy is slow and does not prevent the complications of biliary colic, duct obstruction and pancreatitis which result from the passage of stone fragments. An alternative adjunctive therapy is contact dissolution with MTBE. Experimental studies have shown that combined extracorporeal lithotripsy and MTBE dissolution therapy is feasible, and that with mechanical fragmentation the dissolution time can be reduced by 25–69%.[61,62] In a clinical study of 24 patients with symptomatic gallbladder stones treated by a combination of extracorporeal lithotripsy and MTBE therapy, 8 of 12 patients with pure radiolucent stones and 4 of 12 with calcified stones were stone free within 3–5 days.[63] Oral dissolution therapy was administered for 3 months and at a median follow-up of 5 months, complete stone clearance occurred in 11 (92%) of the radiolucent stone group and 8 (66%) of the calcified stone group. The clearance rate with the combined therapy seems to be greater than either therapy on its own.

Percutaneous cholecystolithotomy

Background

The percutaneous extraction of gallstones was first described in 1985 for the treatment of high risk patients with acute cholecystitis and was performed in up to five stages using a transhepatic tract.[64,65] The technique evolved from the introduction of percutaneous cholecystostomy as an alternative to operative cholecystostomy and utilized well-established techniques for dilating percutaneous tracts and stone extraction. In 1988, Kellett *et al.*[66] described an adaptation of the technique used for percutaneous nephrolithotomy for the extraction of gallbladder stones. The gallbladder was accessed transperitoneally enabling the use of large cannulae for easier stone extraction without traumatizing the liver. The transperitoneal approach to the gallbladder is generally avoided because of the risk of bowel puncture and intraperitoneal bile leakage. It has been postulated from two studies of computed tomography of the gallbladder that because of the interposition of liver and colon, safe peritoneal puncture was not feasible in 34% of patients[67] and that puncture of the gallbladder fundus was only possible in 13%.[68] However, it has been shown in practice that the majority of gallbladders (101 of 113) can be safely punctured by this route.[69] Intraperitoneal bile leakage does not occur if the gallbladder is drained until a tract has formed.

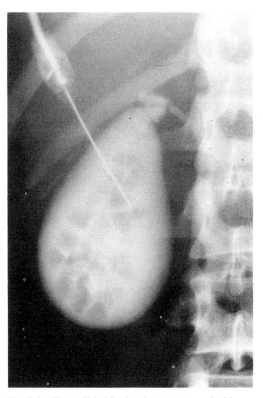

Fig. 7.6   The gallbladder has been punctured with a needle to display the gallbladder and cystic duct.

Selection and contraindications

An ultrasound scan of the fasting gallbladder performed before and after a fatty meal is used to determine the suitability of a patient for percutaneous cholecystolithotomy. Stone composition, number and size do not affect selection. The gallbladder should be thin-walled with a fasting volume of greater than 15 ml. Almost 80% of all patients with symptomatic gallstones fulfil these criteria. The gallbladder that is non-functioning because of a stone impacted in Hartmann's pouch does not constitute a contraindication and patients with acute complications of gallbladder stones, particularly the elderly and high risk, are also suitable. The only patients unsuitable for the procedure are those with contracted, thick-walled gallbladders, not only because the gallbladder is diseased but also because of the technical difficulty in puncturing and dilating a track through a thick, fibrosed, gallbladder wall.

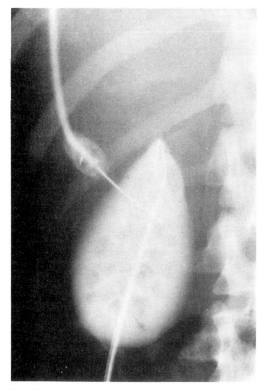

Fig. 7.7 Puncture of the fundus under fluoroscopic control to ensure a fundal puncture and easy dilatation of the track into the gallbladder.

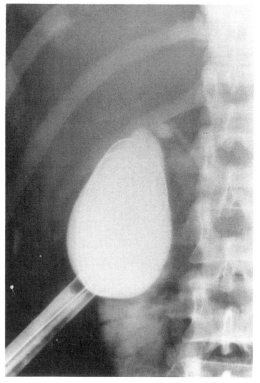

Fig. 7.8 An Amplatz sheath placed in the gallbladder with a guide wire curled up in the gallbladder.

Technique

The procedure is performed under general anaesthesia or local anaesthesia with intravenous sedation. A percutaneous cholecystogram is obtained and then the fundus of the gallbladder is punctured with a Kellett needle (152 mm long dwell sheathed needle, Becton Dickinson, Ontario, Canada), using a combination of ultrasound and fluoroscopic guidance (Figure 7.6). A guide wire is placed in the gallbladder for the entire procedure as a safety measure (Figure 7.7). The track is dilated to 28–30Fr using Teflon® (USCI) and telescoping metal dilators (Keymed, Southend-on-Sea, UK) before inserting an Amplatz Teflon® sheath (Lewis Medical, London, UK) (Figure 7.8). The gallbladder is inspected with a rigid cholecystoscope (Olympus, Keymed, Southend-on-Sea, UK) and stones up to 10 mm in diameter are flushed out or removed with forceps (Figures 7.9 and 7.10a and b). Stones

too large to pass through the Amplatz sheath are fragmented by intracorporeal electrohydraulic or ultrasound lithotripsy and removed piecemeal. The gallbladder is carefully inspected and a spot film taken to ensure that all the stones have been removed. At the end of the procedure, a Foley catheter is introduced through the Amplatz sheath and placed on free drainage. Patients are discharged from hospital after 24–48 hours and a 'tubogram' is performed as an outpatient 10 days later (Figure 7.11). The catheter is removed provided that the biliary tree is clear of stones and that there is no extravasation of contrast along the tract into the peritoneal cavity. Patients are able to return to normal activities as soon as the Foley catheter is removed, although many do so before this.

Most percutaneous cholecystolithotomies are performed in a single stage but in patients with a stone impacted in Hartmann's pouch or with an acutely inflamed gallbladder, the

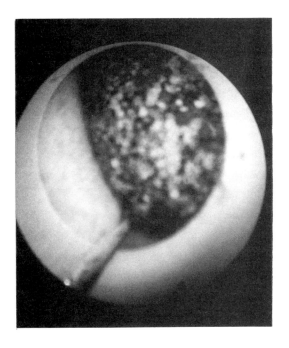

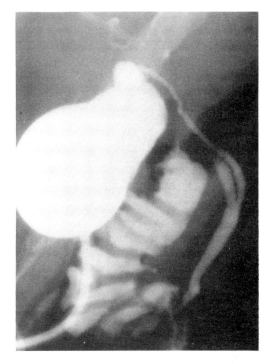

gallbladder clear of stones, with a normal cystic duct and unimpeded flow of contrast into the duodenum.

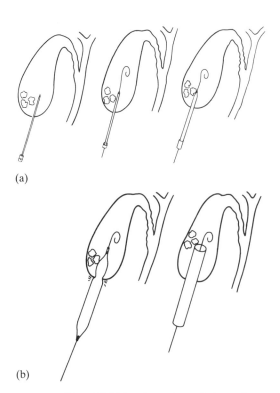

Fig. 7.10   (a) and (b) The alternative techniques for gaining access to gallbladder using a balloon dilator after the initial dilatation to 12F.

gallbladder is electively decompressed by percutaneous cholecystostomy, performed under local anaesthesia, for 7–10 days before the stones are removed. The purpose of this is to allow the stone to disimpact or for the acute inflammation to resolve.

Results

Our experience of percutaneous cholecys-tolithotomy,[69] the largest study to date, is summarized in Table 7.1. The procedure was successful in 100 of 113 patients (89%). Fourteen patients with a median age of 70 years presented with an acute complication of gallstone disease and 24 were regarded as high risk for surgery, classified as ASA III or IV. Failures were due either to failed gallbladder puncture and dilatation or to residual cystic duct stones. Failed puncture and dilatation occurred when the gallbladder wall became invaginated and moved away from the puncturing needle and dilators. To overcome this a special catheter with a removable anchor

Table 7.1 Summary of patients treated by percutaneous cholecystolithotomy at the Middlesex Hospital

	n	%
Clinical presentation		
Biliary colic	89	79
Atypical symptoms	10	9
Acute complications	14	12
Procedure		
Success	100	89
Failed puncture/dilatation	6	
Retained cystic duct stone	7	
Stages		
Single	72	72
Multiple	28	28
Duration of procedure – median (minutes)		
First 10	166	
Last 50	51	
Hospital Stay (from initial stage) – median (days)		
Elective–single	2	
Staged	6	
Acute	12	
Convalescence – median (days)		
Full recovery	12	
Employment	18	
Outcome at median 14 months – ultrasound assessment		
Stone free	83	90
Definite stones	9	10
Residual	5	
De novo	4	

to secure the fundus to the abdominal wall has been developed. Only the first 2 patients with residual cystic duct stones were advised to undergo cholecystectomy and the others have remained symptom free. Cystic duct patency was regained in 15 of 16 patients with Hartmann's pouch stones. Decompression of 13 of 14 acute gallbladders for 7–10 days before stone extraction resulted in resolution of acute cholecystitis (6), mucocoeles (2), perforated empyemas associated with liver abscesses (2) and jaundice alone with empyema or with pancreatitis (3). Endoscopic sphincterotomy was performed to remove duct stones in 2 of the 3 jaundiced patients following successful percutaneous cholecystolithotomy. Chiverton *et al.*[70] report successful stone clearance in 56 of 60 fit patients (93%) with non-acute gallstone disease.

Selection does not depend on the number, size or composition of the stones and in the Middlesex Hospital series patients had a median of five gallstones (range 1–800) with a median diameter of 10 mm (range 3–30 mm). The duration of the procedure gradually reduced with increasing experience (Table 7.1)

and compared favourably with cholecystectomy. The duration of the procedure depended on difficulties encountered during puncturing and dilatating, the stone load and the experience of the operators. Multiple hard stones, greater than 1 cm in diameter, each requiring lithotripsy and removal piecemeal, took much longer to remove than a solitary stone of less than 1 cm in diameter. There were 15 complications which mostly occurred during development of the technique, including transient cholangitis related to the omission of antibiotic prophylaxis and four subhepatic bile collections which were drained percutaneously in 1 patient and managed conservatively in the other 3. Other reported complications are colonic puncture and pancreatitis which were managed conservatively. There were no deaths in either of these studies, although one death has been reported following the development of bile peritonitis in a study of 11 elderly and high risk patients with acute cholecystitis treated by percutaneous cholecystolithotomy using a more protracted technique with 2–4 stages and lasting a mean 21 days.

Outcome

There is very little follow-up reported. In the Middlesex Hospital study, 92 of 100 patients who underwent successful percutaneous cholecystolithotomy were followed up for a median 14 months (range 6–37 months). The majority of patients (90%) were completely cured of their symptoms (79%) or had their major symptoms cured and occasionally experienced minor discomfort (11%). This contrasts with the 30–50% of patients who develop symptoms after open cholecystectomy of whom 34–50% complain of wound pain. Nine of 92 patients have reformed stones although 5 are believed to be due to residual stones or fragments. None have required treatment, 7 remain asymptomatic and the other 2 have minimal symptoms. Even with endoscopic clearance, which should be more thorough than other non-operative treatments, it is often difficult to remove radiologically undetectable, tiny fragments adherent to or embedded in the mucosa and therefore, latterly, patients were given adjuvant bile acid therapy for an arbitrary 3 month period. No patient taking the course of bile acid therapy developed stone recurrence. When gallbladder emptying was assessed 86 (93%) showed a reduction in volume of greater than 30% following a fatty meal and included 8 of 10 patients treated with an acute gallbladder and 11 of 13 patients with non-function due to an obstructing Hartmann's pouch stone.

Laparoscopic cholecystolithotomy

If expertise to access the gallbladder percutaneously is not available, then it can be punctured laparoscopically under direct vision.[71] A rigid cholecystoscope is introduced through a trocar sheath positioned in the right hypochondrium. The stones are pulverized with an ultrasonic lithotripter and flushed out by continuous irrigation and aspiration. Following the procedure the gallbladder is drained for 7 days. Seventeen patients with biliary colic have been treated by this method with minimal morbidity. Experimental work in pigs has shown that the gallbladder incision can be successfully closed using staples and fibrin glue, avoiding the need for post-procedural drainage.[72] The need to provide biliary drainage is a disadvantage of both the laparoscopic and percutaneous techniques.

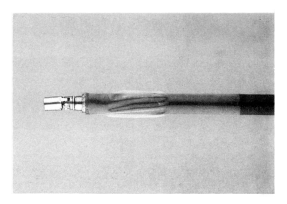

Fig. 7.12 The rotary lithotrite in the closed position.

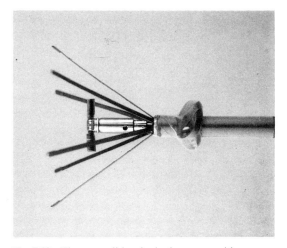

Fig. 7.13 The rotary lithotrite in the open position showing the collar, which prevents withdrawal out of the gallbladder, the impeller and the protective umbrella which prevent the impeller damaging the gallbladder wall.

Minicholecystostomy and radiological stone removal

Ultrasound guided surgical cholecystostomy, under sedation and local anaesthesia, has been described in 36 elderly, high risk patients with acute cholecystitis or severe biliary colic.[73] Stone extraction was performed, on the seventh to tenth post-operative day, using radiological techniques via the 24Fr cholecystostomy tract. Ninety-seven per cent (35 of 36) of gallbladder, 86% (6 of 7) of cystic duct and 63% (5 of 8) of bile duct stones were successfully extracted through the short surgical tract.

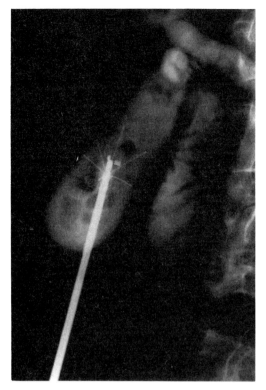

Fig. 7.14 The rotary lithotrite positioned in the gallbladder, the protective umbrella and impeller are clearly seen.

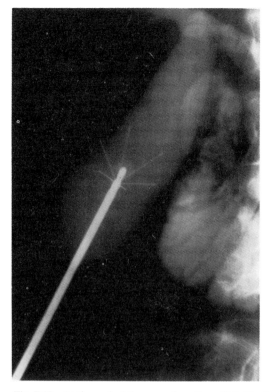

Fig. 7.15 At the end of the procedure the gallbladder is clear of stones.

Minicholecystostomy does not appear to have any advantage over the newer, less invasive technique of percutaneous cholecystolithotomy which can also be performed under local anaesthesia in the high risk patient.

Percutaneous rotary lithotripsy

This method uses the percutaneous rotary lithotrite (Kensey Nash, Exton, Pennsylvania or Rotalith, Baxter, California) which consists of a rotating metal arm (impeller) held within a rigid basket (Figures 7.12 and 7.13). It is introduced into the gallbladder in compressed form through a 10Fr percutaneous catheter. The lithotrite rotates at 30,000 revolutions per minute and generates a vortex sucking the stones into the basket (Figures 7.14 and 7.15). The impeller reduces the stones to a sludge which is flushed out at the end of the procedure (Figure 7.16). Percutaneous rotary lithotripsy is performed under local anaesthesia

and intravenous sedation and can usually be completed in a single stage. This is an advantage over percutaneous cholecystolithotomy in which one or two stages are usually required to dilate a track before stone extraction when local anaesthesia is used. For safe rotary lithotripsy, patients should have a thin-walled, functioning gallbladder of sufficient volume to admit the lithotrite. In the initial report of clinical results with the Kensey Nash lithotrite,[74] stones were cleared from nine of 10 gallbladders, although 5 patients were administered oral bile acid therapy because of residual stones or fragments. Rotation times of 7–39 minutes were required. In our own study 25 patients were treated; 13 patients were considered unfit for conventional therapy (complex group) and 12 elected to have the procedure (non-complex group). In the complex group 9 patients were treated under local anaesthesia. Only 6 of the 13 patients had a clear gallbladder at the end of the first procedure, but after

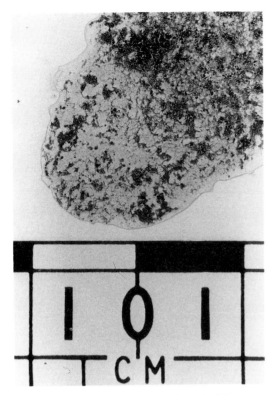

Fig. 7.16 The debris aspirated at the end of the procedure.

further treatments which included cholecystoscopy, endoscopic sphincterotomy and percutaneous cholecystolithotomy 11 patients had a stone-free gallbladder. The morbidity was high, mainly due to pain and bile leaks, causing a prolonged hospital stay (median 18 days). In the non-complex group 6 patients had the procedure performed under local anaesthesia. Ten patients had a successful clearance of the gallbladder and the remaining 2 patients had stones removed at cholecystoscopy. Despite a good clearance of the stones and a smooth technical procedure, the morbidity was high with eight emergency admissions on account of complications, and a prolonged length of stay (median 13 days). Experience in Europe and the United States is similar with numerous local complications suggesting that the technique requires considerable development before it can be applied widely in the clinical setting. The long-term outcome is unknown. Histological examination of pigs' gallbladders

into which human gallstones had been placed and treated with the Kensey Nash lithotrite showed acute haemorrhagic mucosal injury immediately after treatment and extensive mucosal regeneration with some stone fragment granulomata and mural fibrosis when examined at 1 month (28 ± 5 days).[75] Although rotary lithotripsy is a promising new method, it is not without complications; it seems that as with MTBE dissolution therapy complete clearance of stones and fragments is difficult to obtain and recurrent stone formation might be expected to be higher than other non-operative methods.

Endoscopic gallbladder techniques

In the diagnosis of treatment of gallbladder disorders, it appears to be a natural sequence of events that endoscopic techniques have followed percutaneous transhepatic ones. Examples are ERCP and PTC, ERBD and PTCD. The explanation for these developments is that endoscopic techniques are less invasive than percutaneous techniques.

Endoscopic transpapillary catheterization of the gallbladder was first reported in 1984[76] and has now become almost standardized[77] but its indications and benefits have yet to be fully identified. Its diagnostic potential has not yet been established. Direct contrast instillation may provide improved opacification of the gallbladder and peroral cholecystoscopy may become possible. Therapeutically, considered indications for endoscopic transpapillary cannulation of the cystic duct are for the instillation of MTBE in contact dissolution therapy and the treatment of acute cholecystitis.

Contact dissolution

MTBE instillation via a nasovesicular catheter has the advantages that there is no intraperitoneal leakage along the catheter and extravasation into the duodenum is less likely as the catheter occludes the cystic duct. Foerster *et al.*[78] successfully catheterized the gallbladder in 18 of 22 patients (82%) with a special catheter system without the need for endoscopic sphincterotomy. They then performed MTBE dissolution therapy in 14 patients resulting in complete stone clearance in 8 (57%), the other 6 having residual debris in the gallbladder. In

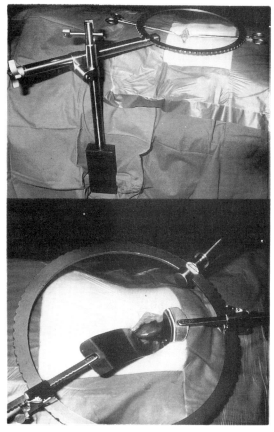

Fig. 7.17   The Bookwalter retractor in position (a) at the beginning and (b) during a minicholecystectomy.

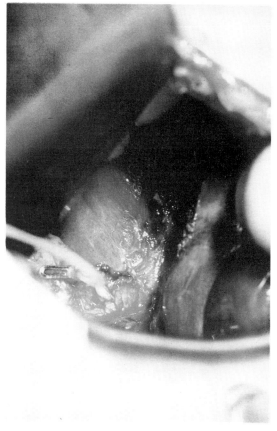

Fig. 7.18   A tantalum clip maintaining the cholangiocatheter securely in the cystic duct for the operative cholangiogram.

another study, although cannulation of the cystic duct was successful in 90% (45 of 50) of patients, MTBE dissolution therapy alone was only successful in 2 of 7 patients despite treating them for a maximum of 14 days. In the remaining 36 patients, combined ESWL and gallstone dissolution with MTBE via the nasovesicular catheter was performed. The treatment lasted a mean 10 days, patients receiving a mean of three ESWL sessions (range 1–9) resulting in complete stone clearance in 20 patients (60%). The complication rate was 10% (pancreatitis 3, cystic duct perforation 1, guide wire impaction 1).

Acute cholecystitis

As there is increased morbidity and mortality following surgery for acute cholecystitis,

particularly in the elderly, endoscopic transcystic cannulation of the gallbladder is another alternative means of decompressing and draining the gallbladder. Soehendra[79] has successfully managed 12 of 13 patients with acute cholecystitis, 9 of whom had stone obstruction of the cystic duct. In 8, stones in the gallbladder were also removed by combined ESWL and MTBE administration via the nasovesicular catheter. The other 4 patients were treated with a 7Fr pigtail endoprosthesis. Tamada *et al.*[80] treated 14 patients with an endoprosthesis in the cystic duct and report that fever resolved in all patients, pain improved in 64% and that 57% of thickened gallbladder walls and 88% of sludge reduced or improved. The endoprosthesis is better tolerated by the patient but the nasovesicular catheter has the advantages that it can be used for irrigation, the instillation of antibiotics or MTBE for direct dissolution of gallstones, to obtain a contrast study and can be flushed when it blocks.

Operative techniques

The introduction of laparoscopic cholecystectomy has overshadowed minicholecystectomy which is another technique of performing cholecystectomy and has many of the advantages of the laparoscopic operation.

Minicholecystectomy

Background

Minicholecystectomy has been performed by a small number of surgeons for several years but has never caught on, probably because of the technical difficulty of the procedure and the unfounded assumption that it is less safe than the traditional open operation.

Technique

The operation is performed through a small transverse incision (4–6 cm).[81,82,83] One method used a stabilized ring retractor (Bookwalter retractor, Codman) (Figure 7.17) which comes with a variety of fixed and malleable blades and provides accurate, fixed retraction with excellent exposure despite the small incision.[83] The surgeon's hand does not enter the abdomen at any stage and the operation can be performed without an assistant. The dissection is similar to conventional cholecystectomy and may be performed antegradely or retrogradely. It is important to maintain haemostasis throughout the operation as even a small amount of bleeding obscures the exposure, and for this purpose the use of Turner–Warwick's diathermy scissors is recommended. Per-operative cholangiography is performed, securing the cholangiocatheter with a titanium clip (Figure 7.18). The cystic duct and artery are also clipped as the application of ligatures is difficult unless these structures are very superficial. Alternatively, the branches of the cystic artery can be divided with diathermy on the gallbladder wall. The wound is closed with three to five absorbable sutures to the abdominal wall and an absorbable subcuticular skin suture. No

modification of the incision is required for the more difficult gallbladder, for exploration of the bile duct or for choledochoduodenostomy. The cosmetic result is excellent and comparable to that of laparoscopic cholecystectomy.

Results

Minicholecystectomy in most patients causes minimal wound pain, early discharge from hospital and early return to work. For example, Ledet performed minicholecystectomy on 200 consecutive patients with an age ranging from 16 to 82 years; all were discharged 3–10 hours post-operatively and subsequently experienced no significant complications.[84] Furthermore, patients with sedentary jobs were able to return to work 4–5 days after the operation. Merrill also reported good results in 82 unselected patients undergoing minicholecystectomy, although he kept his patients in hospital for 2 days after the operation.[85] More recently, McDermott *et al.* compared their first 50 consecutive patients treated by laparoscopic cholecystectomy with their first 55 consecutive patients treated by minicholecystectomy and found that the minicholecystectomy was quicker than the laparoscopic technique yet post-operative stay was similar in both groups.[86] Our own experience is that patients after minicholecystectomy spend 3–4 days in hospital compared with 1–2 days in hospital after the laparoscopic technique and that both groups return to work within 2–3 weeks, although more in the laparoscopic group return to work earlier than in the minicholecystectomy group. It should be emphasized that the differences between the two procedures are not as great as initially perceived and support the concept of open surgery if any problem occurs during the laparoscopic technique.

Minicholecystostomy

For the acutely ill patient it is possible under a local anaesthetic with per-operative ultrasound guidance to localize the fundus of the gallbladder and then to make a small incision over the gallbladder, open the distended gallbladder and extract the stones without leakage of bile or gallbladder contents into the peritoneal cavity. The procedure is completed by placing a Foley catheter into the gallbladder and closing the wound around the Foley catheter. When the patient is better, radiology is undertaken through the catheter in the X-ray department so that adequate screening can be obtained. Residual stones can be removed as for percutaneous cholecystolithotomy. Frequently in these patients no further treatment is necessary unless further symptoms develop.

Discussion

For those who have been engaged in the management of the gallstone patient, the present enthusiasm for laparoscopic cholecystectomy may prove to be an unfortunate drawback preventing a more logical approach to the management of gallstones. Undoubtedly, the prime treatment for gallstones must be prevention yet there are very few studies outlining the factors which predispose to gallstones in a population or studies which attempt to define ways of preventing gallstones. Similarly, the techniques used for dissolution, lithotripsy or percutaneous techniques have become an area of lesser interest. Yet, the ideal must always be to remove the stone from the gallbladder, retain the gallbladder and prevent recurrence of those stones. It must be remembered that up to 40% of patients continue to experience symptoms after cholecystectomy, only a minimum of which are attributable to unsuccessful surgery.[87] Symptoms after cholecystectomy may include persisting pain or dyspepsia, mistakenly attributed to asymptomatic gallstones, an understandable error when abdominal ultrasonography is increasingly the first investigation carried out in patients with epigastric pain. Alternatively, biliary symptoms may have been replaced by new symptoms which have been precipitated or exacerbated by gallbladder removal.

Loss of the reservoir function of the gallbladder results in disturbance of bile metabolism and alterations in the dynamics of the bile release. Bile flow into the duodenum changes from intermittent, meal related, to continuous and its composition also changes, becoming more damaging to gastric and oesophageal mucosa. This leads to increased duodenogastric reflux,[88] which is aggravated further by the impaired function of the antropyloric motor unit that appears to result from a direct effect of bile on the duodenum.[89] Subsequent symptoms have been related to the increased incidence of gastritis (described in up to 50% of patients), to alkaline duodenogastric reflux and to the quality of change in the composition of bile.

It has recently been shown that all gastro-oesophageal reflux markers increase after cholecystectomy.[90] The reason for this is unclear but neural and hormonal mechanisms are proposed. Stuart et al.[91] have shown an inverse relationship between gallbladder distension pressure and lower oesophageal sphincter pressure suggesting a neural link. Bile bathing the antrum has been shown to stimulate gastric acid secretion. Sandler et al. have identified tachykinins in high concentrations in the fundus, which have a profound effect on lower oesophageal sphincter function; their release may be triggered by bile or by gastritis.[92] The bile salt pool is reduced by 50% which may result in subclinical fat malabsorption and post-cholecystectomy diarrhoea which may be attributed to bile catharsis.[93] The presence of fat in the colon is known to excite the release of gastrointestinal hormones, most notably peptide YY which affects the motility of the antrum and pylorus[94] and which may have an effect on the lower oesophagus. More bile is in circulation at any one time and is subject to the effect of bacterial degradation, leading to the formation of secondary bile acids which have been implicated in colonic neoplasia following cholecystectomy. Werner et al.[95] have shown increased risks of carcinoma of the right side of the colon in 1,2-dimethylhydrazinamine-treated mice after cholecystectomy, while case control studies have shown an increase in right-sided colonic tumours in women after cholecystectomy.[96]

In certain circumstances preservation of the gallbladder seems particularly desirable: for example, in the presence of gastro-oesophageal reflux as symptoms following cholecystectomy are even more frequent in such cases; or following vagotomy and pyloroplasty or gastric resection as post-vagotomy diarrhoea may become a significant problem.[97]

Thus, there is a need for caution in considering cholecystectomy and its use for symptoms which are not related to the gallbladder is deprecated not only on the grounds of performing an unnecessary operation but on the possible grounds of doing harm to the patient. Alternative techniques do have a role, not only for technical reasons in avoiding the very difficult laparoscopic cholecystectomy but also for good physiological reasons as outlined above. The quest for the ideal dissolution agent must be continued for the combination of percutaneous puncture of the gallbladder with an appropriate rotary lithotrite and an ideal dissolution agent could well answer the quest for the true outpatient gallstone treatment with preservation of the gallbladder.

References

1. Dodds, W.J., Groh, W.J., Darweesh, R.M.A. *et al.* (1985). Sonographic measurement of gallbladder volume. *American Journal of Radiology, 145*, 1009–10.
2. Rambow, A., Staritz, M. Wosiewitz, U. *et al.* (1990). Analysis of radiolucent gallstones by computed tomography for *in vivo* estimation of stone components. *European Journal of Clinical Investigation, 20*, 475–8.
3. Neoptolemos, J.P., Hofmann, A.F. and Moossa, A.R. (1986). Chemical treatment of stones in the biliary tree. *British Journal of Surgery, 73*, 515–24.
4. Danzinger, R., Hofmann, A.F., Schoenfield, L.J. and Thistle, J.L. (1972). Dissolution of cholesterol gallstones by chenodeoxycholic acid. *New England Journal of Medicine, 286*, 1–8.
5. Fromm, H. (1986). Gallstone dissolution therapy. *Gastroenterology, 91*, 1560–7.
6. Roehrkasse, R., Fromm, H., Malavolti, M. *et al.* (1986). Gallstone dissolution treatment with a combination of chenodeoxycholic and ursodeoxycholic acids. Studies on safety, efficacy and effects on high lithogenicity, bile acid pool and serum lipids. *Digestive Diseases and Sciences, 31*, 1032–40.
7. Walters, J.R.H., Hood, K.A., Gleeson, D. *et al.* (1992). Combination therapy with oral ursodeoxycholic and chenodeoxycolic acids improves gallstone dissolution efficacy. *Gut, 33*, 375–80.
8. Maton, P.N., Iser, J.H. Rueven, A. *et al.* (1982). Outcome of chenodeoxycholic acid (CDCA) treatment in 125 patients with radiolucent gallstones. *Medicine, 61*, 85–96.
9. Fromm, H., Roat, J.W., Gonzalez, V. *et al.* (1983). Comparative efficacy and side effects of ursodeoxycholic acids in dissolving gallstones: a double-blind controlled study. *Gastroenterology, 85*, 1257–64.
10. Schoenfield, L.J., Lachin, J.M. and Steering Committee, The National Cooperative Gallstone Study Group (1981). Chenodiol (chenodeoxycholic acid) for dissolution of gallstones: the National Cooperative Gallstone Study Group. *Annals of Internal Medicine, 95*, 257–82.
11. Gleeson, D., Ruppin, D.C., Saunders, A. *et al.* (1990). Final outcome of ursodeoxycholic acid treatment in 126 patients with radiolucent gallstones. *Quarterly Journal of Medicine, 76*, 711–29.
12. Thistle, J.L. (1989). Postdissolution gallstone recurrence. *Digestive Diseases and Sciences, 34*, 44S–48S.
13. Dowling, R.H., Gleeson, D.C., Hood, K.A. *et al.* (1988). Gallstone recurrence and postdissolution management. In: *Bile Acids and the Liver* (eds Paumgartner, G., Stiehl, A. and Gerok, W.), MTP Press, Lancaster, pp. 355–67.
14. O'Donnell, L.D. and Heaton, K.W. (1988). Recurrence and re-recurrence of gall stones after medical dissolution: a longterm follow up. *Gut, 29*, 655–8.
15. Villanova, N., Bazzoli, F., Taroni, F. *et al.* (1989). Gallstone recurrence after successful oral bile acid treatment. A 12-year follow-up study and evaluation of long-term postdissolution treatment. *Gastroenterology, 97*, 726–31.
16. Dowling, R.H. (1988). Medical treatment of gallbladder stones: good news and bad news. In: *Trends in Bile Acid Research* (eds Paumgartner, G., Stiehl, A. and Gerok, W.), Kluwer Academic, London, pp. 283–305.
17. Hood, K., Gleeson, D., Ruppin, D.C. *et al.* (1988). Prevention of gallstone recurrence by non-steroidal anti-inflammatory drugs. *Lancet, ii*, 1223–5.
18. Broomfield, P.C., Chopra, R., Sheinbaum, R.C. *et al.* (1988). Effects of ursodeoxycholic acid and aspirin on the formation of lithogenic bile and gallstones during loss of weight. *New England Journal of Medicine, 319*, 1567–72.
19. Kurata, J.H., Marks, J and Abbey, D. (1991). One gram of aspirin per day does not reduce risk of hospitalization for gallstone disease. *Digestive Diseases and Sciences, 36*, 1110–5.
20. Chaussy, C., Schmiedt, E., Jocham, D. *et al.* (1982). First clinical experience with extracorporeally induced destruction of kidney stones by shock waves. *Journal of Urology, 127*, 417–20.
21. Brendel, W. and Enders, G. (1983). Shock waves for gallstones: animal studies. *Lancet, i*, 1054.
22. Sauerbruch, T., Delius, M., Paumgartner, G. *et al.* (1986). Fragmentation of gallstones by extracorporeal shock waves. *New England Journal of Medicine, 314*, 818–22.
23. Lubock, P. (1989). The physics and mechanics of lithotripters. *Digestive Diseases and Sciences, 34*, 999–1005.
24. Ferrucci, J.T. (1989). Biliary lithotripsy. *American Journal of Radiology, 153*, 15–22.
25. Forgacs, I.C., Maisey, M.N., Murphy, G.M. *et al.* (1984). Influence of gallstones and ursodeoxycholic acid therapy on gallbladder emptying. *Gastroenterology, 87*, 299–307.

26. Spengler, U., Sackmann, M., Sauerbruch, T. *et al.* (1989). Gallbladder motility before and after extracorporeal shock-wave lithotripsy. *Gastroenterology*, **96**, 860–3.

27. Sackmann, M., Delius, M., Sauerbruch, T. *et al.* (1988). Shock-wave lithotripsy of gallbladder stones. The first 175 patients. *New England Journal of Medicine*, **318**, 393–7.

28. Sackmann, M., Pauletzki, J. and Sauerbruch, T. (1991). The Munich gallbladder lithotripsy study. Results of the first 5 years with 711 patients. *Annals of Internal Medicine*, **114**, 290–6.

29. Brink, J.A., Simeone, J.F., Mueller, P.R. *et al.* (1980). Physical characteristics of gallstones removed at cholecystectomy: implications for extracorporeal shock-wave lithotripsy. *American Journal of Radiology*, **151**, 927–31.

30. Darzi, A., El-Sayed, E., O'Morain, C. *et al.* (1991). Piezoelectric lithotripsy for gallstones: analysis of results in patients with extended selection. *British Journal of Surgery*, **78**, 163–6.

31. Greiner, L., Munks, C., Heil, W. *et al.* (1990). Gallbladder stone fragments in feces after biliary extracorporeal shock-wave lithotripsy. *Gastroenterology*, **98**, 1620–4.

32. Rawat, B. and Burhenne, H.J. (1990). Extracorporeal shock wave lithotripsy of calcified gallstones. Work in progress. *Radiology*, **175**, 667–70.

33. Hood, K.A., Keightley, A., Dowling, R.H. *et al.* (1988). Piezoceramic lithotripsy of gallbladder stones: initial experience in 38 patients. *Lancet*, **i**, 1322–4.

34. Greiner, L., Wenzel, H. and Jakobeit, Ch. (1987). Biliare Stosswellen-Lithotripsie. Fragmentation und Lyse-ein neues Verfahren. *Deutsche Medizinische Wochenschrift*, **112**, 1893–6.

35. Ponchon, T., Barkun, A.N., Pujol, B. *et al.* (1989). Gallstone disappearance after extracorporeal lithotripsy and oral bile acid dissolution. *Gastroenterology*, **97**, 457–63.

36. Burhenne, H.J., Becker, C.D., Malone, D.E. *et al.* (1989). Biliary lithotripsy: early observations in 106 patients. *Radiology*, **171**, 363–7.

37. Burnett, D., Ertan, A., Jones, R. *et al.* (1989). Use of external shock-wave lithotripsy and adjuvant ursodiol for treatment of radiolucent gallstones. *Digestive Diseases and Sciences*, **34**, 1011–15.

38. Fache, J.S., Rawat, B., Burhenne, H.J. (1990). Extracorporeal cholecystolithotripsy without oral chemolitholysis. *Radiology*, **177**, 719–21.

39. Darzi, A., Leahy, A., O'Morain, C. *et al.* (1990). Gallstone clearance: a randomized study of extracorporeal shock wave lithotripsy and chemical dissolution. *British Journal of Surgery*, **77**, 1265–7.

40. Schoenfield, L.J., Berci, G. and Carnovale, R.L. (1991). The effect of ursodiol on the efficacy and safety of extracorporeal shock-wave lithotripsy of gallstones. The Dornier National Biliary Lithotripsy Study. *New England Journal of Medicine*, **323**, 1239–45.

41. Maher, J.W., Summers, R.W., Dean, T.R. *et al.* (1990). Early results of combined electrohydraulic shock-wave lithotripsy and oral litholytic therapy of gallbladder stones at the University of Iowa. *Surgery*, **108**, 648–54.

42. Delius, M., Enders, G., Heine, G. *et al.* (1987). Biological effects of shock waves: lung haemorrhage by shock waves in dogs–pressure dependence. *Ultrasound in Medicine and Biology*, **13**, 61–7.

43. Darzi, A., Reid, I., Kay, E. *et al.* (1990). Piezoelectric lithotripsy and soft tissue injury. Safety limits in the experimental and clinical setting. *Gut*, **31**, 1110–4.

44. Stephenson, T.J., Johnston, A.G. and Ross, B. (1989). Short-term effects of extracorporeal shock wave lithotripsy on the human gallbladder. *Journal of Pathology*, **158**, 239–46.

45. Sackmann, M., Ippisch, E., Sauerbruch, T. *et al.* (1990). Early gallstone recurrence rate after successful shock-wave therapy. *Gastroenterology*, **98**, 392–6.

46. Darzi, A., McCollum, P., Leahy, A. *et al.* (1990). Gallstone recurrence after successful shock wave lithotripsy. *British Journal of Surgery*, **77**, A703.

47. Allen, M.J., Borody, T.J., Bugliosi, R.F. *et al.* (1985). Rapid dissolution of gallstones by methyl tert-butyl ether: preliminary observations. *New England Journal of Medicine*, **312**, 217–20.

48. Allen, M.J., Borody, T.J., Bugliosi, R.F. *et al.* (1985). Cholelitholysis using methyl tertiary butyl ether. *Gastroenterology*, **88**, 122–5.

49. Thistle, J.L., May, G.R., Bender, C.E. *et al.* (1989). Dissolution of cholesterol gallbladder stones by methyl tert-butyl ether administered by percutaneous transhepatic catheter. *New England Journal of Medicine*, **320**, 633–9.

50. Hellstern, A., Leuschner, M., Frenk, H. *et al.* (1990). Gall stone dissolution with methyl tert-butyl ether: how to avoid complications. *Gut*, **31**, 922–5.

51. Zakko, S.F. and Hofmann, A.F. (1990). Microprocessor-assisted solvent-transfer system for gallstone dissolution. *In vitro* and *in vivo* validation. *Gastroenterology*, **99**, 1807–13.

52. Zhou, J., Lee, S.H., Rawat, B. *et al.* (1990). Iodinated contrast medium as an aid to gallstone dissolution with methyl tert-butyl ether: *in vitro* study. *Radiology*, **175**, 479–82.

53. Griffith, S.L., Burney, B.T., Fry, F.J. *et al.* (1990). Experimental gallstone dissolution with methyl tert butyl ether (MTBE) and transcutaneous ultrasound energy. *Investigative Radiology*, **25**, 146–52.

54. Faulkner, D.J. and Kozarek, R.A. (1989). Gallstones; fragmentation with a tunable dye laser and dissolution with methyl tert-butyl ether *in vitro*. *Radiology*, **170**, 185–9.

55. Luschner, U., Hellstern, A., Schmidt, K. *et al.* (1991). Gallstone dissolution with methyl tert-butyl in 120 patients – efficacy and safety. *Digestive Diseases and Sciences*, **36**, 193–9.

56. McCullough, J.E., Stadheim, L.M., Reading, C.C. *et al.* (1990). Gallstone recurrence after methyl tert-butyl ether dissolution. *Gastroenterology*, **98**, A255.

57. Ponchon, T., Baroud, J., Pugol, B. *et al.* (1988). Renal failure during dissolution of gallstones by methyl-tert-butyl ether. *Lancet*, **ii**, 176–7.

58. vanSonnenberg, E., Casola, G., Zakko, S.F. *et al.* (1988). Gallbladder and bile duct stones: percutaneous therapy with primary MTBE dissolution and mechanical methods. *Radiology*, **169**, 505–9.

59. McNulty, J., Chua, A., Keating, J. *et al.* (1991). Dissolution of cholesterol gall stones using methyltert-butyl ether: a safe effective treatment. *Gut*, **32**, 1550–3.

60. vanSonnenberg, E., Zakko, S., Hofmann, A.F. *et al.* (1991). Human gallbladder morphology after gallstone dissolution with methyl tert-butyl ether. *Gastroenterology*, **100**, 1718–23.

61. Peine, C.J., May, G.R., Nagorney, D.M. *et al.* (1990). Safety of same-day sequential extracorporeal shock wave lithotripsy and dissolution of gallstones by methyl tert-butyl ether in dogs. *Mayo Clinic Proceedings*, **65**, 1564–9.

62. Lu, D.S., Ho, C.S. and Allen, L.C. (1990). Gallstone dissolution in methyl tert-butyl ether after mechanical fragmentation. *American Journal of Radiology*, **155**, 67–72.

63. Holl, J., Sauerbruch, T., Sackmann, M. *et al.* (1991). Combined treatment of symptomatic gallbladder stones by extracorporeal shock-wave lithotripsy (ESWL) and instillation of methyl tert-butyl ether (MTBE). *Digestive Diseases and Sciences*, **36**, 1097–1101.

64. Akiyama, H., Nagusa, Y., Fujita, T. *et al.* (1985). A new method for non-surgical cholecystolithotomy. *Surgery Gynecology and Obstetrics*, **161**, 73–4.

65. Kerlan, R.K., La Berge, J.M. and Ring, E.J. (1985). Percutaneous cholecystolithotomy; preliminary experience. *Radiology*, **157**, 653–6.

66. Kellett, M.J., Wickham, J.E.A. and Russell, R.C.G. (1988). Percutaneous cholecystolithotomy. *British Medical Journal*, **296**, 453–5.

67. Hruby, W., Urban, M., Stackl, W. *et al.* (1989). Stonebearing gallbladders: CT anatomy as the key to safe percutaneous lithotropsy. *Radiology*, **173**, 385–7.

68. Warren, L.P., Kadir, S. and Dunnick, N.R. (1988). Percutaneous cholecystostomy: anatomic considerations. *Radiology*, **168**, 615–16.

69. Cheslyn-Curtis, S., Gillam, A., Russell, R.C.G. *et al.* (1992). Selection, management and early outcome of 113 patients with symptomatic gallstones treated by percutaneous cholecystolithotomy. *Gut*, **33**, 1253–9.

70. Chiverton, S.G., Inglis, J.A., Hudd, C. *et al.* (1990). Percutaneous cholecystolithotomy; the first 60 patients. *British Medical Journal*, **300**, 1310–12.

71. Perissat, J., Collet, D.R. and Belliard, R. (1989). Gallstones: laparoscopic treatment, intracorporeal lithotripsy followed by cholecystostomy or cholecystectomy – a personal technique. *Endoscopy*, **21**, 373–4.

72. Frimberger, E. (1989). Operative laparoscopy: cholecystotomy. *Endoscopy*, **21**, 367–72.

73. Gibney, R.G., Fache, J.S., Becker, C.D. *et al.* (1987). Combined surgical and radiological intervention for complicated cholelithiasis in high risk patients. *Radiology*, **165**, 715–19.

74. Miller, F.J., Rose, S.C., Buchi, K.N. *et al.* (1991). Percutaneous rotational contact biliary lithotripsy: initial clinical results with the Kensey Nash Lithotrite. *Radiology*, **178**, 781–5.

75. Dempsey, D.T., Contreras, C., Milner, R. *et al.* (1990). Percutaneous ablation of gallstones. *Journal of Surgical Research*, **49**, 116–20.

76. Kozarek, R.A. (1984). Selective cannulation of the cystic duct at the time of ERCP. *Journal of Clinical Gastroenterology*, **6**, 37–40.

77. Foerster, E-C., Auth, J., Runge, U. *et al.* (1988). Endoscopic retrograde catheterization of the gallbladder. *Endoscopy*, **20**, 30–3.

78. Foerster, E.C., Matek, W. and Domschke, W. (1990). Endoscopic retrograde cannulation of the gallbladder: direct dissolution of gallstones. *Gastrointestinal Endoscopy*, **36**, 444–50.

79. Soehendra, N. (1991). Access to the cystic duct: a new endoscopic therapy for gallbladder diseases? *Endoscopy*, **23**, 36–7.

80. Tamada, K., Seki, H., Sato, K. *et al.* (1991). Efficacy of endoscopic retrograde cholecystoendoprosthesis (ERCCE) for cholecystitis. *Endoscopy*, **23**, 2–3.

81. Goco, I.R. and Chambers, L.G. (1983). 'Minicholecystectomy' and operative cholangiography. A means of cost containment. *American Surgeon*, **49**, 143–5.

82. Dubois, F. and Berthelot, G. (1982). Cholecystectomie par minilaparotomie. *Nouvelle Presse Medicale*, **11**, 1139–41.

83. Russell, R.C.G. and Shankar, S. (1987). The stabilised ring retractor: a technique for cholecystectomy. *British Journal of Surgery*, **74**, 826.

84. Ledet, W.P. (1990). Ambulatory cholecystectomy without disability. *Archives of Surgery*, **125**, 434–5.

85. Merrill, J.R. (1988). Minimal trauma cholecystectomy. *American Surgeon*, **54**, 256–61.

86. McDermott, E.W.M., McGregor, J.R., O'Dwyer, P.J., Murphy, J.J. and O'Higgins, N.J. (1992) Patient outcome following laparoscopic and minilaparotomy cholecystectomy. *Personal communication.*

87. Ruddell, W.S.J., Lintott, D.J., Ashton, M.G. and Axon, A.T.R. (1980). Endoscopic retrograde cholangiography and pancreatography in investigation of post-cholecystectomy patients. *Lancet*, **i**, 444–7.

88. Brown, T.H., Walton, G., Cheadle, W.G. and Larson, G.M. (1989). The alkaline shift in gastric pH after cholecystectomy. *American Journal of Surgery*, **157**, 58–65.

89. Johnson, A.G. (1972). Pyloric function and gall stone dyspepsia. *British Journal of Surgery*, **59**, 449–54.

90. Walsh, T.N., Jazrawi, S., Byrne, P.J. *et al.* (1991). Cholecystectomy and oesophageal reflux. *British Journal of Surgery*, **78**, 753.

91. Stuart, R., Byrne, P.J., Marks, P., Lawlor, P., Gorey, T.F. and Hennessy, T.P.J. (1990). Extrinsic pathology

alters oesophageal motility in the dog. *British Journal of Surgery*, **77**, A709.

92. Sandler, A.D., Maher, J.W., Weinstock, J.V. *et al.* (1991). Tachykinins in the canine gastroesophageal junction. *American Journal of Surgery,* **161**, 165–70.

93. Thaysen, E.H. and Pedersen, L. (1976). Idiopathic bile acid catharsis. *Gut*, **17**, 965–70.

94. Adrian, T.E., Savage, A.P., Bacarese-Hamilton, A.J., Wolfe, K., Besterman, H.S. and Bloom, S.R. (1986). Peptide YY abnormalities in gastrointestinal disease. *Gastroenterology*, **90**, 379–84.

95. Werner, B., deHeer, K. and Mitschke, H. (1977). Cholecystectomy and carcinoma of the colon. *Zeitschrift Krebsporschung Klin. Oncol*, **88**, 223–30.

96. Turunen, M.J. and Kivilaakso, E.O. (1981). Increased risk of colorectal cancer after cholecystectomy. *Annals of Surgery*, **194**, 639–41.

97. Taylor, T.V. (1981). Postvagotomy and cholecystectomy syndrome. *Annals of Surgery*, **194**, 625–9.

8

A review of open cholecystectomy

A.W. Bradbury and J.B. Rainey

Introduction

Although observations on human gallstones date back to ancient times it was not until the middle of the 19th century, when cholecystostomy had been successfully developed and performed on both sides of the Atlantic, that any form of treatment became available. Carl Johann August Langenbuch (1846–1901) performed the first cholecystectomy on 15th July 1882 in Berlin, having stated that 'the gallbladder should be removed, not because it contains stones, but because it forms them'. The patient was a 42 year old man who had suffered from biliary colic for 16 years and had become a morphine addict as a consequence. His gallbladder contained two large cholesterol stones and its removal was reported to have been technically quite straightforward. The man recovered without incident and went home after 6 weeks. A short time later in 1884, J. Knowsley Thornton and Robert Abbe in America performed successful choledocholithotomy. Such was the success of these operations that Tait was moved to comment in 1885 that 'amongst all the advances which modern abdominal surgery has seen, I claim that there is none so certain nor so free from risk and so brilliantly successful as the surgical treatment of gallstones' (Halpert 1982).

Of these methods cholecystostomy long remained the most popular, especially in England and America. However, cholecystectomy soon won favour in Germany and Switzerland due to Langenbuch and after 1890 to Ludwig Courvoisier. The procedure was introduced to America in 1886 and by 1910 it had become accepted by W.J. Mayo as the standard treatment. However, even in the 1930s, less than one-quarter of all patients with symptomatic gallstones were being operated on. This reluctance to operate was due to the relatively high mortality and complication rate arising, in particular, from uncontrolled bleeding and sepsis. The advent of antibiotics, the discovery by Henrik Dam that 'cholemic bleeding' could be prevented by the administration of vitamin K, together with improvements in anaesthesia, quickly reduced the risk to acceptable levels. Currently, cholecystectomy remains one of the most common general surgical operations. In the USA alone between 500,000 and 700,000 cholecystectomies are performed annually (Gliedman and Wilk 1985).

Nevertheless, cholecystectomy does remain associated with a small but significant mortality and morbidity. Thus, even in the absence of complications and following a short hospital stay, two-thirds of patients require to remain off work for more than 6 weeks (Bates et al. 1984) and 27–50% complain of wound pain 1–2 years after their operation (Ros and Zambon 1987). Alternatives to open surgery have been sought including oral and contact dissolution therapy, extracorporeal shockwave lithotripsy, percutaneous cholecystostomy, percutaneous cholecystolithotomy, laproscopic cholecystolithotomy, and minicholecystostomy with radiological stone removal (Cheslyn-Curtis and Russell 1991). Although some of these techniques show promise in selected patients, the long-term results await evaluation. In addition, none of the above methods remove the source of stone formation and cannot eliminate further cholelithiasis or deal with the question of gallbladder malignancy. More recently attempts have been made to reduce the morbidity associated with cholecystectomy by reducing the length of the incision. For example, 'minicholecystectomy' may be performed through a 4–6 cm subcostal incision (Goco and Chambers 1983) using a stabilized ring retractor so that the operator's hands do not enter the abdomen and an assistant is not required (Russell and Shankar 1987). Exponents of the technique claim improved cosmesis, earlier discharge from hospital (usually 3 days), markedly reduced post-operative wound pain and earlier return to work when compared with the routine open cholecystectomy. However, the technique has not been generally accepted as an alternative to standard open cholecystectomy. By contrast laparoscopic cholecystectomy has been welcomed by the surgical community and represents the first significant challenge to open cholecystectomy as the 'gold standard' for symptomatic gallstones (McSherry 1989) in over a century.

Technique

Except in the emergency situation, the diagnosis of cholelithiasis should have been confirmed pre-operatively either by radiological contrast studies or ultrasound examination. Clinical, radiological and biochemical studies also allow the surgeon to ascertain the likelihood of gallstones being present in the common bile duct. The general condition of the patient should be optimized prior to surgery. In particular, jaundiced patients should have abnormal coagulation corrected with vitamin K and adequate urine output should be ensured. The patient should receive pre-operative prophylactic antibiotic intravenously with induction of anaesthesia and should also be considered for some form of thromboembolic prophylaxis depending on their age and coexisting risk factors.

The technique of open cholecystectomy is well described (Gunn 1986; Williamson 1987) and will not be reiterated here in great detail. Most surgeons use a right upper quadrant muscle cutting incision although some prefer an upper midline or paramedian approach. In the emergency situation, where the diagnosis is in doubt, a midline incision is recommended. Such an incision may be easily extended and allows the surgeon maximal access to the abdomen. Full diagnostic laparotomy should be performed. A tense gallbladder that is difficult to handle or at risk of perforation should be decompressed. Exposure is facilitated by packs and retractors. The cystic duct and cystic artery should be carefully identified and it is vital that no structures are divided until the surgeon is absolutely certain about the biliary anatomy. If the anatomy cannot be safely identified then a 'fundus-first' technique may be adopted or the cystic duct cannulated from within the gallbladder. Alternatively the surgeon may elect to perform a cholecystostomy or a subtotal cholecystectomy (Schein 1991).

Opinions differ as to whether an operative cholangiogram should be performed in all or only selected cases (Mirizzi 1937; Kelley and Blumgart 1985; Herman 1990). A history of jaundice or pancreatitis, deranged liver function tests, a dilated common bile duct on ultrasound examination or on direct visualization, small and numerous gallstones, and a functioning gallbladder (as shown by oral cholecystogram) all increase the likelihood of choledocholithiasis. In addition to excluding common bile duct stones a normal cholangiogram is able to reassure the surgeon that the biliary tree is intact following earlier dissection and to help exclude other biliary pathology such as tumour.

Drainage of the peritoneal cavity also remains controversial (Williams *et al.* 1972; Kambouris *et al.* 1973; Gupta *et al.* 1978; Maull *et al.* 1978; Todd and Reemtsama 1978). Proponents claim that drainage alerts the surgeon to excessive post-operative blood loss and to biliary leak (Gunn 1969). The alternative view claims that drainage may provide a false sense of security and may increase infective complications. Saline or tetracycline lavage of the peritoneal cavity is recommended, especially if there has been significant bile contamination (Hancock 1990).

Indications

Although gallstones are extremely prevalent in Western society, post-mortem studies have shown that the natural history of cholelithiasis is usually uncomplicated (Bateson and Bouchier 1975; Gracie and Ransohoff 1982; Thistle *et al.* 1984; McSherry *et al.* 1985). In general, therefore, prophylactic cholecystectomy is not recommended (Ransohoff *et al.* 1987; Way 1989; Gibney 1990). However, there are certain groups at increased risk of developing symptomatic gallstone disease for whom prophylactic surgery might be considered (see below). For patients with symptomatic gallstones, the effectiveness of cholecystectomy is well proved with over three-quarters of patients being completely relieved of their presenting complaints (Gilliland and Traverso 1990). Because the mortality for patients with untreated symptomatic gallstone disease is the same as for those with asymptomatic cholelithiasis, surgery is performed to relieve symptoms not prevent death (Ransohoff *et al.* 1983). The decision to operate is therefore based primarily upon the degree of discomfort being experienced by the patient.

Cholecystectomy is the only treatment for gallstones in which the source of gallstone formation is removed. This has obvious benefits in preventing further stones from forming but also has the advantage of removing asymptomatic gallbladder cancer which may be present in up to 5% of cases (Graham 1931). There is a close epidemiological association between the presence of gallstones (especially those over 3 cm in diameter) and gallbladder cancer. Since 70–80% of cancerous gallbladders contain gallstones, cholelithiasis has been considered a premalignant state (Lund 1960; Diehl 1983; Lowenfels *et al.* 1989; Aldridge and Bismuth 1990). There also appears to be a strong genetic element in gallstone formation and in some ethnic groups there may be an argument for prophylactic cholecystectomy in the presence of otherwise asymptomatic gallstones (Weiss *et al.* 1984; Lowenfels *et al.* 1985, 1989). Even within low risk populations there appears to be an inverse relationship between the numbers of cholecystectomies performed and the risk of death from gallbladder malignancy (Diehl and Beral 1981).

The classical indication for cholecystectomy is acute cholecystitis. Combined analysis of several randomized, controlled trials have now shown that early surgery results in fewer technical complications, fewer deaths and less post-operative morbidity than surgery deferred until after the acute episode has settled (van der Linden and Sunzel 1970; MacArthur *et al.* 1975; Lahtinen *et al.* 1978; Jarvinen and Hasbacka 1980). However, in poor risk patients an expectant policy may be preferred in order to maximize their fitness for surgery. Alternatively, a percutaneous cholecystostomy may be employed followed by interval cholecystectomy (Welch and Malt 1972; Gagic and Frey 1975; Werbel *et al.* 1989). Common bile duct stones detected at the time of cholecystectomy can be cleared from the duct by choledocholithotomy in approximately 98% of cases (Motson and Wetter 1990). A controlled trial comparing the surgeon's ability to find and clear bile duct stones at operation with pre-operative endoscopic retrograde cholangiopancreatography (ERCP) and endoscopic sphincterotomy (ES) showed that the latter method was associated with more complications (Neoptolemus *et al.* 1988). However, patients with bile duct stones who have already had a cholecystectomy or who are considered unfit for surgery may be managed successfully with ERCP and ES rather than with further surgery. However, such endoscopic procedures are also not without significant mortality and morbidity (Worthley and Toouli 1988; Davidson *et al.* 1988; Rosseland and Solhaug 1988; Simon *et al.* 1989).

Gallstone pancreatitis appears to be associated with the passage of small gallstones, formed in the gallbladder, through the sphincter of Oddi. Most attacks are mild and settle with conservative measures. However, patients should be considered for cholecystectomy during the same admission as following discharge, pending readmission for delayed elective surgery, there is a high rate of recurrent pancreatitis (Ranson 1979). In severe attacks or in patients unfit for surgery ERCP and ES may be indicated (Neoptolemus *et al.* 1988).

Mortality and morbidity

Currently, overall mortality from cholecystectomy can be less than 1% (Seltzer *et al.* 1970; Boquist *et al.* 1972; McSherry and Glenn 1980; Ganey *et al.* 1986; Gilliland and Traverso 1990). However, the elderly, those undergoing surgery for the complications of gallstone disease and those with serious pre-existing medical diseases are at increased risk. In the earliest major review of the subject Heuer (1934) reported a 6.6% overall mortality representing 2,453 deaths among a series of 36,623 patients operated upon in 21 European and American hospitals. Deaths were most often related to biliary pathology progressing to liver failure, surgical error and the respiratory complications of relatively unrefined general anaesthesia. Later, Glenn and Hayes (1952) reported a 1.8% mortality following 3,439 cholecystectomies carried out from 1932 to 1950 at the Cornell Medical Centre, New York. An additional 6,011 patients from the same institution operated upon from 1952 to 1978 had a mortality rate of 1.7%. Ohio surgeons reported a mortality rate of 1.8% from more than 28,000 cholecystectomies carried out during the same period (Arnold *et al.* 1973).

Similarly, major morbidity following cholecystectomy has been variously estimated at between 4 and 32% (Meyer *et al.* 1967; Holm *et al.* 1968; Magee and MacDuffee 1968; Haff *et al.* 1969). Such adverse effects may be conveniently placed within three broad categories. Firstly, there are those complications which are general to all abdominal surgery and which are not specifically related to gallstone disease or operations on the biliary tree. Secondly, there is morbidity which is specifically related to cholelithiasis and cholecystectomy. Iatrogenic bile duct injury would be included in the category. Thirdly, there are the possible long-term consequences of cholecystectomy in terms of bile salt metabolism and predisposition to other diseases.

Non-specific morbidity

Cholecystectomy, in common with all other major abdominal operations, leads to a neuro-humoral metabolic stress response and to marked changes in cardiopulmonary function. Both may have a bearing upon the immediate post-operative course and eventual outcome in terms of morbidity and mortality. For example, over 50% of patients undergoing elective cholecystectomy have been shown, electrocardiographically, to develop per-operative myocardial ischaemia associated with significant changes in pulse and blood pressure (Jakobsen *et al.*1989). Furthermore, cholecystectomy performed through either an upper midline or a right subcostal incision can lead to marked impairment of pulmonary function post-operatively due to atelectasis and diaphragmatic splinting (Larsson 1990). It is perhaps not surprising therefore that myocardial events, cerebrovascular accidents, chest infections as well as thromboembolic events are among the most common sources of morbidity following cholecystectomy (Habib *et al.* 1990; Hacker *et al.* 1990). Such morbidity arising from cholecystectomy is particularly increased in elderly patients, especially if surgery is performed in the emergency situation for the complications of gallstone disease and if patients have other medical problems such as chronic obstructive airways disease and ischaemic heart disease. For example, Huber *et al.* (1983) reported an overall mortality of 7.5% and a complication rate of 28% in a series of 93 cholecystectomies performed on patients over the age of 70 years. Of the 50 patients undergoing elective surgery there was only one death and 10 complications, whereas for those undergoing emergency surgery the mortality and morbidity rate was 14% and 33% respectively. In addition, the elderly are more likely to present with the complications of gallstones and in particular with common bile duct stones (Strohl and Diffenbaugh 1953; Morrow *et al.* 1978; Sullivan *et al.* 1982; Edlund 1982; Sheridan *et al.* 1987; Irvin and Arnstein 1988). Incidental gallbladder carcinoma is also more common in the elderly (Strohl *et al.* 1964). This age-related mortality and morbidity is particularly relevant given the increasing proportion of elderly people in the population and the high prevalence of gallstones in that age group. Post-mortem studies indicate that whereas gallstones are present in less than 10% of those aged 30–40 years they are present in over half of those aged over 70 years (Crump 1931). As a result biliary tract disease has for some time been the most common single indication for surgery in those over 65 years of age (Ibach *et al.* 1968; Gaines 1977).

Morbidity specifically related to cholelithiasis and cholecystectomy

It is possible to define groups of patients that appear to be at increased risk specifically from cholelithiasis and cholecystectomy. For example, although diabetics do not have an increased incidence of cholelithiasis, they appear more prone to develop the complications of gallstones and to suffer significantly more morbidity and mortality from the subsequent surgery (Rabinowitch 1932; Turril *et al.* 1961; Mundth 1962; Bennion and Grundy 1978; Walsh *et al.* 1982; Pickleman and Gonzalez 1986; Ransohoff *et al.* 1987; Sandler *et al.* 1986). As a result some authorities have recommended that diabetics undergo prophylactic cholecystectomy but this is not a generally accepted view (Ikard 1990). Thus it has been argued that diabetic morbidity is increased as a consequence of the associated cardiovascular and renal disease rather than to the diabetic state itself. Thus excess morbidity following biliary surgery is seen in those patients suffering from vascular and renal disease regardless of the presence or absence of a diabetic aetiology (Walsh *et al.* 1982). Morbidly obese patients also have a markedly higher incidence of gallstones and their complications, particularly after a period of weight loss (Thiet *et al.* 1984). For this reason prophylactic cholecystectomy is recommended (where appropriate in conjunction with bariatric surgery) (Amaral and Thompson 1985). Similarly, although elective cholecystectomy appears to be a safe procedure in patients who have had a successful cardiac transplant, emergency surgery is associated with a high mortality and morbidity (Sekela *et al.* 1990). This is likely to be, at least in part, a consequence of their immunosuppressive therapy and as such may apply to other groups of immunocompromised patients such as renal transplant recipients and patients receiving cytotoxic chemotherapy.

Although cholelithiasis is rare in children it is nearly always associated with a specific cause such as congenital haemolytic anaemia or cystic fibrosis which may well increase the risk of surgery (MacMillan *et al.* 1974; Pokorny *et al.* 1984). Similarly, emergency surgery for the complications of pigment stones arising as a result of sickle cell disease is associated with a significantly increased risk when compared to the elective situation (Stephens and Scott 1980; Ware *et al.* 1988).

Controversy remains as to whether cholecystectomy performed 'incidentally' at the time of other surgery is associated with increased morbidity (Green *et al.* 1990). Incidental cholecystectomy supplementing a range of other 'clean' abdominal operations would appear significantly to increase the risk of infective complications (Gibney 1990). Early fears, however, that cholecystectomy undertaken at the same time as aortic graft replacement would lead to an increased risk of prosthetic infection, do not appear to have been confirmed (Bickerstaff *et al.* 1984; Ameli *et al.* 1987). Furthermore, patients undergoing a variety of abdominal procedures do show an increased incidence of post-operative cholecystitis when 'incidental' gallstones are left *in situ* (Gately and Thomas 1983; Ameli *et al.* 1987). This may be due to dehydration, the fasting state, vagotomy or opiate analgesia (Jonsson and Andersson 1976; Ottinger 1983). Overall, it is likely that 'incidental' cholecystectomy poses no increased risk to the patient if it is performed by an adequately experienced surgeon with adequate exposure.

Pregnancy appears to be associated with an acceleration in the growth of gallstones (DeVore 1980). Furthermore, complications such as acute pancreatitis and acute cholecystitis (1:1,000–10,000 deliveries) are well recognized (Smoleniec and James 1990). Diagnosis of the acute abdomen during pregnancy can be difficult and as laparotomy, especially in the first trimester, increases the risk of miscarriage, and in the third trimester can be technically difficult, most surgeons would adopt a conservative approach in the first instance (Dixon *et al.* 1983). However, perforation of a viscus, such as the appendix, markedly increases mortality and morbidity for both mother and fetus (Horowitz *et al.* 1985).

Although mortality and major morbidity have been studied in a number of large retrospective series, minor morbidity arising from cholecystectomy is more difficult to define and has received relatively little attention. As with any abdominal operation, control of wound pain immediately post-operatively is a major therapeutic goal. This is not only to ensure patient comfort but also to minimize respiratory complications. Intermittent parenteral boluses of opiate analgesia are probably the most common form of pain control but may be both ineffective and lead to respiratory depression (Hull 1985). Patient-controlled opiate analgesia allows better control of pain and regional (epidural or intrapleural) and local anaesthesia have been used successfully following cholecystectomy (Scott *et al.* 1989). In centres where the aim has been to reduce wound pain to the minimum, patients have been regularly discharged 24–48 hours following cholecystectomy (Moss 1986). Although for the majority of patients cholecystectomy is successful in removing presenting symptoms, up to 25% of patients report no relief and in particular suffer prolonged and severe right upper quadrant pain which may be related to the wound or resemble their initial biliary-type pain (Bates *et al.* 1984; Ros and Zambon 1987). There appears to be no satisfactory method of predicting pre-operatively which patients will develop this so-called 'post-cholecystectomy syndrome'. Despite studies of both bile flow and sphincter of Oddi activity there is as yet no convincing explanation why these patients suffer continuing symptoms, although psychological factors may have an important part to play (Jorgensen *et al.* 1990).

Pain and inadequate analgesia or alternatively epidural anaesthesia, pre-existing bladder outflow problems and impaired mobility can also lead to difficulty in initiating micturition post-operatively. In the authors' series of 246 cholecystectomies up to one-third of patients overall, and over 90% of men over 75 years of age, undergoing cholecystectomy experienced urinary retention and required catheterization (Bradbury *et al.* 1993). Ileus following cholecystectomy usually necessitates the use of an intravenous infusion for 1–2 days post-operatively although it is possible to maintain adequate fluid balance and electrolyte concentration by commencing oral hydration 6 hours post-operatively (Ledet 1990; Salim 1991). Early nasogastric feeding has also been practised in some centres although the clinical benefits remain uncertain (Moss 1986).

Infective complications including wound sepsis, subphrenic abscess and septicaemia are not uncommon following cholecystectomy, particularly in the emergency situation. However, such morbidity can be significantly reduced by appropriate antibiotic prophylaxis (Hancock 1990). Wound infection is more common in the 25–50% of patients who have infected bile (Haw and Gunn 1973). Although bile is more likely to be infected in patients who are over 50 years, have a pyrexia or leucocytosis and have a non-functioning gallbladder

or common bile duct stones, it is not possible to predict pre-operatively with sufficient accuracy which patients are at risk of infection. For this reason all patients should be considered for antibiotic prophylaxis (Wells *et al.* 1989). However, prolonged post-operative courses of antibiotics confer no advantage over a three-dose regimen in terms of wound infection, and indeed can be detrimental (Berne *et al.* 1990). Peritoneal lavage with tetracycline in place of prophylactic systemic antibiotics has also been shown to reduce wound infection rates from 12% to less than 1% (Hancock 1990). Wound dehiscence following cholecystectomy should be a rare event and is the result of technical failure (Arnold *et al.* 1970; Habib *et al.* 1990). Patients undergoing cholecystectomy are also at risk of deep venous thrombosis and should be considered for thromboembolic prophylaxis such as low dose heparin given pre-operatively and continued until full mobility is regained (Gunn 1986).

The principal complications arising specifically from cholecystectomy are bile leak, bile duct damage, retained common bile duct stones and reactionary haemorrhage either from the gallbladder bed or from vessels within the free edge of the lesser omentum.

Although leakage of bile into the general peritoneal cavity from either small bile radicals entering the gallbladder directly or from the duct system occurs following cholecystectomy in up to 31% of cases, the majority of these leaks remain clinically unimportant as bile and blood have both been shown to be readily absorbed by peritoneum (Rayter *et al.* 1989). Persistent or clinically detrimental biliary leakage may be treated by drainage of the collection (by placement of a catheter under radiographic control), or by insertion of a T-tube into the common bile duct at relaparotomy (van Sonnenberg *et al.* 1990).

Small collections of blood in the subhepatic space are also common following cholecystectomy and similarly are of no clinical importance (Elboim *et al.* 1983). By contrast, bleeding from a major artery, usually the right hepatic, constitutes one of the main dangers of the operation. Until the 1960s ligation of the hepatic artery or one of its major branches was considered to be a dangerous, often lethal, error (Graham and Cannell 1933). However, a better understanding of liver anatomy and physiology together with experience of hepatic dearterialization in the course of treatment for hepatic neoplasia and trauma has shown that this is not the case (Brittain *et al.* 1964; Mays 1972; Rappaport and Schneiderman 1976; Bengmark and Jeppsson 1988). Thus in the majority of cases adequate hepatic oxygenation is accomplished by the portal venous circulation and/or by the development of collaterals. Post-mortem studies have shown that during elective cholecystectomy such injuries may occur unnoticed in up to 7% of operations (Halasz 1991). Significant post-operative bleeding from major vessels will be accompanied by hypotension and tachycardia and is an indication for relaparotomy. In the absence of cardiovascular instability, blood loss revealed by falling haemoglobin concentration estimations post-operatively or by excess drainage can be treated expectantly or with transfusion.

Although, overall, 10% of patients undergoing routine cholecystectomy will be harbouring common bile duct stones, this may be much higher in the elderly and in patients presenting as an emergency with the complications of gallstone disease such as pancreatitis, obstructive jaundice and cholangitis. By the ninth decade of life onwards approximately 80% of patients may have choledocholithiasis (Gliedman and Wilk 1985; Hacker *et al.* 1990). There is still debate over whether operative cholangiography should be performed in every case or reserved for when there has been clinical or biochemical evidence of choledocholithiasis (Pernthaler *et al.* 1990). The incidence of retained stones after cholecystectomy and positive bile duct exploration varies from 7 to 10% and after a negative exploration is in the region of 1–2% (Habib *et al.* 1990). There is evidence to suggest that this can be improved by the use of choledochoscopy, fluorocholangiography or post-exploration cholangiography (Motson and Wetter 1990). If present, retained stones may be visualized and treated by endoscopic retrograde cholangiography (ERC), sphincterotomy and stone extraction with further laparotomy being required for only a minority of cases (Gadacz 1991).

Iatrogenic bile duct injury remains the most serious complication of cholecystectomy, leading McSherry (1989) to comment: 'the infrequent but often devastating complication of intra-operative bile duct injury . . . still

occurs despite advances in surgical training. The burden that it frequently imposes is a shortened life span frequented by repeated operations interspersed with bouts of cholangitis. If this disaster could be eliminated, there would be no justification to seek alternatives to cholecystectomy.' More than 80% of all benign bile duct strictures are formed as a result of injury sustained during the course of open cholecystectomy (Lindenauer 1973; Habib *et al.* 1990). The exact incidence of bile duct injury during open cholecystectomy is difficult to assess due to lack of reporting and the fact that many injuries will go initially unrecognized (Pitt *et al.* 1982). However, rates of 0.1–0.4% have been reported in two large series of 1,000 patients (Andren-Sandberg *et al.* 1985; Habib *et al.* 1990). The surgeon may injure the biliary tree by ligating or transecting the wrong duct, by occluding the common duct during 'flush' ligation of the cystic duct, by rendering the bile duct ischaemic or by traumatizing the duct during over-forceful exploration (Northover and Terblanche 1979; Terblanche *et al.* 1983; Moosa *et al.* 1990). Johnston (1986) has proposed a triad of factors contributing to bile duct injury; dangerous anatomy, dangerous pathology and dangerous surgery. Dangerous pathology would include acute cholecystitis and empyema, as well as portal hypertension and obesity. Although such 'difficult' cholecystectomies have often been cited as carrying a greater risk of bile duct injury, recent reviews have demonstrated that bleeding and inflammation play a small part in reported injury, and that injury is most commonly sustained during what otherwise appears to be straightforward elective surgery (Pitt *et al.* 1982). By contrast, obesity was a contributing factor in 83% of Moosa's series of 68 major bile duct injuries (Moosa *et al.* 1990). While dangerous pathology should be readily evident alerting the inexperienced surgeon to seek help, dangerous anatomy may not be recognized until it is too late. Significant anomalies of the extrahepatic biliary tree and adjacent hepatic arteries are rarely recognized prior to surgery but may be present in up to 50% of individuals and frequently involve an unusual junction of the cystic duct with the common hepatic duct (Northover and Terblanche 1982; Andren-Sandberg *et al.* 1985). Dangerous surgery is probably the most common cause of bile duct injury and is perhaps the most readily preventable. Inadequate experience was felt to have contributed to 85% of Lord Smith's (1979) series of 1,554 post-cholecystectomy strictures with only 15% of strictures being produced by consultants. Similarly, in the Lund study 80% of 65 strictures were produced by trainee surgeons who had carried out between 25 and 100 operations (Andren-Sandberg *et al.* 1985). By contrast, in Moosa's series from San Diego, three-quarters of 81 bile duct injuries had been carried out or directly supervised by attending surgeons (Moosa *et al.* 1990). Nevertheless, as bile duct injury can be associated with a 50% mortality rate, it is clear that trainee surgeons must be carefully supervised, perhaps more closely and for longer than for some other operations, while learning to perform cholecystectomy safely (Habib *et al.* 1990). Although less than 20% of bile duct injuries are recognized at the time of surgery, primary repair over a T tube offers the best chance of success in these cases. If this is not possible a biliary enteric anastomosis may be formed (Johnston 1986). Major ductal injuries unrecognized at the time of surgery usually present in a few days with deepening jaundice, biliary ascites or fistula, often with subhepatic abscess and sepsis. At this stage the patient should be immediately referred to a specialist hepatobiliary unit in order that the risk of further complications, such as portal hypertension and biliary cirrhosis, can be minimized (Blumgart *et al.* 1984; Collins and Gorey 1984; Knight and Smith 1985; Johnston 1986; Lillemoe 1990).

Long-term consequences of cholecystectomy

Several long-term adverse effects may be associated with cholecystectomy. For example, cholecystectomy leads to marked changes in bile salt and fat metabolism that may increase the risk of colorectal adenoma and carcinoma particularly in the proximal colon (Moorehead and McKelvey 1989; Sweeting *et al.* 1989; Berkel *et al.* 1990; Soltero *et al.* 1990). Prior to cholecystectomy the bile acid pool circulates two to three times after each meal whereas in the absence of a gallbladder bile salts circulate even during the fasting state. This enhanced enterohepatic circulation leads to increased exposure of bile acids to intestinal bacterial degradation and to an increase in secondary

bile acids that have been postulated to be carcinogenic. Cholecystectomy would also appear to increase the incidence of chemically induced pancreatic carcinoma in rodents, but the evidence in humans is conflicting (Chester *et al.* 1990; Haddock and Carter 1990). Changes in trace metal, iron, copper and transferrin metabolism have also been described but as yet have not been shown to be of any clinical importance (Fraser *et al.* 1989). In addition, cholecystectomy leads to duodenogastric reflux of bile which may in turn cause gastritis and promote the growth of gastric adenomas (Lorusso *et al.* 1990).

Conclusions

Cholecystectomy has stood the test of time as the treatment of choice for symptomatic gallstones. Although in routine practice the open operation is almost inevitably going to be superseded by more technologically advanced laparoscopic procedures, it is unlikely to be rendered totally obsolete. Open surgery will still be indicated where laparoscopic removal proves to be impossible or results in complications, where there is an absence or failure of equipment or when cholecystectomy is required as part of another procedure (Grace *et al.* 1991; Paterson-Brown *et al.* 1991). However, as surgeons will be expected to undertake open cholecystectomy with decreasing frequency, their personal experience and practice at the operation will diminish. As a consequence, they will increasingly come to rely on a sound knowledge of the key points, risks and complications garnered from the extensive literature relating to over a century of open cholecystectomy.

References

Aldridge, M.C. and Bismuth, H. (1990). Gallbladder cancer: the polyp-cancer sequence. *British Journal of Surgery*, **77**, 363–4.

Amaral, J.F. and Thompson, W.R. (1985). Gallbladder disease in the morbidly obese. *American Journal of Surgery*, **149**, 551–7.

Ameli, F.M., Weiss, M., Provan, J.L. *et al.* (1987). Safety of cholecystectomy with abdominal aortic surgery. *Canadian Journal of Surgery*, **30**, 170–6.

Andren-Sandberg, A., Alinder, G. and Bengmark, S. (1985). Accidental lesion of the common bile duct at cholecystectomy. Pre- and perioperative factors of importance. *Annals of Surgery*, **201**, 328–32.

Arnold, D.J., Zollinger, R.W., Barlett, R.M. *et al.* (1970). Twenty-eight thousand six hundred and twenty-one cholecystectomies in Ohio: results of a survey in Ohio hospitals by the gallbladder survey committee, Ohio Chapter, American College of Surgeons. *American Journal of Surgery*, **119**, 714–17.

Barry, R.E. (1988). The pathogenesis of acute pancreatitis. *British Medical Journal*, **296**, 589.

Bates, T., Mercer, J.C. and Harrison, M. (1984). Symptomatic gallstone disease: before and after cholecystectomy. *Gut*, **25**, 579–80.

Bateson, M.C. and Bouchier, I.A.D. (1975). Prevalence of gallstones in Dundee: a necropsy study. *British Medical Journal*, **4**, 427–30.

Bengmark, S. and Jeppsson, B. (1988). Hepatic dearterialization. *Surgical Annals*, **20**, 159–77.

Bennion, L.J. and Grundy, S.M. (1978). Risk factors for the development of cholelithiasis in man (second of two parts). *New England Medical Journal*, **299**, 1221–7.

Berkel, J. *et al.* (1990). Cholecystectomy and colon cancer. *American Journal of Gastroenterology*, **85**, 61–4.

Berne, T.V. *et al.* (1990). Controlled comparison of cefmetazole with cefoxitin for prophylaxis in elective cholecystectomy. *Surgery, Gynecology and Obstetrics*, **170**, 137–40.

Bickerstaff, L.K., Hollier, L.H., Van Peenan, H.J. *et al.* (1984). Abdominal aortic aneurysm repair combined with a second surgical procedure–morbidity and mortality. *Surgery*, **95**, 487–91.

Blumgart, L.H., Kelley, C.J. and Benjamin, I.S. (1984). Benign bile duct stricture following cholecystectomy, critical factors in management. *British Journal of Surgery*, **71**, 836–43.

Boquist, L., Bergdahl, L. and Anderson, A. (1972). Mortality following gallbladder surgery: a study of 3,257 cholecystectomies. *Surgery*, **71**, 616–24.

Bradbury, A.W., Stonebridge, P.A., Wallace, I.W. *et al.* (1993) Open biliary surgery and the use of routine inpatient audit. *Journal of the Royal College of Surgeons of Edinburgh*, **38**, 86–8.

Brittain, R.S., Marchioro, T.L., Hermann, G. *et al.* (1964). Accidental hepatic artery ligation in humans. *American Journal of Surgery*, **107**, 822–32.

Cheslyn-Curtis, S. and Russell, R.C.G. (1991). New trends in gallstone management. *British Journal of Surgery*, **78**, 143–9.

Chester, J.F. *et al.* (1989). Experimental pancreatic cancer in the Syrian hamster: effect of cholecystectomy. *Digestion*, **44**, 36–40.

Collins, P.G. and Gorey, T.F. (1984). Iatrogenic biliary stricture: presentation and management. *British Journal of Surgery*, **71**, 980–2.

Crump, C. (1931). The incidence of gallstones and gallbladder disease. *Surgery, Gynecology and Obstetrics*, **53**, 447–55.

Cuschieri, A. (1990). The laparoscopic revolution. *Journal of the Royal College of Surgeons of Edinburgh*, **34**, 295.

Davidson, B.R., Neoptolemos, J.P. and Carr-Locke, D.L. (1988). Endoscopic sphincterotomy for common bile duct calculi in patients with gallbladder *in situ* considered unfit for surgery. *Gut*, **29**, 114–20.

DeVore, G.R. (1980). Acute abdominal pain in the pregnant patient due to pancreatitis, acute appendicitis, cholecystitis or peptic ulcer disease. *Clinics in Perinatology*, **7**, 349–69.

Diehl, A.K. and Beral, V. (1981). Cholecystectomy and changing mortality from gallbladder cancer. *Lancet*, **2**, 187–9.

Diehl, A.K. (1983). Gallstone size and the risk of gallbladder cancer. *Journal of the American Medical Association*, **250**, 2323–6.

Dixon, N.P., Green, J., Rogers, A. and Rubin, L. (1983). Fetal loss after cholecystectomy during pregnancy. *CMAJ*, **88**, 576–7.

Dubois, F., Icard, P., Beryelot, G. *et al.* (1990). Coelioscopic cholecystectomy. Preliminary report of 36 cases. *Annals of Surgery*, **211**, 60–2.

Edlund, G. and Ljungdahl, M. (1990). Acute cholecystitis in the elderly. *American Journal of Surgery*, **159**, 414–16.

Elboim, C.M., Goldman, L., Hann, L. *et al.* (1983). Significance of post-cholecystectomy subhepatic fluid collections. *Annals of Surgery*, **198**, 137–41.

Fraser, W.D. *et al.* (1989). Changes in iron, zinc and copper concentrations in serum and in their binding to transport proteins after cholecystectomy and cardiac surgery. *Clinical Chemistry*, **35**, 2243–7.

Gadacz, T.R. (1991). Reoperation versus alternatives in retained biliary calculi. *Surgical Clinics of North America*, **21**, 93–108.

Gagic, N. and Frey, C.F. (1975). The results of cholecystostomy for the treatment of acute cholecystitis. *Surgery, Gynecology and Obstetrics*, **140**, 255–7.

Gaines, R.D. (1977). Surgery for gallbladder disease in the elderly. *Geriatrics*, **37**, 71–4.

Ganey, J.B., Johnson, P.A., Prillaman, P.E. *et al.* (1986). Cholecystectomy: clinical experience with a large series. *American Journal of Surgery*, **151**, 352–7.

Gatley, J.F. and Thomas, E.J. (1983). Acute cholecystitis occurring as a complication of other diseases. *Archives of Surgery*, **118**, 1137–41.

Gibney, E.J. (1990). Asymptomatic gallstones. *British Journal of Surgery*, **77**, 368–72.

Gilliland, T.M. and Traverso, L.W. (1990). Modern standards for comparison of cholecystectomy with alternative treatments for symptomatic cholelithiasis with emphasis on long term relief of symptoms. *Surgery, Gynecology and Obstetrics*, **170**, 39–44.

Glenn, F. and Hayes, D.M. (1952). The causes of death following biliary tract surgery for non-malignant disease. *Surgery, Gynecology and Obstetrics*, **94**, 283–7.

Glenn, F. and McSherry, C.K. (1963). Etiological factors in fatal complications following operations upon the biliary tract. *Annals of Surgery*, **157**, 695–706.

Gliedman, M. and Wilk, P. (1985). The present status of biliary tract surgery. *Surgical Annals*, **17**, 76–100.

Goco, I.R. and Chambers, L.G. (1983) "Mini-cholecystectomy" and operative cholangiography. A means of cost containment. *American Surgeon*, **49**, 143–5.

Grace, P.A., Quereshi, A., Coleman, J. *et al.* (1991). Reduced postoperative hospitalization after laparoscopic cholecystectomy. *British Journal of Surgery*, **78**, 160–2.

Gracie, W.A. and Ransohoff, D.F. (1982). The natural history of silent gallstones. The innocent gallstone is not a myth. *New England Journal of Medicine*, **307**, 798–800.

Graham, E.E. (1931). Prevention of carcinoma of the gailbladder. *Annals of Surgery*, **93**, 317–22.

Graham, R.R. and Cannell, D. (1933). Accidental ligation of the hepatic artery. *British Journal of Surgery*, **20**, 566–79.

Green, J.D., Birkhead, G., Hebert, J. *et al.* (1990). Increased morbidity in surgical patients undergoing secondary (incidental) cholecystectomy. *Annals of Surgery*, **211**, 50–4.

Gunn, A.A. (1969). Abdominal drainage. *British Journal of Surgery*, **56**, 274–6.

Gunn, A.A. (1986). Cholecystectomy, cholecystostomy and exploration of the common bile duct. In: *Atlas of General Surgery* (eds Dudley, H., Carter, D.C. and Russell, R.C.G.), Butterworths, London.

Gupta, S., Rauscher, G., Stillman, R. *et al.* (1978). The rational use of drains after cholecystectomy. *Surgery, Gynecology and Obstetrics*, **146**, 191–2.

Habib, N.A., Foo, C.L., El-Masry, R. *et al.* (1990). Complications of cholecystectomy in district general hospitals. *British Journal of Clinical Practice*, **44**, 189–92.

Hacker, K.A., Schultz, C.C. and Helling, T.S. (1990). Choledochotomy for calculous disease in the elderly. *American Journal of Surgery*, **160**, 610–12.

Haddock, G. and Carter, D.C. (1990). Aetiology of pancreatic cancer. *British Journal of Surgery*, **77**, 1159–65.

Haff, R.C., Butcher, H.R. Jr. and Ballinger, W.F. (1969). Biliary tract operations: a review of 1,000 patients. *Archives of Surgery*, **98**, 428–34.

Halasz, N.A. (1991). Cholecystectomy and hepatic artery injuries. *Archives of Surgery*, **126**, 137–8.

Halpert, B. (1982). Fiftieth anniversary of the removal of the gallbladder. *Archives of Surgery*, **117**, 1526–30.

Hancock, B.D. (1990). Audit of major colorectal and biliary surgery to reduce rates of wound infection. *British Medical Journal*, **301**, 911–12.

Haw, C.S. and Gunn, A.A. (1973). The significance of infection in biliary surgery. *Journal of the Royal College of Surgeons of Edinburgh*, **18**, 209–12.

Herman, R.E. (1990). Surgery for acute and chronic cholecystitis. *Surgical Clinics of North America*, **20**, 1263–75.

Heuer, G.J. (1934). The factors leading to death in operations upon the gallbladder and bile ducts. *Annals of Surgery*, **99**, 881–92.

Horgan, P.G., Campbell, A.C., Gray, G.R. and Gillespie, G. (1989). Biliary leakage and peritonitis following removal of T-tubes after bile duct exploration. *British Journal of Surgery*, **76**, 1296–7.

Horowitz, M.D., Gomez, G.A., Santiesteban, R. and Burkett, G. (1985). Acute appendicitis during pregnancy. *Archives of Surgery*, **120**, 1362–7.

Huber, D., Martin, E. and Cooperman, M. (1983). Cholecystectomy in elderly patients. *American Journal of Surgery*, **146**, 719–22.

Hull, C.J. (1985). The case for patient-controlled analgesia. In: *Care of the Postoperative Surgical Patient* (eds Smith, J.A.R. and Watkins, J.), Butterworths, London.

Ibach, J., Hume, H. and Erb, W. (1968). Cholecystectomy in the aged. *Surgery, Gynecology and Obstetrics*, **126**, 523–8.

Ikard, R.W. (1990). Gallstones, cholecystitis and diabetes. *Surgery, Gynecology and Obstetrics*, **171**, 528–31.

Irvin, T. and Arnstein, P. (1988). Management of symptomatic gallstones in the elderly. *British Journal of Surgery*, **75**, 1163–5.

Jakobssen, J., Rehnqvist, N. and Davidson, S. (1989). Computerized evaluation of the electrocardiogram during and for a short period after gall bladder surgery. *Acta Anaesthesiology Scandinavia*, **33**, 474–7.

Jarvinen, H.J. and Hasbacka, J. (1980). Early cholecystectomy for acute cholecystitis. A prospective randomized study. *Annals of Surgery*, **191**, 501–7.

Johnston, G.W. (1986). Iatrogenic bile duct stricture: an avoidable surgical hazard? *British Journal of Surgery*, **73**, 245–7.

Jonsson, R.E. and Andersson, A. (1976). Postoperative acute acalculous cholecystitis. *Archives of Surgery*, **111**, 1097–1101.

Jorgensen, T., Teglbjerg, J.S., Wille-Jorgenssen, P. *et al.* (1991). Persisting pain after cholecystectomy. A prospective investigation. *Scandinavian Journal of Gastroenterology*, **26**, 124–8.

Kambouris, A., Carpenter, W. and Allaben, R. (1973). Cholecystectomy without drainage. *Surgery, Gynecology and Obstetrics*, **137**, 613–17.

Kelley, C.J. and Blumgart, L.H. (1985). Per-operative cholangiography and post-cholecystectomy stricture. *Annals of the Royal College of Surgeons of England*, **67**, 93–5.

Knight, M. and Smith, R. (1985). Benign bile duct stricture following cholecystectomy: critical factors in management. *British Journal of Surgery*, **72**, 327.

Lahtinen, J., Alhava, E.M. and Aukee, S. (1978). Acute cholecystitis treated by early and delayed surgery. A controlled clinical trial. *Scandinavian Journal of Gastroenterology*, **13**, 673–8.

Larsson, A. (1990). Lung mechanics during upper abdominal surgery. *Acta Chirugia Scandanavia*, **156**, 155–62.

Ledet, W.P. (1990). Ambulatory cholecystectomy without disability. *Archives of Surgery*, **125**, 1434–5.

Lillemoe, K.D. (1990). Postoperative bile duct strictures. *Surgical Clinics of North America*, **70**, 1355–80.

Lindenauer, S.M. (1973). Surgical treatment of bile duct strictures. *Surgery*, **73**, 875–80.

Lowenfels, A.B., Walker, A.M., Althaus, D.P. *et al.* (1989) Gallstone growth, size, and risk of gallbladder cancer: an inter-racial study. *International Journal of Epidemiology*, **18**, 50–4.

MacMillan, R.W., Schullinger, J.N. and Santuli, T.V. (1974). Cholelithiasis in childhood. *American Journal of Surgery*, **127**, 689–92.

McSherry, C.K. and Glenn, F. (1980). The instance and cause of death following surgery for non-malignant biliary tract disease. *Annals of Surgery*, **191**, 271–5.

McSherry, C.K., Ferstenberg, H., Calhoun, W.F. *et al.* (1985). The natural history of diagnosed gallstone disease in symptomatic and asymptomatic patients. *Annals of Surgery*, **202**, 59–63.

McSherry, C.K. (1989). Cholecystectomy: the gold standard. *American Journal of Surgery*, **158**, 174–8.

Magee, R.B. and MacDuffee, R.C. (1968). One thousand consecutive cholecystectomies. *Archives of Surgery*, **96**, 858–62.

Maull, K., Daugherty, M.E., Shearer, G.R. *et al.* (1978). Cholecystectomy: to drain or not to drain? *Journal of Surgical Research*, **24**, 259–63.

Mays, E.T. (1972). Lobar dearterialization for exsanguinating wounds of the liver. *Journal of Trauma*, **12**, 397–407.

Meyer, K.A., Capos, N.J. and Mittelpunkt, A.J. (1967). Clinical surgery: personal experiences with 1,261 cases of acute and chronic cholecystitis and cholelithiasis. *Surgery*, **61**, 668–8.

Mirrizi, P.L. (1937). Operative cholangiography. *Surgery, Gynecology and Obstetrics*, **65**, 702–5.

Moosa, A.R.., Mayer, A.D. and Stabile, B. (1990). Iatrogenic injury to the bile duct. Who, how, where? *Archives of Surgery*, **125**, 1028–30.

Moossa, A.R., Mayer, A.D. and Stabile, B. (1990). Iatrogenic injury to the bile duct. Who, how, where? *Archives of Surgery*. **125**, 1028–30.

Moorehead, R.J. and McKelvey, S.T.D. (1989). Cholecystectomy and colorectal cancer. *British Journal of Surgery*, **76**, 250–3.

Morrow, D., Thompson, J. and Wilson, S. (1978). Acute cholecystitis in the elderly. *Archives of Surgery*, **113**, 1149–52.

Moss, G. (1986). Discharge within 24 hours of elective cholecystectomy. *Archives of Surgery*, **121**, 1159–61.

Motson, R.W. and Wetter, L.A. (1990). Operative choledochoscopy: common bile duct exploration is incomplete without it. *British Journal of Surgery*, **77**, 975–80.

Mundth, E.D. (1962). Cholecystitis and diabetes mellitus. *New England Journal of Medicine*, **267**, 642–6.

Nathanson, L.K., Shimi, S. and Cuschieri, A. (1991). Laparoscopic cholecystectomy: the Dundee technique. *British Journal of Surgery*, **78**, 155–9.

Neoptolemos, J.P., Carr-Locke, D.L., London, N. *et al.* (1988). Controlled trial of urgent endoscopic retrograde cholangiopancreatography and endoscopic sphincterotomy versus conservative treatment for acute pancreatitis due to gallstones. *Lancet*, **2**, 979–83.

Neoptolemos, J., Shaw, D. and Carr-Locke, D. (1989). A multivariate analysis of preoperative risk factors in patients with common bile duct stones. *Annals of Surgery*, **209**, 157–61.

Neugebauer, E., Troidl, H., Spangenberger, W. *et al.* (1991). Conventional versus laparoscopic cholecystectomy and the randomized controlled trial. *British Journal of Surgery*, **78**, 150–4.

Norell, S., Ahlbom, A., Erwald, R. *et al.* (1986). Diabetes, gallstone disease and pancreatic cancer. *British Journal of Cancer*, **54**, 377–8.

Northover, J.M.A. and Terblanche, J. (1979). A new look at the arterial supply of the bile duct in man and its surgical implications. *British Journal of Surgery*, **66**, 379–84.

Northover, J.M.A. and Terblanche, J. (1982). Applied surgical anatomy of the biliary tree. *Clinical Surgery International*, **5**, 1–16.

Ottinger, L.W. (1978). Invited commentary: postoperative acute cholecystitis in Japan. *World Journal of Surgery*, **2**, 666.

Paterson-Brown, S., Garden, O.J. and Carter, D.C. (1991). Laparoscopic cholecystectomy. *British Journal of Surgery*, **78**, 131–2.

Pernthaler, H., Sandbichler, P., Schmid, Th. and Margreiter, R. (1990). Operative cholangiography in elective cholecystectomy. *British Journal of Surgery*, **77**, 39–40.

Pickleman, J. and Gonzalez, R.P. (1986). The improving results of cholecystectomy. *Archives of Surgery*, **121**, 930–4.

Pitt, H.A., Miyamoto, T., Parapatis, S.K. *et al.* (1982). Factors influencing outcome in patients with post-operative biliary strictures. *American Journal of Surgery*, **144**, 14–21.

Pitt, H.A., Cameron, J.L., Postier, R.G. and Gadacz, T.R. (1981). Factors affecting mortality in biliary tract surgery. *American Journal of Surgery*, **141**, 66–72.

Pokorny, W.J., Saleem, M. and O'Gorman, R.B. *et al.* (1984). Cholelithiasis and cholecystitis in childhood. *American Journal of Surgery*, **148**, 742–4.

Rabinowitch, I.M. (1932). On the morbidity arising from surgical treatment of chronic gallbladder disease in diabetes mellitus. *Annals of Surgery*, **96**, 70–4.

Ransohoff, D.F., Gracie, W.A., Wolfenson, L.B. *et al.* (1983). Prophylactic cholecystectomy or expectant management for silent gallstones. *Annals of Internal Medicine*, **99**, 199–204.

Ransohoff, D.F., Gracie, W.A., Wolfenson, L.B. *et al.* (1987). Prophylactic cholecystectomy or expectant management for silent gallstones. *Annals of Internal Medicine*, **106**, 829–32.

Ranson, J.H.C. (1979). The timing of biliary surgery in acute pancreatitis. *Annals of Surgery*, **189**, 654–63.

Rappaport, A.M. and Schneiderman, J.H. (1976). The function of the hepatic artery. *Review of Physiology Biochemistry and Pharmacology*, **76**, 130–75.

Rayter, Z., Tonge, C., Bennett, C.E. *et al.* (1989). Bile leaks after simple cholecystectomy. *British Journal of Surgery*, **76**, 1046–8.

Ros, E. and Zambon, D. (1987) Post cholecystectomy symptoms; a prospective study. *Gut*, **28**, 1500–4.

Roslyn, J.J. and Tompkins, R.K. (1991). Reoperation for biliary strictures. *Surgical Clinics of North America*, **21**, 109–16.

Rosseland, A. and Solhaug, J. (1988). Primary endoscopic papillotomy in patients with stones in the common bile duct and gallbladder *in situ*: a 5–8 year follow-up study. *World Journal of Surgery*, **12**, 111–16.

Salim, A.S. (1991). Duration of intravenous fluid replacement after abdominal surgery: a prospective randomized study. *Annals of the Royal College of Surgeons of England*, **73**, 119–23.

Sandler, R.S., Maule, W.F. and Baltus, M.E. (1986). Factors associated with postoperative complications in diabetes after biliary tract surgery. *Gastroenterology*, **91**, 157–62.

Schein, M. (1991). Partial cholecystectomy in the emergency treatment of acute cholecystitis in the compromised patient. *Journal of the Royal College of Surgeons of Edinburgh*, **36**, 295–7.

Scott, N.B., Mogensen, T., Bigler, D. and Kehlet, H. (1989). Comparison of the effects of continuous intrapleural vs epidural administration of 0.5% bupivicaine on pain, metabolic response and pulmonary function following cholecystectomy. *Acta Anaesthesiology Scandanavia*, **33**, 535–9.

Sekela, M.E., Hutchins, D.A., Young, J.B. and Noon, G.P. (1990). Biliary surgery after cardiac transplantation. *Archives of Surgery*, **126**, 571–3.

Seltzer, M.H., Steiger, E. and Rosato, F.E. (1970). Mortality following cholecystectomy. *Surgery, Gynecology and Obstetrics*, **130**, 64–6.

Sheridan, W., Williams, H. and Lewis, M. (1987). Morbidity and mortality of common bile duct exploration. *British Journal of Surgery*, **74**, 1095–9.

Simon, D., Brooks, W. and Hersh, T. (1989). Endoscopic sphincterotomy: a reappraisal. *American Journal of Gastroenterology*, **84**, 213–19.

Smith, R. (1979). Obstructions of the bile duct. *British Journal of Surgery*, **66**, 69–79.

Smoleniec, J. and James, D. (1990). General surgical problems in pregnancy. *British Journal of Surgery*, **77**, 1203–4.

Soltero, E., Cruz, N.I., Nazario, C.M. *et al.* (1990). Cholecystectomy and right colon cancer in Puerto Rico. *Cancer*, **66**, 2249–52.

Sparkman, R.S. (1967). Bobbs centennial. The first cholecystostomy. *Surgery, Gynecology and Obstetrics*, **61**, 965–71.

Stephens, C. and Scott, R. (1980). Cholelithiasis in sickle cell anaemia. Surgical of medical management. *Archives of Internal Medicine*, **140**, 648–51.

Strachan, C.J.L. (1985). Prevention of post-operative sepsis. In: *Care of the Postoperative Surgical Patient* (eds Smith, J.A.R. and Watkins, J.), Butterworths, London.

Sullivan, D., Hood, T. and Griffen, W.O. (1982). Biliary tract surgery in the elderly. *American Journal of Surgery*, **143**, 218–20.

Strohl, E.C. and Diffenbaugh, W.G. (1953). Biliary tract surgery in the elderly patient. *Surgery, Gynecology and Obstetrics*, **97**, 467–70.

Strohl, E.C., Diffenbaugh, W.G. and Anderson, R.E. (1964). Biliary tract surgery in the elderly patient. *Geriatrics*, **24**, 275–9.

Sweeting, J. *et al.* (1989). Effect of cholecystectomy on bile acid kinetics. *Gastroenterology*, **97**, 1593–4.

Terblanche, J., Allison, H.H. and Northover, J.M.A. (1983). An ischaemic basis for biliary strictures. *Surgery*, **94**, 52–7.

Thiet, M.D., Mittelstaedt, C.A., Herbst, C.A. *et al.* (1984). Cholelithiasis in morbid obesity. *Southern Medical Journal*, **77**, 415–17.

Thistle, J.L., Cleary, P.A., Lachin, J.M. *et al.* (1984). The natural history of cholelithiasis: the national cooperative gallstone study. *Annals of Internal Medicine*, **101**, 171–80.

Todd, G. and Reemtsama, K. (1978). Cholecystectomy with drainage. *American Journal of Surgery*, **135**, 622–3.

Turril, F.L., McCarron, M.M. and Mikkelsen, W.P. (1961). Gallstones and diabetes: an ominous association. *American Journal of Surgery*, **102**, 184–90.

van der Linden, W. and Sunzel, H. (1970). Early versus delayed operation for acute cholecystitis. A controlled clinical trial. *American Journal of Surgery*, **120**, 7–13.

van Sonnenberg, E., Casola, G., Wittich, G.R. *et al.* (1990). The role of interventional radiology for complications of cholecystectomy. *Surgery*, **107**, 632–8.

Walsh, D.B., Eckhauser, F.E., Ramsburgh, S.R. *et al.* (1982). Risk associated with diabetes mellitus in patients undergoing gallbladder surgery. *Surgery*, **91**, 254–7.

Ware. R., Filston, H.C. and Schultz, W.H. (1988). Elective cholecystectomy in children with sickle haemoglobinopathies. *Annals of Surgery*, **208**, 17–22.

Way, L.W. (1989). Trends in the treatment of gallstone disease: putting the options into context. *American Journal of Surgery*, **158**, 251–3.

Weiss, K.M., Ferrell, R.E., Hanis, C.L. *et al.* (1984). Genetics and the epidemiology of gallbladder disease in new world native peoples. *American Journal of Human Genetics*, **36**, 1259–64.

Welch, J.P. and Malt, R.A. (1972). Outcome of cholecystostomy. *Surgery, Gynecology and Obstetrics*, **135**, 717–20.

Wells, G.R., Taylor, E.W., Lindsay, G. *et al.* (1989). Relationship between bile colonization, high-risk factors and postoperative sepsis in patients undergoing biliary tract operations while receiving a prophylactic antibiotic. *British Journal of Surgery*, **76**, 374–7.

Werbel, G.B., Nahrwold, D.L., Joehl, R.J. *et al.* (1989). Percutaneous cholecystostomy in the diagnosis and treatment of acute cholecystitis in the high-risk patient. *Archives of Surgery*, **124**, 782–6.

Wetter, L.A. and Way, L.W. (1991). Surgical therapy for gallstone disease. *Gastroenterology Clinics of North America*, **20**, 157–69.

Williams, C., Halpin, D. and Knox, A. (1972). Drainage following cholecystectomy. *British Journal of Surgery*, **59**, 293–6.

Williamson, R.C.N. (1987). Surgery of the biliary tract and pancreas. In: *General Surgical Operations* (eds Kirk R.M. and Williamson R.C.N.), Churchill Livingstone, Edinburgh.

Worthley, C.S. and Toouli, J. (1988). Gallbladder nonfilling: an indication for cholecystectomy after endoscopic sphincterotomy. *British Journal of Surgery*, **75**, 796–8.

9

Laparoscopic appendicectomy

G. Bell and D.S. Byrne

This chapter details the current techniques used for laparoscopic appendicectomy. It should be emphasized that the overall principles that apply to open appendicectomy also apply to the laparoscopic approach.

Laparoscopic appendicectomy was first described by the German gynaecologist Semm[1] in 1983. He did not recommend that the technique be used for acute appendicitis, and it was several years before other surgeons explored this possibility. Schreiber[2] in 1987 produced the first report of laparoscopic appendicectomy for acute appendicitis in 24% of 70 female patients included in a study of acute and chronic right iliac fossa pain. He encountered few complications and suggested that this was a suitable alternative to open appendicectomy. Since then, there have been numerous reports of laparoscopic appendicectomy.[3-17] The consistent finding from these early studies is that, laparoscopic appendicectomy is technically simple, can be achieved in over 90% of cases and is associated with a low complication rate. Now that the laparoscopic approach to surgery is being widely accepted, more and more general surgeons are evaluating this technique.

Technique

Several operative techniques are described using two basic approaches. In the first, the appendix is mobilized within the peritoneal cavity and then excised extraperitoneally as in open appendicectomy. In the second approach, the appendicectomy is performed entirely within the peritoneal cavity and the appendix is then retrieved through one of the abdominal cannulae.

The operation is carried out under general anaesthesia. Peri-operative antibiotic prophylaxis is used in all cases where acute appendicitis has been diagnosed, and this may be administered rectally 1 hour before surgery or intravenously at induction of anaesthesia. Although not routinely necessary, a urinary catheter may be inserted to drain the bladder initially. If used, this should be done as an 'in–out' procedure.

A Veress needle is inserted immediately below the umbilicus, its correct position being confirmed by the 'saline drop test'. A pneumoperitoneum is established, the intra-abdominal pressure being automatically regulated to a maximum of 15 mmHg. If intra-abdominal adhesions are suspected or the abdomen is distended, the Hasson technique[18] can be used to enter the peritoneal cavity. After withdrawing the Veress needle, a 10 mm trocar and cannula are inserted through an infraumbilical incision. An end-viewing 10 mm laparoscope is introduced through this cannula to inspect the peritoneal cavity and confirm the diagnosis. The view of the structures in the right iliac fossa and pelvis may be improved by placing the patient in a minor Trendelenburg position with 15° of left-sided tilt.

The position of the other cannulae is variable and depends on the appendicectomy technique selected. This will usually be determined by the pathology encountered.

Extraperitoneal appendicectomy

In a small number of cases where the appendix is minimally inflamed and where the caecum and appendix are mobile, only one more cannula is required. A small incision is made in the right iliac fossa at a site closest to the pole of the caecum and, using transillumination to avoid blood vessels in the abdominal wall, a 10 mm trocar and cannula are inserted under direct vision. The tip of the appendix is picked up with grasping forceps and is drawn inside the cannula. The cannula and appendix are then withdrawn together to deliver the appendix onto the skin surface where it is manipulated through the wound until the pole of the caecum becomes visible. This manoeuvre is facilitated by evacuation of the pneumoperitoneum, allowing the anterior abdominal wall to fall back onto the caecum. The mesoappendix is ligated and divided; the appendix may be ligated or stapled as in open appendicectomy, according to personal preference. The caecum is returned to the peritoneal cavity and, after reintroducing the right iliac fossa cannula, the appendix stump and surrounding area can be inspected for haemostasis. Irrigation of the stump and any areas involved in the inflammatory process is carried out routinely using an antibiotic solution. The right iliac fossa cannula is removed under direct vision and the gas is evacuated from the peritoneal cavity. The wounds are then closed with sutures to the linea alba and skin.

Where the appendix is firmly bound down by inflammatory adhesions or is retrocaecal in position, it is necessary to mobilize the appendix within the peritoneal cavity. A third trocar and cannula (5 mm) are inserted in the left iliac fossa for the dissection. More medial placement of this cannula in the suprapubic region results in instrument crowding and may impede the dissection. Forceps are passed through the right iliac fossa cannula to grasp the tip of the appendix. If the appendix is very oedematous, a preknotted ligature can be placed round its tip to provide traction. The tip of the appendix is then drawn up towards the right iliac fossa cannula placing the mesoappendix under slight tension and stretching it

like a 'sail'.[12] The mesentery is dissected using diathermy, keeping close to the appendix. Large vessels may be individually secured using clips. The dissection is usually started at the tip of the appendix working towards the base but it can equally be performed in the opposite direction and the appendix mobilized in a retrograde fashion.

The retrocaecal appendix is mobilized by dividing the lateral peritoneal reflection of the caecum. The appendix can then be manipulated to allow dissection of its mesentery down to the pole of the caecum.

Once fully mobilized, the appendix is drawn inside the right iliac fossa cannula and dealt with as described previously.

As the appendix is delivered onto the surface of the abdomen, a degree of wound contamination is inevitable. This can be minimized by withdrawing the appendix as far as possible inside the cannula.

The appendix may on occasion be too swollen to fit into the 10 mm cannula. In such cases, the right iliac fossa incision can be enlarged slightly or the cannula replaced by a larger one (12 mm).

Intraperitoneal appendicectomy

This is the most frequently used approach to laparoscopic appendicectomy. With this technique, the risk of wound contamination is reduced as all the dissection is performed within the peritoneal cavity. The positions of the cannulae are the same as described previously: 10 mm cannulae in the subumbilical and right iliac fossa positions and a 5 mm cannula in the left iliac fossa. The mesoappendix is divided using diathermy or clips for large vessels and the appendix is mobilized down to its base. Preknotted ligatures are then used to ligate the appendix. The ligatures are introduced through the left iliac fossa cannula and the appendix is drawn through the loop of the ligature which is then firmly applied at the junction of the appendix and caecum. Three ligatures are applied in this way and the appendix is then divided leaving two ligatures on the stump. Where the neck of the appendix is narrow, Hulka clips can be used as an alternative method of occluding the appendicular stump.[19]

The appendix is retrieved through the 10 mm right iliac fossa cannula.

Alternatively, the appendicectomy can be performed using a laparoscopic stapling device which divides tissue after applying staples to both sides of the line of resection (Endo GIA, Auto Suture Co., UK). It is essential to use a 12 mm cannula to accommodate the broad shaft of the Endo GIA. This should be placed in the right upper quadrant of the abdomen or in the left iliac fossa in order to allow sufficient room to open the instrument in the abdomen. Two sizes of staple are available, the size required being dependent on the thickness of the tissue to be stapled. This is determined using a specific measuring device (Endo Gauge, Auto Suture Co., UK).

The appendix is picked up near its base and a window is created in the mesoappendix close to the appendix using the diathermy hook or dissecting scissors. The Endo Gauge is then applied successively to the base of the appendix and its mesentery. The Endo GIA, loaded with the appropriate cartridge, is then introduced through the mesenteric window and is applied to the appendix and mesoappendix in turn to complete the appendicectomy. The appendix is then retrieved through the 12 mm cannula.

When applying the Endo GIA, the tips of the stapler should be clearly visible to ensure that no other tissue is incorporated into the staple line. Slight haemorrhage may arise from the appendicular staple line but this usually subsides spontaneously. If necessary, a suture can be placed to control this. Diathermy should be avoided in this area as this may disrupt the staple formation.

If the appendix is perforated at its base, the Endo GIA can be applied to the pole of the caecum and a cuff of caecum excised with the appendix.

Peritoneal lavage is particularly important in such cases and should be directed not only at the appendix stump and right iliac fossa, but also at the pelvis and subdiaphragmatic areas where infected fluid may have drained.

If required the appendicular stump can be buried in the caecum using a purse-string or Z suture. This is more easily done when the appendicectomy is completed extra-abdominally but, with a little experience of intra-abdominal suturing and knot tying, can also be readily achieved in the intraperitoneal approach. Many surgeons now regard this step as unnecessary.[20,21]

In children, the smaller size of the abdomen necessitates the placement of the cannula at a greater distance from the right iliac fossa to avoid instrument crowding. It may be particularly advantageous to introduce the laparoscope in the left iliac fossa in order to provide a wider view of the appendix and caecum.

Intraoperative complications

Conversion to open procedure

It is important that conversion to the open procedure should not be regarded as a failure, but as the most sensible decision when the difficulties encountered make the procedure dangerous. The need to convert from the laparoscopic procedure to the open procedure is probably less than 5%. In a series of 915 laparoscopic appendicectomies for both acute and recurrent appendicitis, Pier et al.[16] reported an overall conversion rate of only 2%. In fact, most of these conversions occurred in the first 50 cases (24%) and the authors attributed this to the 'learning curve' effect. This pattern has been confirmed by Byrne et al.[14,22]

Obesity may cause difficulties, particularly if attempting to deliver the pole of the caecum onto the skin surface. However, unless the patient is morbidly obese, the appendicectomy can usually be completed using one of the techniques described above. Indeed, obese patients may derive the greatest benefit from the laparoscopic procedure as they otherwise often require large wounds and are at increased risk of wound complications.

Previous lower abdominal surgery need not preclude the use of the laparoscopic approach, provided access to the peritoneal cavity can be obtained safely.

Occasionally, the appendix may be concealed by omental adhesions. In this situation, gentle traction on the omentum using atraumatic forceps will usually reveal the appendix. The view of the appendix may also be obscured by small bowel dilatation secondary to local or generalized peritonitis. Although tilting the patient in the manner described above will usually displace the small bowel sufficiently to expose the appendix, this may not always be the case. In such circumstances, conversion to the open procedure may be necessary.

The position of the appendix is seldom a problem. When the appendix is retrocaecal, a well-defined peritoneal fold attaching the appendix and caecum to the lateral abdominal wall can usually be identified. Once this is divided, the appendix can be fully mobilized and removed. In cases where the inflammatory reaction surrounding the appendix results in its adhesion to the posterior wall of the caecum, the dissection may be more difficult due to the limited view of this area.[7,14] More extensive mobilization of the caecum and ascending colon will improve the visualization of the appendix and facilitate the dissection.

Bleeding may occur from the cannula sites if care is not taken to avoid blood vessels in the abdominal wall. Bleeding may also occur from the mesoappendix, especially if it is oedematous. Such bleeding can usually be controlled with diathermy, clips or ligatures and seldom requires conversion to the open procedure.

Perforation of the base of the appendix may create difficulties in applying ligatures to the appendix[12,23] and this has been quoted as a contraindication to the procedure.[24] With the use of the Endo GIA stapling device, this is no longer the case as the stapler can easily be applied across the pole of the caecum.

Post-operative complications

Similar complications to those encountered after open appendicectomy can be expected after laparoscopic appendicectomy. The principal complication is wound infection. In spite of the use of antibiotic prophylaxis, the incidence of wound infection following open appendicectomy remains in the region of 4–7%.[25,26] Most reports of laparoscopic appendicectomy so far have noted low wound infection rates but these are usually based on selected cases. However, McAnena et al.[23] in a series of 40 patients comparing the two approaches, reported a statistically significant reduction in wound infection rates after the laparoscopic operation. Pier et al.[16] report only 14 cases of mild omphalitis (1.5%) and no serious wound infections in 915 cases, and Nowzaradan et al.[24] report none in 35 patients. Without more objective data, the true incidence of wound infection is difficult to establish but it would appear to be no higher than after open appendicectomy.

Care should be taken when using diathermy as thermal injury to surrounding tissues can occur. Gotz et al.[12] and Schreiber[2] have each reported one case of peritonitis from stump ischaemia due to thermal injury.

There have been isolated reports of herniation of the omentum or small bowel through the subumbilical cannula site after laparoscopic procedures;[10,27] this can be avoided by suturing the defect in the linea alba in all cases.

Clinical implications

Laparoscopic appendicectomy has not been accepted by general surgeons with the same enthusiasm as other laparoscopic procedures. Most surgeons claim to perform open appendicectomy through a small transverse incision in less than 30 minutes and with few operative or post-operative complications. This, of course, only applies to thin, young, healthy patients. Many obese patients require much longer incisions with a concomitant increase in wound complications. Furthermore, most appendicectomies are performed by surgical trainees and this probably results in larger wounds and an increase in complications.[28]

The major advantage of the laparoscopic approach is that it affords a better view of the appendix and pelvic organs. This leads to greater diagnostic accuracy and a potential reduction in the number of unnecessary appendicectomies.[29–31] Furthermore, in infected cases, the peritoneal cavity can be more thoroughly irrigated and free fluid and purulent collections aspirated under direct vision.

Laparoscopic appendicectomy requires two or three small puncture wounds rather than the muscle-splitting or muscle-cutting incision of open appendicectomy. One can therefore expect less post-operative wound pain. Indeed, several studies have revealed that post-operative analgesic requirements are significantly less after laparoscopic appendicectomy than after open appendicectomy.[14,22,23,32] This results in more rapid mobilization and discharge from hospital.

It is frequently claimed that laparoscopic surgery produces fewer intra-abdominal adhesions than open surgery and there is some recent evidence to support this. According to Semm,[1] adhesions between the caecum or omentum and the deep surface of an appendicectomy scar occur in 90% of patients after appendicitis. De Wilde,[33] comparing patients after open and laparoscopic appendicectomy, found adhesions in 80% of open cases and in only 10% of laparoscopic cases. He concluded that the risk of late adhesive obstruction might therefore be reduced by the laparoscopic approach. Infertility problems in female patients might also be reduced by this method.

Many patients with lower abdominal peritonitis of uncertain aetiology, subsequently found to be suffering from appendicitis, initially undergo laparotomy as a diagnostic procedure. In a retrospective study of a population of 700,000 over a period of 1 year, Byrne and Bell[22] identified 40 such patients, 80% of whom were found to have uncomplicated acute appendicitis. If this is representative of the national practice, as many as 2,500 'unnecessary' laparotomies may be performed for simple acute appendicitis each year in the United Kingdom. This type of procedure is associated with a high morbidity 'atelectasis/respiratory infection; wound pain, infection and dehiscence; adhesions) which could be substantially reduced by more widespread use of the laparoscope, if only for diagnostic purposes.[34]

Young female patients with recurrent right iliac fossa pain frequently present diagnostic and therapeutic dilemmas in surgical practice. There is no doubt that in some cases the pain is appendicular in origin, but these cases are difficult to identify. Many patients undergo laparoscopy while being investigated by gynaecologists and, in the absence of pelvic pathology, are then referred to a surgeon for appendicectomy. As the range of laparoscopic surgical procedures increases, both in the general and gynaecological fields, a combined approach to the problem may be an advantage.

Financial implications

The financial implications of laparoscopic appendicectomy have not been fully evaluated.

Although the operation takes longer to complete during the initial learning phase, most reports suggest that the typical duration of the operation is about 30 minutes. Several comparative studies of laparoscopic and open appendicectomy have found no difference in the operating times for laparoscopic and open appendicectomy.[14,22,23,32]

With the use of disposable instruments and stapling devices, the theatre costs can undoubtedly rise. However, apart from the Endo GIA stapler, all of these can be replaced by reusable materials. This additional expenditure is therefore in most cases avoidable. The shorter post-operative hospital stay reported in most recent series should help to offset any increase in the theatre costs. In the long run, one can expect similar savings to be achieved by laparoscopic appendicectomy as have been demonstrated in laparoscopic cholecystectomy.[35] The earlier return to normal activity for this young population (typically 7–14 days[22]) represents a benefit to the community which, though difficult to quantify, should not be overlooked.

Implications for surgical training

Traditionally, surgical trainees have gained their initial experience of emergency surgery performing appendicectomies. Although the increasing use of the laparoscopic approach will reduce this, the better visualization of the appendix and its surrounding structures afforded by this method should improve the appreciation of the anatomy of this region and should therefore enable the surgeon to cope with the open procedure, should conversion prove necessary.

As laparoscopic surgery becomes more widespread, experience in this approach will become an essential part of junior surgeons' training. Laparoscopic appendicectomy is a relatively easy operation to perform and may provide the necessary practice for trainees to develop their skills before proceeding to more major procedures.

Summary

Laparoscopic appendicectomy can be safely performed in the majority of patients with acute appendicitis. It has the particular advantage of improved diagnostic accuracy and may reduce the number of unnecessary appendicectomies. It allows more thorough peritoneal lavage, gives rise to less wound pain, and is associated with earlier discharge from hospital and a more rapid return to normal activities. The cosmetic result is excellent and it reduces the need for large incisions in obese patients. Furthermore, it could substantially reduce the need for laparotomy in cases of lower abdominal peritonitis of uncertain aetiology.

References

1. Semm, K. (1983). Endoscopic appendectomy. *Endoscopy*, **15**, 59–64.
2. Schreiber, J.H. (1987). Early experience with laparoscopic appendectomy in women. *Surgical Endoscopy*, **1**, 211–16.
3. Fleming, J.S. (1985). Laparoscopically directed appendicectomy. *Australian and New Zealand Journal of Obstetrics and Gynaecology*, **25**, 238–40.
4. Wilson, T. (1986). Laparoscopically-assisted appendicectomies. *Medical Journal of Australia,* **145**, 551.
5. Gangal, H.T. and Gangal, M.H. (1987). Laparoscopic appendicectomy. *Endoscopy*, **19**, 127–9.
6. Leahy, P.F. (1989). Technique of laparoscopic appendicectomy. *British Journal of Surgery*, **76**(6), 616.
7. Browne, D.S. (1990). Laparoscopic-guided appendicectomy. A study of 100 consecutive cases. *Australian and New Zealand Journal of Obstetrics and Gynaecology*, **30**(3), 231–3.
8. McKernan, J.B. and Saye, W.B. (1990). Laparoscopic techniques in appendectomy with argon laser. *Southern Medical Journal*, **83**, 1019–20.
9. Schreiber, J.H. (1990). Laparoscopic appendectomy in pregnancy. *Surgical Endoscopy*, **4**, 100–2.
10. Gotz, F., Pier, A. and Bacher, C. (1990). Modified laparoscopic appendectomy in surgery: a report on 388 operations. *Surgical Endoscopy*, **4**, 6–9.
11. Pier, A., Gotz, F. and Bacher, C. (1991). Laparoscopic appendectomy in 625 cases: from innovation to routine. *Surgical Laparoscopic and Endoscopy*, **1**, 8–13.
12. Gotz, F., Pier, A. and Bacher, C. (1991). Die laparoskopische Appendektomie. Indikation, Technik und Ergebnisse bei 653 Patienten. *Chirurg*, **62**, 253–6.
13. O'Regan, P.J. (1991). Laparoscopic appendectomy. *Canadian Journal of Surgery*, **34**, 256–8.
14. Byrne, D.S., Bell, G., Morrice, J.J. and Orr, G. (1992). Technique for laparoscopic appendicectomy. *British Journal of Surgery*, **79**, 574–5.
15. Bryant, T.L. (1992). Laparoscopic appendectomy: a simplified technique. *Journal of Laparoendoscopic Surgery*, **2**, 343–50.
16. Pier, A., Gotz, F., Bacher, C. and Ibald, R. (1993). Laparoscopic appendicectomy. *World Journal of Surgery*, **17**, 29–33.
17. Tate, J.J.T., Dawson, J.W., Chung, S.C.S., Lau, W.Y. and Li, A.K.C. (1993). Laparoscopic versus open appendicectomy: prospective randomised trial. *Lancet*, **342**, 633–7.
18. Hasson, H.M. (1971). Modified instrument and method for laparoscopy. *American Journal of Obstetrics and Gynaecology*, **110**, 886–7.
19. Schultz, L.S., Pietrafitta, J.J., Graber, J.N. and Hickok, D.F. (1991). Retrograde laparoscopic appendectomy: report of a case. *Journal of Laparoendoscopic Surgery*, **1**, 111–14.
20. Engstrom, L. and Fenyo, G. (1985). Appendicectomy: assessment of stump invagination. A prospective randomized trial. *British Journal of Surgery*, **72**, 971–2.
21. Dass, H.P., Wilson, S.J., Khan, S., Parlade, S. and Uy, A. (1989). Appendicectomy stumps: 'to bury or not to bury'. *Tropical Doctor*, **19**, 108–9.
22. Byrne, D.S. and Bell, G. (1992). Appendicectomy: laparoscopic or open? Presentation to the 2nd European Congress of Viscero-synthesis (Minimally Invasive Surgery and New Technology), Luxembourg, September 11.
23. McAnena, O.J., Austin, O., O'Connell, P.R., Hederman, W.P., Gorey, T.F. and Fitzpatrick, J. (1992). Laparoscopic versus open appendicectomy: a prospective evaluation. *British Journal of Surgery*, **79**, 818–20.
24. Nowzaradan, Y., Westmoreland, J., McCarver, C.T. and Harris, R.J. (1991). Laparoscopic appendectomy for acute appendicitis: indications and current use. *Journal of Laparoendoscopic Surgery*, **5**, 247–59.
25. Krukowski, Z.H., Irwin, S.T., Denholm, S. and Matheson, N.A. (1988). Preventing wound infection after appendicectomy: a review. *British Journal of Surgery*, **75**, 1023.
26. Seco, J.L., Ojeda, E., Requilon, C., Serrano, S.R. and Santamaria, J.L. (1990). Combined topical and systemic antibiotic prophylaxis in acute appendicitis. *American Journal of Surgery*, **159**, 226–30.
27. McMillan, J. and Watt, I. (1993). Herniation at the site of cannula insertion after laparoscopic cholecystectomy. *British Journal of Surgery*, **80**, 915.
28. Gilmore, O.J.A. and Martin, T.D.M. (1974). Aetiology and prevention of wound infection in appendicectomy. *British Journal of Surgery*, **61**, 281–7.
29. Paterson-Brown, S., Thompson, J.N., Eckersley, J.R.T., Ponting, G.A. and Dudley, H.A.F. (1988). Which patients with suspected appendicitis should undergo laparoscopy? *British Medical Journal*, **296**, 1363–4.
30. Spirtos, N.M., Eisenkop, S.M., Spirtos, T.W., Poliakin, R.I. and Hibbard, L.T. (1989). Laparoscopy–a diagnostic aid in cases of suspected appendicitis. Its use in women of reproductive age. *American Journal of Obstetrics and Gynaecology*, **156**, 90–4.
31. Paterson-Brown, S. (1991). The acute abdomen: the role of laparoscopy. In: *Gastrointestinal Emergencies*, Part I (eds Williamson, R.C.N. and Thompson, J.N.) Bailliere Tindall, London, pp. 691–703.
32. Attwood, S.E.A., Hill, A.D.K., Murphy, P.G., Thornton, J. and Stephens, R.B. (1992). A prospective randomized trial of laparoscopic versus open appendectomy. *Surgery*, **112**, 497–501.
33. De Wilde, R.L. (1991). Goodbye to late bowel

obstruction after appendicectomy (letter). *Lancet*, **338**, 1012.

34. Reiertsen, O., Rosseland, A.R., Hoivik, B. and Solheim, K. (1985). Laparoscopy in patients admitted for acute abdominal pain. *Acta Chirurgia Scandanavia*, **151**, 521–4.

35. Fullarton, G.M., McMillan, R. and Bell, G. (1991). Evaluation of the cost of laparoscopic and open cholecystectomy. Proceedings of the Society for Minimally Invasive Therapy. International Meeting. Mary Ann Liebert Inc. (Publishers), New York, p. 49.

10

Endoscopic control of major gastrointestinal haemorrhage

R.J.C. Steele and S.C.S. Chung

Introduction

Fibre-optic endoscopy of the gastrointestinal tract is a necessary skill in surgical gastro-enterology, and the control of gastrointestinal haemorrhage is one of the major roles of this specialty. Endoscopic therapy for upper gastrointestinal bleeding is a rapidly advancing and expanding field, and it is important for the surgeon who is likely to be operating for bleeding to be aware of the potential benefits and limitations of this type of treatment. We also believe that surgeons should be involved in the delivery of endoscopic haemostasis, not least because it may often prove to be the definitive means of obtaining control of the bleeding, but also because it is very important to recognize when conventional surgery becomes necessary and to be able to act promptly. Lives can be lost by inappropriate persistence with endoscopic treatment.

Another good reason for surgeons being involved with therapeutic fibre-optic endoscopy is that it demands similar skills to those needed for other types of endoscopic surgery. In particular it is necessary to estimate depth from two-dimensional visual cues, and if a surgeon has mastered this ability for one type of procedure, it is relatively simple to translate it to another. In addition, with the advent of high resolution chip cameras and videoendoscopy, both endoscopist and surgeon are well used to seeing the operating field on a video monitor.

Endoscopic haemostasis can be divided conveniently into two major areas: therapy for bleeding oesophageal varices and the control of haemorrhage from peptic ulcers. This chapter is structured accordingly, with two sections dealing with variceal and non-variceal upper gastrointestinal bleeding respectively. Emphasis is placed on the practical aspects of treatment, but short reviews of the key literature are also provided.

Variceal bleeding

Background

Injection sclerotherapy is well established as the most effective endoscopic means of controlling bleeding from oesophageal varices, and although other promising methods are being developed, evidence of their efficacy in the literature is still scanty. Sclerotherapy for varices was first performed in 1936 by Crafoord and Frenckner,[1] but it is only since enthusiasm for portosystemic shunting waned in the 1970s that it has really gained favour. There is no doubt that endoscopic sclerotherapy is successful in the control of acute haemorrhage; although only 25% of patients admitted with bleeding varices will be seen to be bleeding at the time of urgent endoscopy, about 60% of the remainder will have further bleeding during the same hospital admission,[2] and several studies testify to the ability of sclerotherapy greatly to improve on these figures.[3-5] Acute sclerotherapy has also been shown to be more effective than balloon tamponade in a randomized, controlled trial.[6]

Opinion regarding the exact timing of injection for the acute bleed is divided. Some favour immediate injection, whereas others prefer a period of resuscitation combined with vasoactive therapy and/or balloon tamponade as appropriate followed by semi-elective injection. Objective evidence supports the former approach; Prindiville and Trudeau[7] found that immediate emergency injection provided significantly better control of bleeding than delayed endoscopic treatment, and these findings have been substantiated in a similar study by Shemesh *et al.*[8] Unfortunately, however, a single session of injection at the time of bleeding carries a high rate of recurrent bleeding,[9] and continued sclerotherapy aimed at obliteration of the varices is necessary to obtain acceptable recurrence rates.[10,11] Even then, recurrence of bleeding is a major problem, and there has been a recent swing of opinion back to elective portosystemic shunting when long-term control is a problem.[12]

It is generally accepted, however, that all patients who have bled from varices should be treated initially with sclerotherapy, with the exception of those with isolated gastric varices; these patients require early shunting.[13] It is less clear how often the injections should be repeated, although in two studies comparing weekly with 3 weekly treatments, the more frequent schedule seemed to be preferable. Westaby *et al.*[14] found that the weekly injections resulted in more rapid obliteration of the varices, and Sarin's group also demonstrated a significant reduction in rebleeding for the more frequent treatment.[15] Both studies showed more oesophageal ulceration in the weekly group, but this did not seem to be a significant clinical problem.

Which sclerosant to use is also a subject of some debate. Kitano *et al.*[16] found that 5% ethanolamine was better than 2% sodium tetradecyl sulphate (STD) in terms of early rebleeding and ulceration, but Rose and Smith[17] could find no difference between the two compounds. Ethanolamine has also been compared with 1% polidocanol, and the former was superior in controlling acute bleeding and in preventing rebleeding.[18] Absolute alcohol has been used to good effect,[19] but no comparisons with other substances have been carried out. As yet, therefore, there is little evidence to support strongly one sclerosant for universal use.

It is also worth touching on the controversy over the precise placement of the sclerosing injections. Most workers favour intravariceal injections, but some advocate paravariceal injection or oesophageal wall sclerosis in the belief that thrombosis of the oesophageal varices may precipitate the development or rupture of gastric varices.[20] In fact, a relatively high proportion of intended intravariceal injections end up being paravariceal,[21,22] and the paravariceal component may be useful in compressing the varices. Comparisons between the two techniques have been made, and these have come down quite strongly in favour of the intravariceal technique.[21,23]

Finally, there are two recent developments which must be mentioned as they look set to have a significant impact on the endoscopic treatment of varices. Firstly, injection of cyanoacrylate glue has been employed with excellent results; consistent control of bleeding with elimination of the need for emergency surgery has been reported.[24,25] Secondly, elastic 'O' rings similar to those used to band haemorrhoids have been applied successfully to oesophageal varices, and preliminary results suggest that this technique may be as effective as sclerotherapy but with fewer complications.[26,27]

Technique of endoscopic sclerotherapy

When a patient is admitted with gastrointestinal bleeding, it is possible to estimate the likelihood of variceal bleeding on past history and clinical grounds. If there is documented previous evidence of varices, or if there is a clear history of excessive alcohol intake combined with signs of liver decompensation (liver palms, spider naevi, bruising, encephalopathy, jaundice) or portal hypertension (ascites, caput medusa), then the endoscopist must be prepared to carry out sclerotherapy. Obviously, resuscitation should be initiated immediately, and securing adequate vascular access is a major priority. Hypovolaemia should be corrected, initially with plasma expander if the situation demands it, and then with blood. Using large amounts of crystalloid should be avoided, as this will exacerbate peripheral oedema and ascites. A clotting screen must be obtained rapidly, as many of these patients will have a coagulation disorder due to defective hepatic synthesis of clotting factors, and hyperplenism may lead to thrombocytopenia. Fresh frozen plasma or factor concentrate and platelets should then be ordered as appropriate.

There is, however, no merit in delaying endoscopy for any significant length of time, and as soon as resuscitation has been initiated, the patient with suspected varices should be transferred urgently to the endoscopy room. We find that the most suitable endoscope for injecting varices is a double channel fibre-optic instrument, and although others find overtubes (such as the Williams tube) to be useful, we prefer to use the free-hand method. We also favour intravariceal injection rather than paravariceal, as it leads to more rapid oblitera-tion of the varices. The double channel endoscope is useful for various reasons; excel-lent suction and irrigation are maintained with the injection needle in place, the large diame-ter of the instrument shaft gives some degree of tamponade which can be used during the procedure and, finally, the two channels provide an extra degree of flexibility for precise positioning of the needle.

As indicated above, there is little concrete evidence to support one sclerosant over another, but we tend to favour 3% STD. Needles come in a bewildering range of sizes and makes, but the main choice is between a reusable metal coil type and a disposable Teflon® or plastic sheathed device (Figure 10.1). The disposable needle is preferable because it is possible to create a slight bend on the tip by deforming the needle shaft before inserting it into the endoscope. This gives an additional degree of rotational control over the position of the needle in the oesophagus.

Before starting, it is important that the patient is adequately sedated. The pharynx should be sprayed with 15% lignocaine, and an intravenous injection of a benzodiazepine such as midazolam or diazemuls given. Unfortunately, if the patient has been a heavy drinker, this type of sedation may have little effect, and it is then advisable to use pethidine as well. If the bleeding is torrential, and there is clearly a significant risk of aspiration, it is as well to consider carrying out the endoscopy under general anaesthesia with the airway protected by cuffed endotracheal intubation.

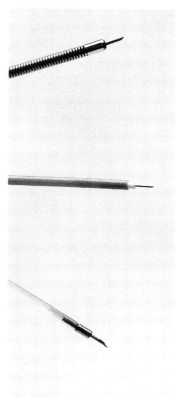

Fig. 10.1 Injector needles. Top: metal, reusable. Middle and bottom: plastic, disposable.

Alternatively, a pharyngeal overtube system used over the endoscope allows safe endoscopy in a patient with a stomach full of blood.

The majority of patients will have stopped actively bleeding at the time of endoscopy, and because about 30% of patients with varices may be bleeding from another lesion, it is important to carry out as complete an endoscopy as possible to rule out this eventu-ality. However, if oesophageal varices are the only abnormalities to be found (Figure 10.2), and there is evidence of recent bleeding such as fresh blood or coffee ground in the stomach, then the varices should be assumed to be the source of bleeding and immediate sclerother-apy carried out. Further evidence of recent bleeding in the form of a cherry red or white spot may be seen on a varix, and, of course, active bleeding may be seen as a jet of blood from the site of rupture, placing the diagnosis beyond doubt.

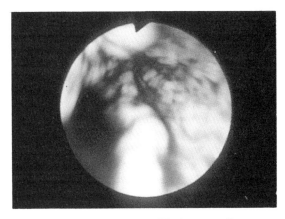

Fig. 10.2 Oesophageal varices. The brown 'coffee ground' liquid indicates fairly recent upper gastrointestinal haemorrhage.

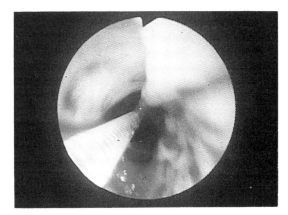

Fig. 10.3 Injection of varix.

The injection of the varices should be attempted at the initial endoscopy in all cases, whether or not there is active bleeding, as there is no benefit in an initial period of balloon compression. The needle assembly is inserted into the channel of the endoscope with the sharp tip withdrawn into the sheath, and the needle primed with sclerosant. If the needle tip is exposed during passage along the endoscope it may damage the wall of the channel at the bending section of the instrument and cause leakage into the fibre bundle. When the needle emerges from the end of the channel, it is safe to expose the sharp tip and to withdraw the whole needle just inside the endoscope. This prevents the needle from

damaging the oesophageal wall, but allows the endoscopist to bring it into the field of vision at a moment's notice, ready to inject.

If active haemorrhage is seen, the bleeding varix should be dealt with first by puncturing it just proximal to the bleeding site and instructing the endoscopy assistant to inject 1–2 ml of sclerosant. Further injections should then be carried out at 2 cm intervals along the same variceal column and along the other columns, starting at the gastro-oesophageal junction (Figure 10.3). If no bleeding is seen, the variceal column at 11–2 o'clock should be injected first, as this is the most awkward to reach. Changing the position of the needle by torqueing the shaft of the endoscope and by swapping the needle over to the other channel will allow access to all the varices. In between injections, the needle should be withdrawn into the endoscope channel to prevent laceration of the varices when the patient struggles or retches.

If massive bleeding obscures the view, the best policy is to insert the endoscope into the stomach, suck out as much blood as possible and leave the instrument in this position for about 5 minutes to tamponade the varices. During this time, it is useful to give a bolus of 250 µg of somatostatin to reduce the portal pressure, and 10 mg of metoclopramide to increase the pressure of the lower oesophageal sphincter. If the blood pressure is well maintained, it is also useful to tip the patient head up to prevent blood from refluxing back up the oesophagus from the stomach. The endoscope should then be withdrawn slowly, and it will often be possible to obtain a clear enough view to inject with sufficient precision.

Another common problem is bleeding from the injection sites, and if this occurs it is important to avoid depositing too much sclerosant in the same place as this will cause deep ulceration or even perforation. It is best merely to insert the endoscope into the stomach and wait as described above. Occasionally, despite using all the tricks available, the bleeding will be too vigorous to control by acute sclerotherapy. Under these circumstances, there is no option but to insert a Sengstaken–Blakemore tube (or equivalent), and to repeat the procedure 12–24 hours later. If this fails, then the patient must be considered for emergency oesophageal transection.

Table 10.1 The range of methods employed in endoscopic haemostasis for non-variceal bleeding

1. Thermal methods
   Laser
     –Argon
     –Nd:YAG
   Diathermy
     –Monopolar
     –Bipolar (BICAP®)
   Heater probe
2. Injection methods
   Adrenaline
   Alcohol
   Sclerosant
     –STD
     –Polidocanol
   Clotting factors
3. Topical applications
   Collagen
   Clotting factors
   Cyanoacrylate glue
   Ferromagnetic tamponade
4. Mechanical methods
   Balloon tamponade
   Clips
   Staples
   Sutures

If the acute bleeding is controlled by sclerotherapy, then repeat injection sessions should be carried out weekly until the varices have been obliterated. After this, 3–6 monthly endoscopies are advisable, so that recurrent varices can be treated. Portosystemic shunting should be considered in the good-risk patient with reasonable liver function who has recurrent bleeding despite an intensive programme of sclerotherapy.

Non-variceal bleeding

Background

Endoscopic haemostasis for non-variceal bleeding is currently attracting a lot of interest, but it is certainly less well established than sclerotherapy for varices. One of the reasons for this is the fact that although there are several techniques available, a clear method of choice has yet to emerge. However, if the endoscopic treatment of bleeding peptic ulcers can be refined and widely adopted, it should prove to be more satisfactory than variceal sclerotherapy; if active bleeding can be controlled without recourse to potentially dangerous emergency surgery, the underlying pathology can be effectively treated either by medical means or by elective operation.

To date, there are five endoscopic methods for treating non-variceal bleeding which have been demonstrated to be useful in clinical trials: laser photocoagulation, bipolar diathermy, heater probe treatment, injection sclerotherapy and injection of vasoconstrictor substances. Various other techniques have been tried (Table 10.1), but sufficient experience of these has not yet accrued to warrant further discussion in this chapter. When considering endoscopic haemostasis, it must be appreciated that about 80% of patients with upper gastrointestinal bleeding will stop bleeding spontaneously, and it is therefore important that any haemostatic method be subjected to a controlled clinical trial. In this section, the techniques for the mainstream methods of endoscopic haemostasis are first discussed, and the current evidence relating to their relative merits is then reviewed.

Techniques of endoscopic haemostasis for non-variceal bleeding

Success in controlling bleeding depends not so much on the precise method used, but more on the ability and experience of the endoscopist in acute gastrointestinal haemorrhage, and having the appropriate equipment to hand. As with variceal haemorrhage, resuscitation must take priority, but if the patient remains haemodynamically unstable, emergency endoscopy must not be delayed. Even if the patient is stable urgent endoscopy (within 24 hours of admission) is strongly advised because, haemostasis aside, the chances of making a diagnosis diminish rapidly with time.

Endoscopy for bleeding is usually performed under benzodiazepine sedation, but again general anaesthesia must be seriously considered in the patient who is having copious haematemeses. Monitoring of the patient during the examination is very important, for the endoscopist will be engrossed in the procedure, and while an experienced endoscopy nurse will be able to detect marked changes in the clinical condition, objective measurements provide a more sensitive index of the patient's well-being. As a minimum, pulse and blood pressure should be measured regularly, preferably using an automatic device such as the 'Dinamap' monitor which incorporates an alarm system triggered by preset values. Pulse oximetry is also advisable as arterial desaturation is liable to occur during endoscopy, and this is a particular risk when a large diameter therapeutic instrument is being used for a relatively prolonged period. In any case, it is wise to administer oxygen via nasal prongs during any interventional endoscopy procedure. It may also be necessary to measure the central venous pressure in a patient with cardiorespiratory problems.

Usually the endoscopy will take place in the endoscopy room with the patient lying on a trolley, and it is important that the trolley is suitable. It should be capable of tipping the patient head up as well as head down, and it should have rails which can be moved to allow easy access to the patient but prevent him or her from falling off. To start off the examination, a strict left lateral position should be ensured as this allows blood to pool in the fundus of the stomach where bleeding lesions are uncommon (Figure 10.4). It is important that the patient is not allowed to slip into a supine posture during the procedure, and this can be prevented by placing one or two pillows between the patient's back and the rails of the trolley. If it becomes necessary to view the fundus, this can usually be achieved by a combination of tipping the head of the trolley up and turning the patient to the right lateral position. This will have the effect of pooling blood into the antrum. In the massively bleeding patient, or when blood clots in the stomach obscure the view, the use of a pharyngeal overtube is advisable. The overtube protects the airway from the dangers of aspiration, facilitates the use of a wide-bore lavage tube and simplifies multiple endoscope insertions. The overtube is preloaded onto the shaft of the endoscope, and the instrument is passed in the usual manner; once the stomach has been entered, the overtube is slid over the endoscope until the mouthpiece is at the level of the incisors. The airway is now protected and the endoscope can be removed leaving the overtube in place. Stomach lavage can now take place in safety, and the endoscope replaced with ease.

The choice of endoscope is crucial in the bleeding patient, for both diagnostic and therapeutic reasons. In general, it is best to avoid videoendoscopes as they produce a very

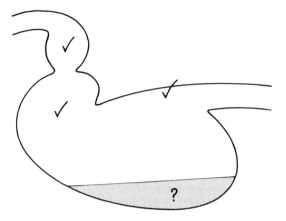

Fig. 10.4 Pool of blood in stomach with patient in the left lateral position. Note that the lesser curve and antrum will be visible at endoscopy.

dark, fuzzy image in the presence of blood owing to saturation of the 'red channel' of the chip camera–although the latest generation of videoscope incorporates a much improved chip which has been specifically designed for gastrointestinal endoscopy, and these instruments may prove to be suitable for acute haemorrhage. The best 'all round' endoscope for bleeding is an instrument with a single wide channel (3.7 mm) with a separate, relatively narrow, forward washing channel. This permits simultaneous washing and therapy, and the wide channel allows good suction when unoccupied and retains some suction even when a therapeutic device is in action. Such an endoscope has excellent optical properties and has a high degree of manoeuvrability. The double channel instrument as recommended for variceal bleeding is also very useful, but may cause difficulties in gaining access to awkwardly placed lesions owing to its large size. The slim or 'paediatric' endoscope is limited by its small-diameter channel, but in some circumstances its extra flexibility can be invaluable, e.g. for injecting an ulcer high on the lesser curve of the stomach.

Washing is a very important part of endoscopy in the presence of active bleeding, as it is vital to obtain a good view of the bleeding point if there is to be any hope of haemostatic intervention. The normal washing channel is designed to clean the lens at the tip of the endoscope, and is of no value in clearing away blood and debris. To do this, it is necessary to use a powerful forward jet of water through either the working channel or a special forward washing channel. The simplest method is to connect a 20 ml syringe full of water to the appropriate channel, but this requires the endoscopist to take one hand off the controls just at a time when fine adjustments of the endoscope tip are needed. A better device is a dental irrigator (a water toothbrush or water-pik) which can be modified by the provision of a foot switch and by attaching the water outlet to the endoscope channel. This system delivers a jet of water of variable force at rates of up to 500 ml per minute, and the foot control frees the hands of the endoscopist during the examination. It is also worth noting that some heater probe and bipolar diathermy devices have integral washing channels which are useful in the single channel endoscope.

When a view of the bleeding lesion has been obtained, a decision has to be made regarding treatment. The most definite indication for endoscopic treatment is active bleeding from an ulcer, either arterial or simple oozing. The only situations where endoscopic treatment should not be attempted are those where the haemorrhage is so fierce that a view of the source cannot be obtained or where the lesion is not accessible to the type of equipment being used. In these cases, struggling to control the bleeding is pointless and will waste precious time which would be better used transferring the patient to the operating theatre.

After successful initial endoscopic haemostasis, the endoscopy ideally should be repeated within 24 hours and any recurrent bleeding treated. If, however, there is clinical evidence of rebleeding before this re-endoscopy, surgery is the treatment of choice unless there is very good reason to avoid operation. It is vital that patients who have had endoscopic haemostasis are monitored carefully until there is endoscopic evidence that the risk of rebleeding is low. Rebleeding is most common for lesions on the posterior wall of the duodenum or high on the lesser curve of the stomach, regardless of the haemostatic method used.

The endoscopic treatment of non-bleeding lesions is more controversial, but there are some guidelines which can be given. An ulcer with a clean base or with a flat black or red

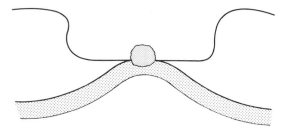

Fig. 10.5 Vessel looping up to ulcer base, with defect in its wall plugged by a 'sentinel clot'.

spot should not be treated as the risk of rebleeding is very low. If there is an adherent clot obscuring the base of the ulcer, this should be left strictly alone as laser or probe treatment will be impossible, and injecting through a clot is very imprecise. A definite visible vessel (a raised red or blue spot) in the base of an ulcer poses a more difficult problem, however, as the risk of rebleeding is in the region of 40%, and there is some evidence that endoscopic treatment of such lesions may be of value.

This so-called visible vessel usually represents a 'sentinel' clot or thrombus which is plugging an artery of any diameter between 0.1 and 2 mm which is looping up to the base of the ulcer[28] (Figure 10.5). The direction in which this vessel is running is often impossible to estimate, however, which makes precise delivery of endoscopic treatment difficult. The techniques required are given in the appropriate subsections of this chapter, but the alternative approach is to observe the patient very carefully and repeat the endoscopy 24 hours later. If active bleeding is then seen, it can be treated accordingly. One important point relating to the conservative treatment of non-bleeding ulcers should be stressed. If adherent clot or a visible vessel is seen but does not rebleed, vigilance should not be relaxed without a further endoscopy demonstrating resolution of the lesion. Although most rebleeding occurs within 72 hours, this is not invariable, and it can occur after more than a week has elapsed from the original episode.

Laser photocoagulation

Laser stands for *l*ight *a*mplification by *s*timulated *e*mission of *r*adiation, and the light produced carries energy which is converted to heat on contact with tissue. The two types of laser which have been used with fibre-optic endoscopes are the argon ion and the neodymium yttrium aluminium garnet (Nd:YAG), and these have somewhat different properties. The argon ion laser has a wavelength of 440–520 nm, and as the penetration into tissue tends to be low, the coagulation effect is consequently superficial. The Nd:YAG laser, on the other hand, has a wavelength of 1,060 nm, and has a greater depth of tissue penetration. This difference means that the Nd:YAG laser is much more effective for controlling haemorrhage from large vessels, and the argon ion laser is now rarely used in the treatment of gastrointestinal bleeding.

Most laser systems available are 'non-contact', and the heat generated causes thermal contraction of the tissue and the vessel wall leading to immediate haemostasis. Endothelial damage stimulates the deposition of platelet and fibrin thrombus which is responsible for the permanent effect. Recently, however, a 'contact' laser probe consisting of a synthetic sapphire crystal has been developed which allows coaptation of the vessel. This principle will be described in the sections dealing with diathermy and heater probe therapy.

A suitable laser unit is a Nd:YAG capable of delivering 60–100 watts. The fibre delivery system consists of a core of quartz fibres enclosed within a catheter which provides protection and a coaxial channel. CO_2 is infused down this channel during operation of the laser to cool and clean the tip of the fibre and to clear blood away from the treatment site. As the Nd:YAG beam is invisible, a helium neon (red) laser beam is incorporated for aiming.

For laser therapy, a double channel endoscope is preferable; one channel is needed for the delivery fibre and one for venting. Venting is necessary to prevent gaseous over-distension of the stomach caused by the CO_2 and to allow escape of the smoke which is generated by the vaporization of tissue and which will otherwise obscure the view. The second channel is also useful for washing the ulcer.

When the decision to treat an ulcer has been made, the laser fibre should be passed down

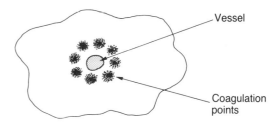

Fig. 10.6 'Ring' of coagulation produced by laser pulses around a visible vessel in the base of an ulcer.

the most convenient channel and the ulcer washed clear of blood and debris. This will allow location of the bleeding point and prevent overlying clot from absorbing energy. The helium neon aiming beam is then activated and passed over the ulcer to check that the target is accessible, and a 0.5 second pulse at 70 watts delivered as a 'test' to the mucosa at the edge of the ulcer. If the settings are correct, the single pulse should blanch the mucosa but not cause ulceration. Ideally, the fibre should be held about 1 cm from the tissue, and this is best achieved by advancing the fibre tip through the biopsy channel so that it is almost touching the target and then withdrawing it to the desired point.

The techniques for treating active arterial bleeding and a visible vessel are similar. The aim is to surround the exposed vessel with coagulated tissue by placing about eight pulses in a tight ring around the bleeding point or protuberant lesion (Figure 10.6). The reason for doing this is to maximize the chance of causing heat damage to the intact vessel both upstream and downstream of the exposed point. If active bleeding is not stopped immediately by the first few laser pulses it may be difficult to complete the 'ring' and it is worth waiting for a few minutes as the bleeding will often slow or stop allowing completion of the procedure. The treatment of simple oozing consists of direct photocoagulation of the appropriate areas until no further bleeding is seen. It is important, however, to make sure that there is no visible vessel associated with the oozing or, if there is, to treat it accordingly.

The main hazards of laser treatment for the patient are exacerbation or induction of bleeding and perforation of the stomach or duodenal wall, although these can be minimized by good technique. The Nd:YAG laser can also be dangerous for the endoscopist and other staff; if the laser beam hits a pool of fluid enough light can be reflected back up the endoscope to cause retinal damage unless a video system is used. In addition, if the laser is activated outside the patient, eye damage can be inflicted on anyone in the vicinity. For this reason all staff members involved with Nd:YAG laser endoscopy should wear specific filter goggles, the room should have all reflective surfaces dulled or removed, windows should be covered and there should be an appropriate warning system to indicate when the laser is in use. Expense is another disadvantage of laser, and the basic unit will cost in the region of £70,000, with additional cost of replacing the laser fibres. The equipment is essentially non-portable, which makes its use in different parts of the hospital awkward, and its complexity makes it relatively difficult to operate and difficult to repair when failure occurs. For all these reasons, photocoagulation for the control of gastrointestinal bleeding is likely to be superseded by the simpler methods described below.

Diathermy coagulation

Diathermy, also known as electrocoagulation, operates by means of heat generated by electrical current flowing through tissue near an electrode. This can be achieved via a monopolar system where the current flows from the active probe through the patient to a ground plate or via a bipolar system where the two electrodes are incorporated into the probe and current is therefore confined to the intended site of coagulation. The former system has the disadvantage of causing unpredictably deep thermal injury, and adherence of the probe tip to the coagulated tissue is a problem. Bipolar diathermy avoids these difficulties to a degree, and the rest of this section will deal only with this system.

Both diathermy and heat probes rely on the principle of coaptive coagulation, in which the walls of the vessel to be treated are brought together by the external pressure of the probe, thus interrupting the blood flow while the heat is being applied (Figure 10.7). This means that dissipation of heat by blood is minimized, and in active bleeding effective mechanical tamponade will confirm that the heat is being delivered to the correct spot.

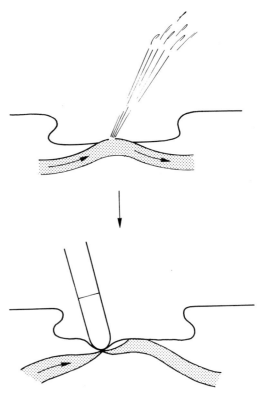

Fig. 10.7 Coaptive coagulation. The bleeding vessel is tamponaded by the diathermy or heater probe, and permanent haemostasis is produced by a combination of pressure and heat.

The bipolar probe most widely used is the BICAP® device, which consists of three pairs of longitudinal bipolar electrodes separated by insulators and arranged in a radial pattern around the tip (Figure 10.8). This arrangement allows current to be delivered to tissue irrespective of whether the probe is placed directly or tangentially onto the target. The probes are available in three diameter sizes–1.6 mm, 2.3 mm and 3.2 mm–and as the best reported results have been achieved with the largest probe, this is to be preferred. The larger probes also incorporate a central washing channel which means that they can be used easily down an endoscope with a single biopsy channel.

The power output settings vary from 5 to 50 watts, and it is possible to set the time of application in pulses of 1–2 seconds, or to have continuous current. It must be appreciated that the current delivered to the tissue

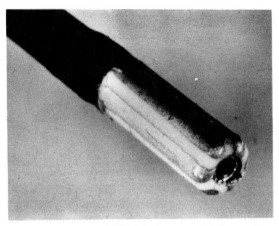

Fig. 10.8 Bipolar or BICAP® electrocoagulation probe. The central channel is used for washing.

depends partly on the electrical resistance, and that this increases with desiccation. Thus, as the contacted tissue heats up and dries out, the current flow is reduced, limiting the degree of damage.

Before use, the probe must be tested by setting the power to 10 watts and the time to 1 second, and activating in a few drops of normal saline. This should cause the saline to sizzle and evaporate. The probe should also be checked for kinks, as these will reduce current flow and make insertion through the endoscope difficult.

After washing the ulcer through the biopsy channel of the endoscope, the probe is passed and supplementary washing through the probe employed as necessary. If there is active arterial bleeding, the bleeding point should be compressed firmly with the probe to achieve as much control as possible. If the bleeding continues, the position of the probe should be changed until the best result is obtained. Then, and only then, a 50 watt (power setting 10) 2 second pulse is delivered two or three times by pressing the footswitch, and the probe withdrawn to observe the result. If there is still active bleeding a further series of pulses can be applied in a slightly different position. More recently it has been suggested that using a lower power and applying the probe for a longer time produces better results by allowing deeper energy penetration of the tissue. The ideal settings have yet to be fully resolved.

In the case of the non-bleeding visible vessel, the 'clue' provided by tamponading the haemorrhage is not available, and it is therefore necessary to produce a ring of coagulation immediately around the vessel by multiple applications of the probe. When this is complete, the vessel itself is treated, with the aim of flattening any protruding lesion. With simple oozing, a lower power setting should be used, and the probe placed directly onto the affected site.

As with laser, perforation is a remote possibility if too much pressure is applied to an area which has been overtreated. Precipitation of bleeding can also occur with direct treatment of a non-bleeding lesion, but this can be largely avoided by preliminary 'ringing'. Sticking of the probe to coagulated tissue can be a problem, although this is more likely with monopolar electrodes.

Heat probe

The heat probe is a device which can be heated rapidly to 150°C, a temperature which has been shown to be effective for coagulation but which avoids excessive tissue vaporization. In some ways it is similar in principle to the BICAP® probe, but it has two theoretical advantages. Firstly, because the temperature produced by the heat probe is independent of tissue desiccation, the delivery of energy is not interrupted by the formation of coagulum, and the strength of tissue bonding may be correspondingly greater. Secondly, because no electrical energy has to pass into the tissue, the probe can be coated by electrically insulating material which prevents adherence to coagulated tissue. In essence, however, the haemostatic effect is achieved in the same way as with diathermy, i.e. using coaptation of the vessel during heating.

The heat probe consists of a hollow metal tip coated with a non-stick material (Teflon®) which minimizes adherence to coagulated tissue (Figure 10.9). The tip contains an inner heating coil, and as the metal used has a high thermal conductivity, a uniform distribution of heat is rapidly achieved. The probe also incorporates water jet channels which terminate proximal to the probe tip. This allows washing during coaptation and coagulation, making it easier to see if the treatment is having the desired effect.

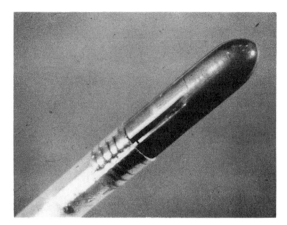

Fig. 10.9 Heater probe. Washing channels are situated proximal to the probe tip.

The probe is available in two sizes–2.5 mm and 3.2 mm–and as the larger probe is generally more effective, the only reason for using the smaller one is not having an endoscope with an appropriately sized channel. The power settings allow delivery of up to 30 joules per pulse, and the duration of the pulse is governed by the preset energy requirement and the amount of energy sensed by a silicon chip in the probe.

To check the probe before use, it is placed in a drop of distilled water and activated at a power of 20 joules. A warning tone should sound, indicating that heat energy is being produced, and the water should boil. The washing system should also be tested and the probe examined for kinks.

The technique is virtually identical to that described for BICAP® with the exception that the settings are graded as energy required in joules rather than wattage and pulse duration. The probe is positioned with firm pressure in order to control active bleeding, and three to four pulses of 25–30 joules are delivered without changing position. If the bleeding is not completely controlled, further pulses in different sites are applied.

Perforation and exacerbation of bleeding can occur with the use of the heater probe, just as with BICAP®. Perforation is more likely with retreatment of a lesion which has already been controlled, and acute duodenal ulcers are particularly at risk.

Adrenaline injection

The precise mechanism whereby adrenaline can bring about permanent haemostasis is not entirely clear, but it is probably the combined result of increased tissue pressure from the injected fluid and active vasospasm encouraging the formation of platelet and fibrin thrombus within the vessel lumen. This process may be aided by the action of adrenaline in activating platelets.

A solution of 1 in 10,000 is used, delivered by means of a standard endoscopic injection needle of the type used to sclerose varices. The metal needle is usually preferable to the Teflon® or plastic variety as it is stiffer and therefore better for injecting chronic ulcers. However, it must be carefully cleaned and sterilized after use to prevent the transmission of disease. Before using, the device should be checked to make sure that the needle tip can easily be pushed out from and withdrawn into the sheath. It should then be tested for patency and primed with the adrenaline solution.

When active arterial bleeding is identified, the lesion is washed, and the needle assembly passed through the biopsy channel of the endoscope with the tip withdrawn just as for variceal injection. It is then best to have the needle assembly, still with the needle inside, protruding just far enough to be included in the field of vision while the endoscope is manoeuvred into the ideal position. Having the needle tip withdrawn at this stage prevents accidental tearing of the mucosa. The needle is then protruded by the assistant who is holding the syringe by pushing the central needle into the sheath, and the tip will be seen to emerge from the end of the sheath by the endoscopist. It is important for the assistant and the endoscopist to agree on wording, because instructions such as 'needle in' and 'needle out' can be very confusing.

The needle is then advanced into the base of the bleeding point, and the assistant asked to inject 0.5 ml of the adrenaline solution. Considerable force may be needed, and if the injection is very easy, the needle is probably not actually in the tissue. If the bleeding does not stop almost immediately, a further 0.5 ml should be injected into the same position, the needle removed and reinserted into a slightly different point. When the bleeding has stopped (Figure 10.10a and b), more

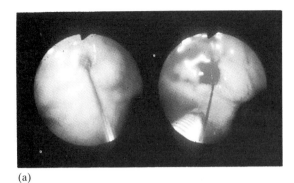

(a)

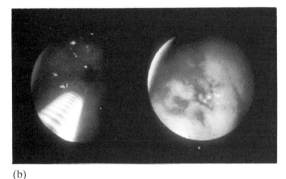

(b)

Fig. 10.10   Adrenaline injection for arterial bleeding.

adrenaline, in 0.5 ml aliquots, should be injected around the bleeding point until it has been surrounded, just as with thermal coagulation methods. Where there is oozing, with or without a visible vessel, the adrenaline should be delivered directly to the bleeding site until the bleeding is seen to stop. The non-bleeding visible vessel can be treated with adrenaline in just the same way as active arterial bleeding, but there is as yet little concrete evidence to support its use in this situation.

Injection can be used in fairly inaccessible sites. For example, the posterior aspect of the duodenum can be treated by advancing the needle through the pylorus and pushing the pyloric wall aside with the sheath; this is more satisfactory with the rigid reusable needle. If there is a high lesser curve ulcer which calls for an acute J manoeuvre, it can be helpful to use a small diameter endoscope and a small needle.

One situation in which injection treatment is particularly useful is where there is active bleeding associated with an adherent clot. This is very difficult to treat using thermal coagula-

tion methods, but with injection it is possible to pass the needle through clot to allow injection of the base of the ulcer. Injection into the right place is demonstrated by cessation of the bleeding.

Exacerbation of bleeding does not seem to be a problem with adrenaline injection, presumably due to the rapid vasospasm induced by treatment, and perforation has never been reported. It is possible, however, that undue force with the needle in a friable ulcer base might induce this latter complication.

Tachycardia and hypertension can occur, and although a fatal arrhythmia has not been reported, it is a wise precaution to use continuous ECG and blood pressure monitoring throughout the procedure.

Injection treatment is by far the cheapest and simplest means of endoscopic haemostasis; a reusable needle costs about £50, and the cost of adrenaline (or any of the other commonly used substances) is negligible. There is also relatively little risk of equipment failure, although it is important always to have at least one extra needle in reserve.

Injection sclerotherapy

The most common types of sclerosant which have been used in non-variceal haemorrhage are absolute alcohol and 1% polidocanol, but 5% ethanolamine and 3% sodium tetradecyl sulphate (STD) can be used. Alcohol causes rapid dehydration and fixation of tissue with subsequent thrombosis, whereas the others are detergents which damage the endothelium of the vessel. It should be noted that ethanolamine is more viscous than the other substances and difficult to inject with a small needle. The equipment required is identical to that used for adrenaline injection, although it may be useful to have a high-pressure injector gun depending on the solution being used. It is also important to have a luer-lock system for the syringe, as sprayed sclerosant may cause eye damage to the endoscopy staff or the patient.

If there is active bleeding, it is now usual to control this with adrenaline injection as described above. The bleeding point is then surrounded with injections of sclerosant using 0.1 ml aliquots of alcohol or 0.5 ml aliquots of the other sclerosants. Alcohol causes intense mucosal necrosis and no more than a total of 1 ml should be injected at any one site; the volume of the other sclerosants should be limited to 5 ml. Sclerotherapy of a non-bleeding visible vessel does not require prior adrenaline injection, although this may become necessary if the injection stimulates active bleeding.

As discussed below, current evidence would suggest that, in active bleeding, adrenaline alone is as effective as adrenaline plus sclerosant. Sclerosants undoubtedly cause mucosal necrosis leading to extension of ulceration and extensive necrosis of the stomach after injection of the left gastric artery has been reported. In general, however, this is a safe technique if the guidelines as to the maximum amount injected are observed, and it may be of particular value in the large visible vessel.

What to use

To decide on which method to use, it is necessary to look critically at the literature concerning the controlled trials which have been carried out to compare the various methods with conventional treatment. In addition, several trials designed to compare different techniques with one another have been completed recently, and these also provide important information.

Laser photocoagulation

First introduced by Kiefhaber *et al.*[29] in the 1970s, laser photocoagulation for bleeding peptic ulcers has been widely studied, and there have been at least 12 randomized, controlled trials comparing this technique with no endoscopic therapy.[30,31] Two types of laser have been used—the argon ion and the neodymium yttrium aluminium garnet (Nd:YAG). The Nd:YAG provides deeper penetration of tissue, and because it is therefore more useful in treating large vessels, it has superseded the argon laser.

To date, there have been nine trials of the Nd:YAG laser, but four of these were poorly designed or failed to give adequate definitions of the type of lesion being treated. Of the remainder, two have shown a significant reduction in rebleeding rates,[31,32] one has shown a significant reduction in the need for

emergency surgery,[33] and one has purported to demonstrate a reduction in mortality.[34] The fourth study, from Krejs *et al.*,[35] could not show any benefit whatsoever from the laser treatment. Of the 12 trials, therefore, although seven have claimed benefit, only four have shown a reduction in the need for emergency surgery, and only two have demonstrated an effect on mortality. Furthermore, these results have to be set against the relatively large numbers of patients excluded from randomization in several of the studies.

Bipolar diathermy

Three controlled trials of bipolar diathermy have shown no benefit for this technique,[36–38] and although O'Brien and colleagues found less rebleeding,[39] there was no difference in the rate of emergency surgery. However, in two separate studies Laine produced a significant reduction in the need for emergency surgery in patients with both active bleeding[40] and non-bleeding visible vessels.[41] It should be said that Laine used the larger 10 Fr probe, and carried out all the procedures himself, which may have accounted for his success.

Heat probe

To date, there have been four trials which have compared heat probe therapy with no active endoscopic treatment. The first, from Fullarton *et al.*, showed a significant reduction in rebleeding when compared with sham treatment,[42] and the 'CURE' study by Jensen (1990) also demonstrated a significant reduction in the need for emergency surgery in high risk patients.[43] However, two other groups have reported no benefit from the use of the heat probe.[31,44]

Injection sclerotherapy

Sclerosants used for ulcer haemostasis include absolute alcohol, 1% polidocanol and 3% STD. There have been no randomized trials of the use of alcohol, although spectacular results have been reported from Japan,[45] and one comparative study has suggested that alcohol injection can reduce the need for surgical intervention.[46] There have been two controlled trials of polidocanol injection, and although a reduction in emergency surgery rate for

Table 10.2. Comparative trials of different techniques for endoscopic haemostasis in non-variceal haemorrhage

Study	Methods Compared	Best result	Difference Statistically Significant
Johnston 1985[55]	Laser vs heat probe	Heat probe	Yes
Goff 1986[56]	Laser vs BICAP®	BICAP®	No
Rutgeerts 1989[57]	Laser vs BICAP®	No difference	–
Rutgeerts 1989[58]	Laser vs adrenaline vs adrenaline (plus) sclerosant	Adrenaline (plus) sclerosant	Yes
Mattewson 1990[31]	Laser vs heat probe	Laser	No
Loizou 1991[59]	Laser vs adrenaline	No difference	–
Hui 1991[60]	Laser vs heat probe vs BICAP®	No difference	–
Lin 1988[61]	Heat probe vs alcohol	No difference	–
Jensen 1990[43]	Heat probe vs BICAP®	Heat probe	Yes
Chung 1991[62]	Heat probe vs adrenaline	No difference	–
Laine 1990[63]	BICAP® vs alcohol	No difference	–
Waring 1991[64]	BICAP® vs alcohol	No difference	–
Chung 1990[53]	Adrenaline vs adrenaline + sclerosant	No difference	–

patients with active bleeding or a visible vessel was achieved in one[47] the other study could only show a significant effect on rebleeding.[48] It has to be stressed, however, that both of these groups used pre-injection with adrenaline before the sclerosant was administered.

Adrenaline injection

Injection of actively bleeding ulcers with adrenaline has been widely used in combination with sclerotherapy[49] and laser therapy,[50] and indeed the effectiveness of laser seems to be greatly enhanced by the initial adrenaline.[51,51] It is difficult to know which of the components of such combined therapy exerts the major therapeutic effect, but in a controlled trial, Chung *et al.* found that adrenaline injection alone reduced the need for emergency surgery in patients with actively bleeding ulcers.[52]

In a subsequent study, the same group of randomized patients had adrenaline injection or adrenaline plus sclerosant (3% STD), and were unable to demonstrate any difference.[53] It must be said, however, that the studies on adrenaline as the sole agent have concentrated on active bleeding, and its effect on rebleeding from a quiescent visible vessel is unknown.

Comparison between different methods

When comparing the different methods of endoscopic haemostasis for non-variceal bleeding, it is important to take into account the type of lesion which is being treated. The reason for this emerges by studying blinded trials in which the control patients are treated conservatively until they fulfil criteria which are independent of the endoscopic appearances. If this is done, it is found that patients with active arterial (pulsatile) bleeding come to surgery in about 60% of cases, whereas the figures for active non-arterial bleeding (oozing) and non-bleeding visible vessels are about 25% and 40% respectively.[54] When the adequately documented studies of the various types of therapy are put together, it is found that laser photocoagulation for active arterial bleeding is associated with an emergency surgery rate of around 40%, whereas both diathermy and injection techniques can reduce this to 15%.[54] For the other types of lesion, the different techniques produce roughly similar results.

Recently, the results of a number of trials comparing different methods have been published, and these are summarized in Table 10.2. One of the problems in the interpretation of such studies is the possibility (probability?) that the workers are more familiar with one of the techniques under examination than with the other. In this case, the results will be dependent on the skill of the operator rather than on the intrinsic qualities of the technique. This aside, however, examination of the table tends to suggest that laser photocoagulation produces less favourable results than any of the other methods, and this goes part of the way towards explaining the recent decline of laser as a therapeutic medium in this context.

In summary, although no definite guidelines can yet be given, it does appear that adrenaline injection is proving to be effective, in active bleeding at least. It is an inexpensive technique which is not prone to equipment failure, and adverse effects have not been reported. It is also easy to use for any competent endoscopist who is accustomed to dealing with acute bleeding. We would therefore commend adrenaline injection for actively bleeding ulcers, and suspend judgement as to the ideal means for preventing rebleeding from high-risk lesions.

References

1. Crafoord, C. and Frenckner, P. (1939). New surgical treatment of varicose veins of the oesophagus. *Acta Oto-laryngologica*, **27**, 422–9.
2. Mitchell, K.A., MacDougall, B.R.D., Silk, D.B.A. and Williams, R. (1982). A prospective reappraisal of emergency endoscopy in patients with portal hypertension. *Scandinavian Journal of Gastroenterology*, **17**, 965–8.
3. Johnston, G.W. and Rodgers, H.W. (1973). A review of 15 years' experience in the use of sclerotherapy in the control of acute haemorrhage from oesophageal varices. *British Journal of Surgery*, **60**, 797–800.
4. Soderlund, C. and Ihre, T. (1985). Endoscopic sclerotherapy versus conservative management of bleeding oesophageal varices: a 5 year prospective controlled trial of emergency and long-term treatment. *Acta Chirurgia Scandanavia*, **151**, 449–56.
5. Terblanche, J., Northover, J.M.A., Bornman, P. *et al.* (1979). A prospective evaluation of injection sclerotherapy in the treatment of acute bleeding from oesophageal varices. *Surgery*, **85**, 239–45.
6. Paquet, K.J. and Feussner, H. (1985). Endoscopic sclerosis and esophageal balloon tamponade in acute haemorrhage from esophageal varices: a prospective controlled randomised trial. *Hepatology*, **5**, 580–3.
7. Prindiville, T. and Trudeau, W. (1986). A comparison of immediate versus delayed endoscopic injection sclerosis of bleeding esophageal varices. *Gastrointestinal Endoscopy*, **32**, 385–8.
8. Shemesh, E., Czerniak, A., Klein, E., Pines, A. and Bat, L. (1990). A comparison between emergency and delayed endoscopic injection sclerotherapy of bleeding oesophageal varices in non-alcoholic portal hypertension. *Journal of Clinical Gastroenterology*, **12**, 5–9.
9. Terblanche, J., Northover, J.M.A., Bornman, P. *et al.* (1979). A prospective controlled trial of sclerotherapy in the long-term management of patients after esophageal variceal bleeding. *Surgical Gynecology and Obstetrics*, **148**, 323–38.
10. Clark, A.W., MacDougall, B.R.D., Westaby, D. *et al.* (1980). Prospective controlled trial of injection sclerotherapy in patients with cirrhosis and recent variceal haemorrhage. *Lancet*, **2**, 552–4.
11. Larson, A.W., Cohen, H., Zweiban, B. *et al.* (1986). Acute oesophageal variceal sclerotherapy: results of a prospective randomised controlled trial. *JAMA*, **255**, 497–500.
12. Sheilds, R. (1991). Bleeding oesophageal varices and the surgeon. *British Journal of Surgery*, **78**, 513–15.
13. Hosking, S.W. and Johnson, A.G. (1988). Gastric varices: a proposed classification leading to management. *British Journal of Surgery*, **75**, 195–6.
14. Westaby, D., Melia, W.M., MacDougall, B.R.D., Hegarty, J.E. and Williams, R. (1984). Injection sclerotherapy for oesophageal varices: a prospective randomised trial of different treatment schedules. *Gut*, **25**, 129–32.
15. Sarin, S.K., Sachdev, G., Nanda, R., Batra, S.K. and Anand, B.S. (1980). Comparison of the two time schedules for endoscopic sclerotherapy: a prospective randomised controlled study. *Gut*, **27**, 710–13.
16. Kitano, S., Iso, Y., Yamaga, H., Hashizume, M., Higashi, H. and Sugimachi, K. (1988). Trial of sclerosing agents in patients with oesophageal varices. *British Journal of Surgery*, **75**, 751–3.
17. Rose, J.D.R. and Smith, P.M. (1985). Oesophageal ulceration after extravasation of sodium tetradecyl

sulphate and ethanolamine oleate during endoscopic sclerotherapy. *Gut*, **26**, A1105.

18. Kitano, S., Koyanagi, N., Iso, Y., Higashi, H. and Sugimachi, K. (1987). Ethanolamine oleate is superior to polidocanol (aethoxysclerol) for endoscopic injection sclerotherapy of esophageal varices: a prospective randomised trial. *Hepato-gastroenterology*, **34**, 19–23.

19. Sarin, S.K., Sachdeva, G.A., Nanda, R., Vij, J.C. and Anand, B.S. (1985). Endoscopic sclerotherapy using absolute alcohol. *Gut*, **26**, 120–4.

20. Paquet, K.J., Busing, U. and Kliems, G. (1977). Wandsklerosierung der Speiserohre wegen Akuter, Konservativ-Unstillbarer und Drohender Varizenblutung. *Deutsche Medizinische Wochenschrift*, **102**, 59–61.

21. Rose, J.D.R., Smith, P.M. and Crane, M.D. (1983). Factors affecting successful endoscopic sclerotherapy for oesophageal varices. *Gut*, **24**, 946–9.

22. Grobe, J.L., Kozarek, R.A., Sanowski, R.A., Le Grand, J. and Kovak, A. (1984). Venography during endoscopic injection sclerotherapy of oesophageal varices. *Gastrointestinal Endoscopy*, **30**, 6–8.

23. Sarin, S.K., Nanda, R., Sachdev, G., Chari, S., Anand, B.S. and Broor, S.L. (1987). Intravariceal versus paravariceal sclerotherapy: a prospective, controlled, randomised trial. *Gut*, **28**, 657–62.

24. Gotlib, J. (1990). Endoscopic obturation of esophageal and gastric varices with a cyanoacrylic tissue adhesive. *Canadian Journal of Gastroenterology*, **4**, 637–8.

25. Grimm, H., Maydeo, A., Noar, M. and Soehendra, N. (1991). Bleeding esophagogastric varices: is endoscopic treatment with cyanoacrylate the final answer? *Gastrointestinal Endoscopy*, **37**, 275.

26. Stiegmann, G.V., Goff, J.S., Sum, J.H., Davis, D. and Bozdech, J. (1989). Endoscopic variceal ligation: an alternative to sclerotherapy. *Gastrointestinal Endoscopy*, **35**, 431–4.

27. Stiegmann, G., Goff, J., Korula, J., Lieberman, D., Reveille, M. and Sun, J. (1990). Endoscopic variceal ligation vs sclerotherapy for bleeding oesophageal varices: early results of a prospective randomised trial. *Gastrointestinal Endoscopy*, **36**, 118.

28. Swain, C.P., Storey, D.W. and Bown, S.G. (1986). Nature of the bleeding vessel in recurrently bleeding gastric ulcers. *Gastroenterology*, **90**, 595–608.

29. Kiefhaber, P., Nath, G. and Moritz, K. (1977). Endoscopical control of massive gastrointestinal haemorrhage by irradiation with a high power neodymium-YAG laser. *Progress in Surgery*, **15**, 140–55.

30. Laurence, B.H. and Cotton, P.B. (1987). Bleeding gastroduodenal ulcers: nonoperative treatment. *World Journal of Surgery*, **11**, 295–303.

31. Mattewson, K., Swain, C.P., Bland, M., Kirkham, J.S., Bown, S.G. and Northfield, T.C. (1990). Randomised comparison of NdYAG laser, heater probe and no endoscopic therapy for bleeding peptic ulcers. *Gastroenterology*, **98**, 1239–44.

32. Rutgeerts, P., Van Trappen, G., Broeckhaert, L.,

Janssens, J., Coremans, G., Geboes, K. and Schurmans, P. (1982). Controlled trial of YAG laser treatment of upper digestive haemorrhage. *Gastroenterology*, **83**, 410–16.

33. MacLeod, I.A., Mills, P.R., Mackenzie, J.F., Joffe, S.N., Russell, R.I. and Carter, D.C. (1983). Neodymium yttrium aluminium garnet laser photocoagulation for major haemorrhage from peptic ulcers and single vessels: a single blind controlled study. *British Medical Journal*, **286**, 345–8.

34. Swain, C.P., Kirkham, J.S., Salmon, P.R., Bown, S.G. and Northfield, T.C. (1986). Controlled trial of Nd-YAG laser photocoagulation in bleeding peptic ulcers. *Lancet*, **1**, 1113–16.

35. Krejs, G.J., Little, K.H., Westergaard, H., Hamilton, J.K., Spady, D.K. and Polter, D.E. (1987). Laser photocoagulation for the treatment of acute peptic ulcer bleeding. *New England Journal of Medicine*, **316**, 1618–21.

36. Goudie, B.M., Mitchell, K.G., Birnie, G.G. and Mackay, C. (1984). Controlled trial of endoscopic bipolar electrocoagulation in the treatment of bleeding peptic ulcers. *Gut*, **25**, A1185.

37. Kernohan, R.M., Anderson, J.R., McKelvey, S.T.D. and Kennedy, T.L. (1984). A controlled trial of bipolar electrocoagulation in patients with upper gastrointestinal bleeding. *British Journal of Surgery*, **71**, 889–91.

38. Brearly, S., Hawker, P.C., Dykes, P.W. and Keighley, M.R. (1987). Per-endoscopic bipolar diathermy coagulation of visible vessels using a 3.2 mm probe–a randomised clinical trial. *Endoscopy*, **19**, 160–3.

39. O'Brien, J.D., Day, S.J. and Burnham, W.R. (1986). Controlled trial of small bipolar probe in bleeding peptic ulcers. *Lancet*, **1**, 464–7.

40. Laine, L. (1987). Multipolar electrocoagulation in the treatment of active upper gastrointestinal tract haemorrhage. *New England Journal of Medicine*, **316**, 1613–17.

41. Laine, L. (1988). Multipolar electrocoagulation for the treatment of ulcers with non-bleeding visible vessels: a prospective, controlled trial. *Gastroenterology*, **94**, A246.

42. Fullarton, G.M., Birnie, G.O., MacDonald, A. and Murray, W.R. (1989). Controlled trial of heater probe treatment in bleeding peptic ulcers. *British Journal of Surgery*, **76**, 541–4.

43. Jensen, D.M. (1990). Heat probe for hemostasis of bleeding peptic ulcers: techniques and results of randomised controlled trials. *Gastrointestinal Endoscopy*, **36**, S42–49.

44. Avgerinos, A., Rekoumis, G., Argirakis, G., Gouma, P., Papadimitriou, N. and Karamanolis, D. (1989). Randomised comparison of endoscopic heater probe electrocoagulation, injection of adrenaline and no endoscopic therapy for bleeding peptic ulcers. *Gastroenterology*, **98**, A18.

45. Asaki, S. (1984). Endoscopic haemostasis by local absolute alcohol injection for upper gastrointestinal tract bleeding–a multicentre study. In: *Endoscopic*

Surgery (eds Okabe, H., Honda, T. and Ohshiba, S.), Elsevier, New York, pp. 105–16.

46. Pascu, O., Draghki, A. and Acalovachi, I. (1989). The effect of endoscopic haemostasis with alcohol on the mortality rate of nonvariceal upper gastrointestinal haemorrhage: a randomised prospective study. *Endoscopy*, **36**, S53–55.

47. Panes, J., Viver, J., Forne, M., Garcia-Olivares, E., Marco, C. and Garau, J. (1987). Controlled trial of endoscopic sclerosis in bleeding peptic ulcers. *Lancet*, **2**, 1292–4.

48. Balanzo, J., Sainz, S., Such, J. *et al.* (1988). Endoscopic haemostasis by local injection of epinephrine and polidocanol in bleeding ulcer. A prospective randomised trial. *Endoscopy*, **20**, 289–91.

49. Soehendra, N., Grimm, H. and Stenzel, M. (1985). Injection of nonvariceal bleeding lesions of the upper gastrointestinal tract. *Endoscopy*, **17**, 129–32.

50. Rutgeerts, P., Van Trappen, G., Broekaert, L. *et al.* (1984). A new and effective technique of Yag laser photocoagulation for severe upper gastrointestinal bleeding. *Endoscopy*, **16**, 115–17.

51. Heldwein, W., Lehnert, P., Martinoff, S. and Loeschke, K. (1988). Local epinephrine injection improves the therapeutic effect of Nd-YAG laser treatment of arterial peptic ulcer bleeding. *Endoscopy*, **20**, 2–4.

52. Chung, S.C.S., Leung, J.W.C., Steele, R.J.C., Crofts, T.J. and Li, A.K.C. (1988). Endoscopic adrenaline injection for actively bleeding ulcers: a randomised trial. *British Medical Journal*, **296**, 1631–3.

53. Chung, S.C.S., Leung, J.W.C., Leong, H.T., Lo, K.K., Griffin, S.M. and Li, A.K.C. (1990). Does adding a sclerosant improve the results of endoscopic epinephrine injection in actively bleeding ulcers? Interim report of a randomised trial. *Gastrointestinal Endoscopy*, **36**, 94.

54. Steele, R.J.C. (1989). Endoscopic haemostasis for non-variceal upper gastrointestinal haemorrhage. *British Journal of Surgery*, **76**, 219–25.

55. Johnston, J.H., Sones, J.Q., Long, B.W. and Posey, L.E. (1985). Comparison of heater probe and YAG laser in endoscopic treatment of major bleeding from peptic ulcers. *Gastrointestinal Endoscopy*, **31**, 175–80.

56. Goff, J.S. (1986). Bipolar electrocoagulation versus Nd-YAG laser photocoagulation for upper gastro-intestinal bleeding lesions. *Digestive Diseases and Sciences*, **31**, 906–10.

57. Rutgeerts, P., Van Trappen, G., Van Hootegem, P. *et al.* (1987). Neodymium-YAG laser photocoagulation versus multipolar electrocoagulation for the treatment of severely bleeding peptic ulcers: a randomised comparison. *Gastrointestinal Endoscopy*, **33**, 199–202.

58. Rutgeerts, P., Van Trappen, G., Broeckaert, L., Coremans, G., Janssens, J. and Hiele, M. (1989). Comparison of endoscopic polidocanol injection and YAG laser therapy for bleeding peptic ulcers. *Lancet*, **1**, 1164–7.

59. Loizou, L.A. and Bown, S.G. (1991). Endoscopic treatment for bleeding peptic ulcers: randomised comparison of adrenaline injection and adrenaline injection + Nd:YAG laser. *Gut*, **32**, 1100–3.

60. Hui, W.M., Ng, M.M.T., Lok, A.S.F., Lai, C.L., Lau, Y.N. and Lam, S.K. (1991). A randomised comparative study of laser photocoagulation, heater probe and bipolar electrocoagulation in the treatment of actively bleeding ulcers. *Gastrointestinal Endoscopy*, **37**, 299–304.

61. Lin, H.J., Tsai, V.T., Lee, D.S. *et al.* (1988). A prospectively randomised trial of heat probe thermocoagulation versus pure alcohol injection in non-variceal peptic ulcer haemorrhage. *American Journal of Gastroenterology*, **83**, 283–6.

62. Chung, S.C.S., Leung, J.W.C., Sung, J.Y., Lo, K.K. and Li, A.K.C. (1991). Injection or heat probe for bleeding ulcer. *Gastroenterology*, **100**, 30–37.

63. Laine, L. (1990). Multipolar electrocoagulation versus injection therapy in the treatment of bleeding peptic ulcers. *Gastroenterology*, **99**, 1303–6.

64. Waring, J.P., Sanowski, R.A., Sawyer, R.L., Woods, C.A. and Foutch, P.G. (1991). A randomised comparison of multipolar electrocoagulation and injection sclerosis for the treatment of bleeding peptic ulcer. *Gastrointestinal Endoscopy*, **37**, 295–8.

11

The acute abdomen

Simon Paterson-Brown

Introduction

In 1942 William Estes, in a paper discussing the problems related to non-penetrating abdominal trauma, mentioned the possible role of laparoscopy, but concluded that it had not been in use long enough for adequate evaluation (Estes 1942). It took many more years and a group of surgeons who were experienced in gynaecological laparoscopy before the benefits of its use as a prelaparotomy investigation for acute abdominal pain were demonstrated. Sugarbaker *et al.* (1975) showed that in 56 patients with acute abdominal pain, 6 of the 27 (22%) who went straight to laparotomy because of their clinical signs did not require an operation, whereas 18 of 29 patients in whom the need for operation was uncertain were discovered at laparoscopy not to require surgery. Since then the use of laparoscopy in the management of the acute abdomen has not only gained in popularity, but has also diversified and can now be divided into three main areas: diagnosis of acute (non-traumatic) abdominal pain; evaluation of abdominal trauma; and therapeutic use (such as laparoscopic appendicectomy).

Diagnostic laparoscopy in the acute abdomen

The case for laparoscopy in diagnostic decision making in the acute abdomen has been strongly supported by a number of studies which have usually considered specific problems such as acute right iliac fossa or pelvic pain (Anteby *et al.* 1975; Leape and Ramenofsky 1980; Anderson and Bridgewater 1981; Deutsch *et al.* 1982; Clarke *et al.* 1986). There is good evidence that selective laparoscopy in patients with acute abdominal pain, and in whom the need for operation is uncertain, alters surgical decision making and significantly improves patient management (Paterson-Brown *et al.* 1989). Patients with suspected appendicitis are particularly suitable for laparoscopy and there is now strong support for the view that all women with suspected appendicitis should undergo laparoscopy because of the high potential diagnostic error rate in this group (Paterson-Brown *et al.* 1988; Spirtos *et al.* 1987). Even when the appendix cannot be seen adequately, signs of right iliac fossa inflammation will usually indicate the presence of underlying acute appendicitis or alternatively another cause may be found at laparoscopy for the patient's symptoms. Acute gynaecological conditions will be recognized which do not require surgery and an early diagnosis of pelvic inflammatory disease can be made. This is important if early treatment is to prevent recurrent episodes with potentially serious sequelae (Pearce 1990). In addition the Curtis–Fitz-Hugh syndrome may be recognized. This syndrome was first reported in the early 1930s (Curtis 1930; Fitz-Hugh 1934) and described as gonococcal salpingitis which tracts up the right paracolic gutter to produce 'perihapatitis' which can be recognized by filmy adhesions running between the upper surface of the liver and the diaphragm. Chlamydia trachomatis has now been shown to produce the same syndrome (Muller-Schoop *et al.* 1978) and patients may present with signs and symptoms suggestive of acute biliary disease (Wood *et al.* 1982). Other conditions may also be mimicked by the Curtis–Fitz-Hugh syndrome (Gatt *et al.* 1986) and reflect the possible widespread nature of the transperitoneal spread of infection. The diagnosis is readily made at laparoscopy and the condition is treated by the appropriate antibiotic (Gatt *et al.* 1986). The difficulty of establishing a diagnosis of pelvic inflammatory disease in general strongly supports the case for laparoscopy in all women in whom it is suspected (Pearce 1990) as it not only confirms the diagnosis but also allows bacteriological samples to be taken so that the correct antibiotic may be prescribed.

More recently laparoscopy has been used in the acute abdomen specifically to investigate suspected intestinal ischaemia following aortic reconstruction and may be performed at the bedside (Iberti *et al.* 1989). In patients with abdominal pain of unknown origin who are ill from other non-related medical conditions such as cardiorespiratory failure, haematological disorders and renal failure, a negative laparotomy or an incorrect decision to observe may have serious and far-reaching consequences. Although there are alternative techniques to help the surgeon decide whether to operate or not (including ultrasonography (Davies *et al.* 1991) and peritoneal cytology (Vipond *et al.* 1990)), it is laparoscopy which provides the surgeon with the last chance to avoid an innappropriate surgical decision.

Laparoscopy for abdominal trauma

Laparoscopy has also been used to assess intra-abdominal injury in patients with blunt abdominal trauma (Gazzaniga *et al.* 1976; Sherwood *et al.* 1980; Berci *et al.* 1983). In a randomized, controlled multicentre comparison of peritoneal lavage and minilaparoscopy under local anaesthesia identification of those patients with minor injuries which did not require laparotomy was easier in the group undergoing laparoscopy where only 1 in 13 unnecessary

laparotomies were performed compared to 3 in 11 in the group undergoing peritoneal lavage, although this difference was not significant (Cuschieri *et al.* 1988). In this study the sensitivity of both techniques was 100% but laparoscopy had a specificity of 94% compared to 83% for lavage. Traumatic diaphragmatic hernia, often a difficult condition to diagnose using standard investigations, can be confirmed by laparoscopy (Adamthwaite 1984). In 10 such cases where herniation was suspected following CT scan or barium meal in addition to routine chest radiographs, laparoscopy revealed a ruptured diaphragm with herniation in 6 patients, without herniation in 2 and no abnormality in 2. These last 2 patients were spared an unnecessary laparotomy.

Therapeutic laparoscopy in the acute abdomen

Recent developments in laparoscopic surgery whereby laparoscopic appendicectomy (Leahy 1989) and closure of perforated peptic ulcers (Mouret *et al.* 1990) are possible, introduces a new dimension to the overall role of laparoscopy in the acute abdomen. However, the logistics of emergency laparoscopic surgery are much more complicated than for simple diagnostic laparoscopy as, not only does the video monitoring and surgical equipment have to be available at night in the emergency theatre, but the nursing staff must also be familiar with the different techniques and procedures required. These problems are likely to be overcome rapidly as more units start performing elective laparoscopic surgery and thereby train the appropriate staff in the techniques and instrumentation required.

Laparoscopic appendicectomy

Although removal of the appendix using laparoscopic techniques is not new (Semm 1986) there remains little evidence that the recovery period following laparoscopic appendicectomy for acute appendicitis is significantly shorter than following the open procedure. What would appear to be true so far, and evidence remains largely anecdotal, is that in the majority of cases the inflamed appendix is easier to find by laparoscopy, particularly when it lies in an awkward

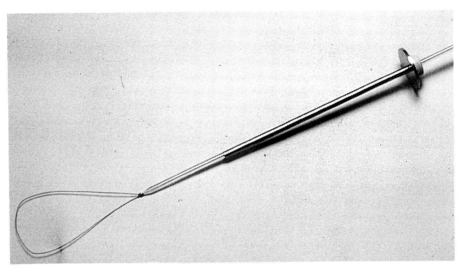

Fig. 11.1 The Endoloop (Ethicon Ltd, UK) which has been passed through a reducing sleeve, which in turn is placed down a 5 mm port. The Endoloop consists of a catgut loop using a pretied Roeder knot complete with introducer which pushes down the knot to close the loop.

position and access through a standard appendicectomy incision is limited. When laparoscopy is performed the ports can be inserted into the most appropriate positions for best access. A technique whereby diagnostic laparoscopy is performed, acute appendicitis confirmed and a small incision directed over the appendix to allow appendicectomy (Fleming 1985) is a compromise which is gaining in popularity (Byrne *et al.* 1992). A comparison between the three methods (standard appendicectomy, laparoscopically guided appendicectomy and laparoscopic appendicectomy) would be timely. In performing laparoscopic appendicectomy ligation of the appendix stump is greatly facilitated by the use of Endoloops (Ethicon Ltd, UK – Figure 11.1) although the ability to tie knots within the peritoneal cavity or by using the Roeder technique is important. Reports are now emerging of large series of laparoscopic appendicectomies with excellent results (Pier *et al.* 1991) and two recent studies comparing standard open appendicectomy with the laparoscopic procedure have both confirmed the advantages of the laparoscopic procedure (McAnena *et al.* 1992; Attwood *et al.* 1992).

Laparoscopic closure of perforated peptic ulcers

A recent study from Hong Kong has demonstrated that a non-operative approach to perforated peptic ulcers can be successful in up to 70% of patients (Crofts *et al.* 1989), with potential non-responders being identified on the basis of a water-soluble contrast meal. The majority of complications in this study were associated with sepsis demonstrating the importance of peritoneal irrigation, which can be performed effectively by laparoscopy without resorting to laparotomy. Whether the surgeon chooses to close the perforation and plug the defect with omentum using suture–and specially designed 'ski' needles are available (Figure 11.2)–clip or tissue glue (Mouret *et al.* 1990) will depend on individual preferences, but a pre-operative contrast meal should be performed as this will help to identify those patients in whom only a peritoneal toilet is required. The same treatment can be used to treat gastric perforations or alternatively the perforation may be converted into a gastrostomy at laparoscopy (Mouret *et al.* 1990).

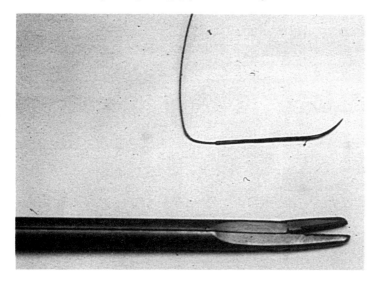

Fig. 11.2   The 'ski' needle and laparoscopic needle holder (both from Ethicon Ltd, UK). The curve of the needle tip is specially designed to allow it to be passed down a 5 mm port.

Laparoscopy and acute cholecystitis

Over the past decade or so early cholecystectomy for acute cholecystitis has become established (McArthur *et al.* 1975; Fowkes and Gunn 1980; Addison and Finan 1988) even in the elderly (van Rensburg 1984; Edlund and Ljungdahl 1990). In patients with acute acalculous cholecystitis, particularly following trauma, sepsis and critically illness, early diagnosis and surgery is essential (Johnson 1987). However, the diagnosis of acute acalculous cholecystitis may not be easy to establish by current techniques (Shuman *et al.* 1984) and it is in these patients that early laparoscopy may be helpful. Even if laparoscopic cholecystectomy cannot be performed due to the severity of the inflammation, external drainage of the gallbladder can be achieved by cholecystostomy (Perissat *et al.* 1990), which may be used as an initial life-saving procedure in the treatment of critically ill patients (Winkler *et al.* 1989).

Laparoscopic cholecystectomy for acute cholecystitis is gaining in popularity as surgeons become more experienced in cholecystectomy for chronic cholecystitis and recurrent biliary colic. However, the surrounding inflammation may make dissection more difficult and the conversion rate to 'open' cholecystectomy has been reported to be as high as 1 in 3 in some series (Flowers *et al.* 1991). Both operating time and hospital stay are also prolonged (Domergue *et al.* 1991) and even though decompression of the acutely inflamed gallbladder is usually required before it can be grasped for retraction, very thick-walled and oedematous gallbladders may still be difficult to grasp with standard instruments. There is little doubt that elective laparoscopic cholecystectomy following a previous attack of acute cholecystitis may be a formidable undertaking, and when this is considered alongside the other advantages of early cholecystectomy, there is no reason to suppose that early laparoscopic cholecystectomy for acute cholecystitis will not soon become standard practice in most units.

The way ahead

The field of laparoscopic surgery for the acute abdomen remains uncharted, but as surgeons and theatre staff become familiar with the techniques possible during elective laparoscopic surgery, the range of emergency procedures will increase. In the first instance the use of diagnostic laparoscopy in the acute abdomen should be encouraged; not only will it improve surgical decision making and overall management (particularly in the young

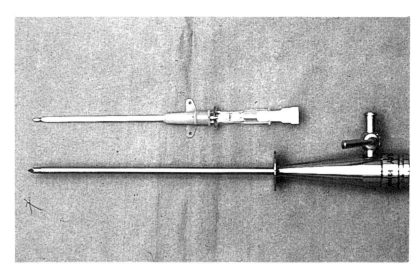

Fig. 11.3   A 2.7 mm diameter 'minilaparoscope' (Thackray Bros, UK) which is demonstrated here alongside a 14G venous cannula.

female) but it will also allow the surgeon to perform the surgery required through smaller and more accurately placed incisions. This does not just apply to acute appendicitis, but also to gynaecological conditions such as bleeding ovarian cysts and ectopic pregnancies, as well as acute diverticulitis, ischaemic bowel and band adhesions. If necessary diagnosis could be made by minilaparoscopy (Figure 11.3) under local anaesthesia with those patients who require further surgery proceeding to general anaesthesia.

As in elective abdominal surgery, the encroachment of laparoscopic procedures into the emergency arena will reduce still further the training opportunities for young surgeons who must now learn their open surgical skills hand-in-hand with those required for laparoscopic techniques. However, the advantages of a more widespread use of laparoscopy and laparoscopic surgery to the patient with acute abdominal pain, namely early diagnosis combined with minimally invasive surgery, must not be ignored.

References

Adamthwaite, D.N. (1984) Traumatic diaphragmatic hernia: a new indication for laparoscopy. *British Journal of Surgery*, **71**, 315.

Addison, N.V. and Finan, P.J. (1988). Urgent and early cholecystectomy for acute gall bladder disease. *British Journal of Surgery*, **75**, 141–3.

Anderson, J.L. and Bridgewater, F.H.G. (1981). Laparoscopy in the diagnosis of acute lower abdominal pain. *Australian and New Zealand Journal of Surgery*, **51**, 462–4.

Anteby, S.O., Schenker, J.G. and Polishuk, W.Z. (1975). The value of laparoscopy in acute pelvic pain. *Annals of Surgery*, **181**, 484–6.

Attwood, S.E.A., Hill, A.D.K., Murphy, P.G., Thornton, J. and Stephens, R.B. (1992). A prospective randomized trial of laparoscopic versus open appendectomy. *Surgery*, **112**, 487–501.

Berci, G., Dunkelman, D., Michel, S.L., Sanders, G., Wahlstrom, E. and Morgenstern, L. (1983). Emergency minilaparoscopy in abdominal trauma. *American Journal of Surgery*, **146**, 261–5.

Byrne, D.S., Bell, G., Morrice, J.J. and Orr, G. (1992). Technique for laparoscopic appendicectomy. *British Journal of Surgery*, **79**, 574–5.

Clarke, P.J., Hands, L.J., Gough, M.H. and Kettlewell, M.G. (1986). The use of laparoscopy in the management of right iliac fossa pain. *Annals of the Royal College of Surgeons of England*, **68**, 68–9.

Crofts, T.J., Park, K.G.M., Steele, R.J.C., Chung, S.S.C. and Li, A.K.C. (1989). A randomized trial of nonoperative treatment for perforated peptic ulcer. *New England Journal of Medicine*, **320**, 970–3.

Curtis, A.H. (1930). Cause of adhesions in right upper quadrant. *Journal of the American Medical Association*, **94**, 1221–2.

Cuschieri, A., Hennessy, T.P.J., Stephens, R. and Berci, G. (1988). Diagnosis of significant abdominal trauma after road traffic accidents: preliminary results of a multicentre trial comparing minilaparoscopy with peritoneal lavage. *Annals of the Royal College of Surgeons of England*, **70**, 153–5.

Davies, A.H., Mastorakou, I., Cobb, R., Rogers, C., Lindsell, D. and Mortensen, N.J.Mc. (1991). Ultrasonography in the acute abdomen. *British Journal of Surgery*, **78**, 1178–80.

Deutsch, A.A., Zelikovsky, A. and Reiss, R. (1982). Laparoscopy in the prevention of unnecessary appendicectomies: a prospective study. *British Journal of Surgery*, **69**, 336–7.

Domergue, J., Fabre, J.M., Guillon, F., Deseguin, C.H., Lepage, B., Zaragoza, C. and Baumel, H. (1991). Laparoscopic cholecystectomy in acute and non-acute cholecystolithiasis. *Research in Surgery*, **3**, 147–9.

Edlund, G. and Ljungdahl, M. (1990). Acute cholecystitis in the elderly. *American Journal of Surgery*, **159**, 414–16.

Estes, W.L. (1942). Nonpenetrating trauma of the abdomen. *Surgery, Gynecology and Obstetrics*, **74**, 419–24.

Fitz-Hugh, T.Jr. (1934). Acute gonococcic peritonitis of right upper quadrant in women. *Journal of the American Medical Association*, **102**, 2094–6.

Fleming, J.S. (1985). Laparoscopically directed appendicectomy. *Australian and New Zealand Journal of Obstetrics and Gynaecology*, **25**, 238–40.

Flowers, J.L., Bailey, R.W., Scovill, W.A. and Zucker, K.A. (1991). The Baltimore experience with laparoscopic management of acute cholecystitis. *American Journal of Surgery*, **161**, 388–92.

Fowkes, F.G.R. and Gunn, A.A. (1980). The management of acute cholecystitis and its hospital cost. *British Journal of Surgery*, **67**, 613–17.

Gatt, D., Heafield, T. and Jantet, G. (1986). Curtis Fitz-Hugh syndrome: the new mimicking disease? *Annals of the Royal College of Surgeons of England*, **68**, 271–4.

Gazzaniga, A.B., Stanton, W.W. and Bartlett, R.H. (1976). Laparoscopy in the diagnosis of blunt and penetrating injuries to the abdomen. *American Journal of Surgery*, **131**, 315–23.

Iberti, T.J., Salky, B.A. and Onofrey, D. (1989). Use of bedside laparoscopy to identify intestinal ischaemia in postoperative cases of aortic reconstruction. *Surgery*, **105**, 686–9.

Johnson, L.B. (1987). The importance of early diagnosis of acute acalculus cholecystitis. *Surgery, Gynecology and Obstetrics*, **164**, 197–203.

Leahy, P.F. (1989). Technique of laparoscopic appendicectomy. *British Journal of Surgery*, **76**, 616.

Leape, L.L. and Ramenofsky, M.L. (1980). Laparoscopy for questionable appendicitis–can it reduce the negative appendectomy rate? *Annals of Surgery*, **191**, 410–13.

McAnena, O.J., Austin, O., O'Connell, P.R., Hederman, W.P., Gorey, T.F. and Fitzpatrick, J. (1992). Laparoscopic versus open appendicectomy: a prospective evaluation. *British Journal of Surgery*, **79**, 818–20.

McArthur, P., Cuschieri, A., Sells, R.A. and Shields, R. (1975). Controlled clinical trial comparing early with interval cholecystectomy for acute cholecystitis. *British Journal of Surgery*, **62**, 850–2.

Mouret, P., Francois, Y., Vignal, J., Barth, X. and Lombard-Platet, R. (1990). Laparoscopic treatment of perforated peptic ulcer. *British Journal of Surgery*, **77**, 1006.

Muller-Schoop, J.W., Wang, S.P., Munzinger, J., Schlapfer, H.U., Knoblauch, M. and Ammann, R.W. (1978). Chlamydia trachomatis as a possible cause of peritonitis and perihepatitis in young women. *British Medical Journal*, **1**, 1022–4.

Paterson-Brown, S., Thompson, J.N., Eckersley, J.R.T., Ponting, G.A. and Dudley, H.A.F. (1988). Which patients with suspected appendicitis should undergo laparoscopy? *British Medical Journal*, **296**, 1363–4.

Paterson-Brown, S., Vipond, M.N., Simms, K., Gatzen, C., Thompson, J.N. and Dudley, H.A.F. (1989). Clinical decision-making and laparoscopy versus computer prediction in the management of the acute abdomen. *British Journal of Surgery*, **76**, 1011–13.

Pearce, J.M. (1990). Pelvic inflammatory disease. *British Medical Journal*, **300**, 1090–1.

Perissat, J., Collet, D. and Belliard, R. (1990). Gallstones: laparoscopic treatment–cholecystectomy, cholecystostomy and lithotripsy. *Surgical Endoscopy*, **4**, 1–5.

Pier, A., Gotz, F. and Bacher, C. (1991). Laparoscopic appendectomy in 625 cases: from innovation to routine. *Surgical Laparoscopy and Endoscopy*, **1**, 8–13.

Semm, K. (1986). Operative pelviscopy. *British Medical Bulletin*, **42**, 284–9.

Sherwood, R., Berci, G., Austin, E. and Morgenstern, L. (1980). Minilaparoscopy for blunt abdominal trauma. *Archives of Surgery*, **115**, 672–3.

Shuman, W.P., Rogers, J.V., Rudd, T.G., Mack, L.A., Plumley, T. and Larson, E.B. (1984). Low sensitivity of sonography and cholescintigraphy in acalculous cholecystitis. *American Journal of Roentgenology*, **142**, 531–4.

Spirtos, N.M., Eisenkop, S.M., Spirtos, T.W., Poliakin, R.I. and Hibbard, L.T. (1987). Laparoscopy–a diagnostic aid in cases of suspected appendicitis. Its use in women of reproductive age. *American Journal of Obstetrics and Gynecology*, **156**, 90–4.

Sugarbaker, P.H., Bloom, B.S., Sanders, J.H. and Wilson, R.E. (1975). Preoperative laparoscopy in diagnosis of acute abdominal pain. *Lancet*, **i**, 442–4.

van Rensburg, L.C.J. (1984). The management of acute cholecystitis in the elderly. *British Journal of Surgery*, **71**, 692–3.

Vipond, M.N., Paterson-Brown, S., Tyrrell, M.R. *et al.* (1990). Evaluation of fine catheter aspiration cytology as an adjunct to decision making in the acute abdomen. *British Journal of Surgery*, **77**, 86–7.

Winkler, E., Kaplan, O., Gutman, M., Skornick, Y. and Rozin, R.R. (1989). Role of cholecystostomy in the management of critically ill patients suffering from acute cholecystitis. *British Journal of Surgery*, **76**, 693–5.

Wood, J.J., Bolton, J.P. and Cannon, S.R. (1982). Biliary-type pain as a manifestation of genital tract infection: the Curtis–Fitz-Hugh syndrome. *British Journal of Surgery*, **69**, 251–3.

12

Abdominal adhesions

Mohan C. Airan and Sung-Tao Ko

Indications and contraindications for abdominal adhesiolysis

One of the most perplexing problems that the general surgeon has faced in the last century is the understanding of formation of intra-abdominal adhesions. Hertzler[1] in 1919, stated that to prevent adhesions one would necessarily have to prevent healing. Because adhesions do form after intra-abdominal surgery, the general surgeon, the infertility specialist, and the gynaecologist are all concerned with the prevention and treatment of intra-abdominal adhesions. Each may be required to divide into peritoneal adhesions.

The indications for adhesiolysis in the abdomen are as follows:

1. Adhesions causing intermittent small bowel obstruction.
2. Adhesions interfering with the performance of a chosen intra-abdominal procedure.
3. Chronic intractable abdominal pain, thought to arise from adhesions.
4. Intractable pelvic pain and dyspareunia.
5. Infertility due to tubal and fimbrial adhesions.[2]
6. Solitary bands in the abdomen, secondary to previous abdominal surgery.

There are some absolute contraindications to abdominal adhesiolysis. These are:

1. Bleeding diathesis.
2. Lack of consent for performing an open adhesiolysis.
3. Previous Noble's plication.

Basic considerations

The goals of intra-abdominal adhesiolysis vary with the indications. If a patient is being operated on for infertility due to past appendicectomy adhesions, the goal would be merely to free the fimbriated ends of the tubes and straighten the fallopian tubes. The rest of the intra-abdominal adhesions would be inconsequential. However, if the patient had, for example, concomitant pelvic pain or dyspareunia then a total pelvic adhesiolysis should be carried out.

Similarly, during a laparoscopic cholecystectomy on a patient with asymptomatic adhesions, adhesiolysis is not indicated unless they prevent access. Adhesions in the upper abdomen due to previous upper abdominal surgery frequently justify an adhesiolysis in order to allow the safe entry of the visualizing umbilical port into the abdomen. If adhesions are suspected around the umbilical area then an alternate site entry would be appropriate to facilitate introduction of pneumoperitoneum and an adhesiolysis carried out in the umbilical area to free the umbilical port area only.

Anatomical considerations (Figures 12.1 and 12.2)

When choosing an alternate site, we prefer to avoid the previous incision site and try to use the lower border of the costal margin. In a supine position, the costal arch always tents the abdominal wall up. The rectus muscle sags downwards from this point in almost all the

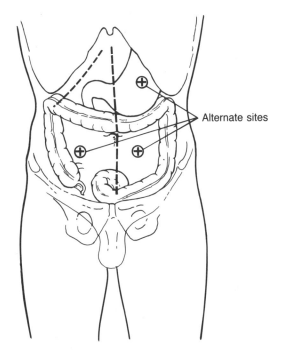

Fig. 12.1. Choice of alternate sites.

patients except the extremely obese, or patients with very protrudent abdomens. We use this anatomic arch to place a standard Veress needle next to the lowest rib in the midclavicular line and advance it with an open

stopcock. The patient is positioned with the head of the table slightly elevated. The three fascial planes, namely, the anterior rectus sheath, the posterior rectus sheath and the peritoneum, are usually palpable in the course of insertion of the needle into the peritoneal cavity. The negative pressure in the peritoneal cavity usually results in an audible hiss of air entering the peritoneum through the Veress needle. This air then forms a small cushion to facilitate further advancement of the needle.

Physiology

Adhesions are usually formed after trauma to the serosal surfaces of the viscera. After injury, peritoneal exudates from the injured site seal the area of injury. These contain fibrin, neutrophils and macrophages. Fibroblasts and primitive mesenchymal cells are drawn to the site of chemotaxis. The new cells are derived from the underlying mesenchyme, as well as from the periphery of the injury. Because the healing occurs from all sides of the injury, the size of the injury is immaterial, and healing takes place in 7 to 8 days irrespective of the size of the injury.[3]

Tissue reorganization begins in 3 days, with invasion of fibroblasts and capillaries. Adhesions are firmly established in 3 weeks. By the time serosal repair has occurred, adhesion formation is firmly established. This

Fig. 12.2. Anatomy.

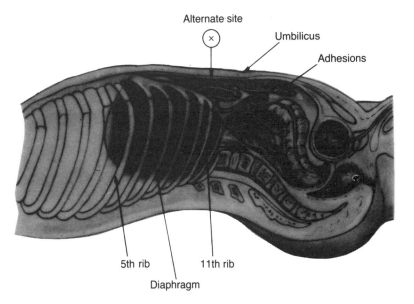

is the basis for recommending that second-look laparoscopy should take place around the eighth post-operative day. This allows filmy adhesions to be broken up prior to the formation of firm collagen.

Positioning of the patient

To prevent pulmonary embolism, the patient should have antiembolic stockings covered with pneumatic compression devices placed on the lower limbs prior to the induction of anaesthesia.[4] If the operation is to be carried out in the upper abdomen the operating table is tilted with the head up position and vice versa for the lower abdominal operation. If the adhesiolysis is to be carried out in the right side of the abdomen the table should be tilted towards the left and vice versa. This allows the underlying viscera to shift out of the way of dissection.

Operative considerations in initial pneumoperitoneum

Placement of Veress needle

The location of scars in the abdomen determines the placement of the Veress needle. Generally speaking, one must go as far away as possible from the previous abdominal incision sites.

The most frequently used alternative entry site is usually just below the costal arch in either midclavicular line. The left side is preferred to the right (Figure 12.1). The reason for this choice is explained above. Where the alternative entry site is in the lower abdomen it is important to avoid the line of the inferior epigastric arteries.

Initial insufflation

The following steps are to be followed when establishing the pneumoperitoneum in a patient with adhesions.

1. Stabilize the skin at the point of entry of the Veress needle (for example, by using sharp towel clips).

2. Use a No. 11 sharp point blade to make a stab incision at the chosen point of entry.

3. Insert the Veress needle–feel the three layers during insertion and, if possible, listen for the hiss of air as it enters the peritoneal cavity.

4. Attach a 5 ml syringe containing 2 ml saline and aspirate.

5. Inject slowly and reaspirate. If blood or bile-stained fluid returns into the syringe then withdraw the needle immediately.

6. Flush the Veress needle and re-enter at a different alternative site. To check that the Veress needle is in the peritoneal cavity, connect to the insufflator and start the flow of CO_2 at 1.2–1.5 litres per minute. Check the intra-abdominal pressure after the first cycle of CO_2 gas. This should usually register between 5 and 7 mmHg on Storz and Wisap machines, and slightly higher on the Wolf machine.

7. The needle should be slightly rotated around its fulcrum to see whether it feels free, and during this movement the intra-abdominal pressure should drop or stay the same.

8. If the intra-abdominal pressure is consistently higher than 9 mmHg then it should be withdrawn and another attempt made at a different site.

9. During the insufflation of CO_2 gas into the abdominal cavity, the relationship between the depth of the Veress needle and the skin should remain constant. In other words, the Veress needle should not be left unattended.

10. As soon as the optical port is introduced into the abdomen, the structures underlying the previous Veress needle entry points, if present, should be thoroughly investigated.

Palmer tests[5]

Once the initial pneumoperitoneum is established a size 21 spinal needle attached to a 5 ml syringe containing 2 ml saline is introduced into the abdomen at the point where a 5 mm trocar cannula is to be placed (Figure 12.3). As soon as the needle enters the peritoneal cavity aspiration yields small air bubbles. The needle can be reintroduced at different angles to determine whether there are adhesions present underneath the peritoneum. Failure to aspirate air readily is a sure indication of underlying adhesions.

Placement of initial 5 mm exploratory trocar cannula

A 5 mm (disposable preferred) trocar cannula is then placed into the abdomen at the Palmer

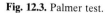

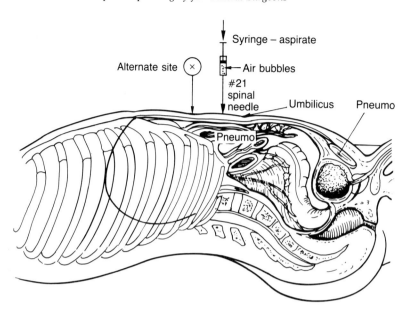

Fig. 12.3. Palmer test.

test site. A 5 mm telescope is then introduced and a quick inspection of the underlying peritoneal cavity is carried out. Special attention should be paid to the site of Veress needle entry point. Where multiple attempts have been made to enter the abdominal cavity, the underlying structures at those entry points are carefully checked. An assessment of the amount of adhesiolysis required to achieve the goals of the operation is now made. At this stage careful consideration to the sites of the other visualizing and operating ports must be made.

Principles of placement of operative ports and monitors

Once the initial pneumoperitoneum has been established and a survey of the intra-abdominal adhesions carried out a detailed plan of the operation of adhesiolysis is formulated. To plan this the following principles should be followed.

Ports

Site of visualizing port (Figure 12.4)

This should almost always be at right angles to the site of dissection. This port should also be as far away as possible from the dissection site.

Site of operating ports (Figure 12.4)

These ports should be located as laterally as possible and should be ideally at a 45° angle to the work to be performed.

Size of operating ports (Figure 12.4)

If electrosurgery is the primary energy source, then conductive cannulae should be used especially if 5 mm ports are used. Five millimetre ports have a narrower dielectric (air) space resulting in a higher capacitance charge build-up. For this reason a 10 mm port is safer in this respect than a 5 mm port.

The choice of port size is in part determined by whether a stapler is to be used. In this case a 10 mm or 12 mm port is required.

We prefer 10 mm operating lateral ports, if extensive adhesiolysis is to be carried out. There are three reasons for this. The first and foremost reason is that the electrical safety is enhanced when a larger dielectric space is available in the 10 mm cannula. The second reason is the ability to change the optical ports at will. This gives the ability to see around adhesions. We prefer a 30° telescope for this purpose. The third and final reason is the

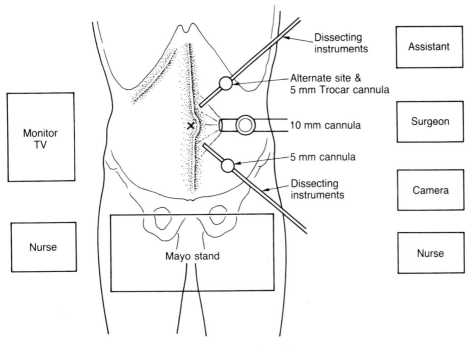

Fig. 12.4. Principles of placement of operative ports and monitors.

ability to use stapling devices through any of the ports.

Video monitors (Figure 12.4)

The video monitors should be placed directly in front of the operating surgeon to reduce operating fatigue. If the monitor cannot be located directly in front it should be in a 20–30° range in front of the operator. The dissection site should be between the monitor and the operator.

If the monitor is placed behind the work area the problem of mirror image resolution is created. For the same reason the assistant should stand on the same side as the surgeon during adhesiolysis. However, for dissection in the lower abdomen (pelvic lymph node dissection, hernia, etc.), a single large monitor at the foot of the table with the surgeon and assistant standing on either side of the operating table is satisfactory. The same applies to work in the upper abdomen (e.g. vagotomy, hiatus hernia repair). In this case a single large monitor may be placed at the head end of the table. This usually results in problems for the anaesthesiologists and, therefore, we prefer two smaller monitors at the upper end of the table on either side of the anaesthesiologist.

If the work to be performed is mainly in the right side of the abdomen, the monitor should be on the right side of the patient and vice versa. Centrally located adhesions due to midline scars can be managed from either side, but in this case the surgeon, assistant and camera operator should be on the same side of the operating table.

Principles of safe use of electrosurgical techniques

It is extremely important that during adhesiolysis the current output of the generator should never exceed 30 watts. The total energy delivered to the tissues depends on the pedal depressing time or the pencil key in-time. The activation time in the pencil key or the foot-pedal should never exceed a tap, measuring a second or less. Very rarely, a current may be turned on for several seconds. If a vascular bundle in an adhesion requires more than 2 to 3 seconds of current application, then use of a staple or an Endoloop should be considered instead. If a vascular pedicle needs to be ligated in continuity, then an extracorporeal knot may be used to ligate and divide the vascular bundle. The audible tone which sounds when current is switched on should be clearly audible and mechanism should always be in the 'on' position.

The grounding (earthing) pad should always be of the return electrode monitoring (REM) type such pads have eliminated pad site burns.

The use of a larger 10 mm port in relation to the capacitative charge that a radio frequency current generates around an insulated current conduit has been discussed above. When this conduit is placed in another hollow tubular structure, a charge is built up on the surface of the tubular structure. When monopolar electro-surgery is used this current will discharge into adjacent tissues. Therefore, the cannulae should be conductive in nature. This enables the electrons to be discharged into the ground (earth) return pad through the abdominal wall.

Every effort should be made to limit the use of irrigating fluid and it should always be aspirated prior to the use of electrical energy. Saline and Ringer-lactate solution are electrolytic fluids and conduct electricity with little resistance compared to tissues. They may thus cause alternate site burns.

As long as the pedal/pencil activation time is restricted to 1–2 seconds and the generator wattage set between 25 and 30 watts, damage to underlying structures can be avoided. When wire electrodes are used to electrocoagulate a structure, care must be taken to cool the tip prior to the second application. Thin wire electrodes can perforate intestinal structure (even when the electrical generator is off) if the tip is hot. It is safest to assume that the tip is always hot.

Bipolar forceps may be used safely on larger vascular structures and their use is recommended for electrocoagulation of larger vessels.

Monopolar scissors can be used to coagulate and cut but the mechanical cutting action of the scissors dulls very soon with repeated use. Disposable scissors are an alternative.

Techniques of adhesiolysis

There are three basic techniques of adhesiolysis.

Wire loop dissection

Wire 'J' and 'L'-shaped loops are satisfactory for lysis of adhesions at the junction of the parietal peritoneum with the underlying viscera. Using back and forth movements the tissues to be lysed are either gently brushed (to divide tissues under tension) or coagulated when tissues are hugged by bowel loops. To effect a cut the tissues have to be distracted and put under tension. It is worth bearing in mind that the smaller the surface area of electrode contact, the greater the current density. Conversely, the greater the contact surface area of the electrode, the smaller the current density. The higher the current density the greater the chance of a clean cut. It is recommended that only coagulating current set between 25–30 watts should be used. To achieve higher current density thinner wire electrodes should be used. The shape of the electrode is a matter of individual preference.

Scissors dissection

Electrified scissors are the preferred instrument for mechanical dissection. The tip of these scissors when closed can be used to cut with electrical energy using the principle of high current density. Coagulation can be achieved with a larger contact area using the back surface of the scissors' blades. The back surface of the scissors blades can also be used to divide the tissues by coagulating under tension. Generally, the scissors are a more satisfactory instrument for adhesiolysis.

Blunt dissection

Blunt dissection is used mainly in laparoscopic cholecystectomy and is less favoured for adhesiolysis. In this technique, fine grasping forceps are used to tear adhesions off the gallbladder. The grasper is electrified for coagulation. This type is probably more dangerous because the tip of the grasper becomes hot and when tissues are pulled towards the duodenum possible thermal or electrical burns can result. It is suspected that this may be one of the mechanisms of reported duodenal perforations.

Prevention of reformation of adhesions

Anthony Luciano[6] in 1989, demonstrated that in the murine experimental model, laparotomy but not laparoscopy, results in formation of *de novo* adhesions. He further concluded that laser laparoscopic adhesiolysis was effective in reducing intraperitoneal adhesions. However, his study did not compare electrosurgery versus laser in a similar setting. Furthermore, the same author 2 years earlier had published a paper stating that there was no significant difference between electrosurgery and laser when comparing thermal injury rates. Filmar[7], in 1986, demonstrated that both lasers and electrosurgery were equally effective in adhesiolysis. It is the impression of the authors that either energy source can be used for adhesiolysis without significant reformation of adhesions. We believe, however, that laparoscopic adhesiolysis would probably be more effective in preventing reformation than open adhesiolysis.

A wide variety of agents used intraperitoneally have not significantly affected reformation of adhesions. These include corticosteroids, antibiotics, antihistamines, Hyskon (32% dextran, 70 in dextrose). Jansen[8] has shown that a properly timed 'second-look' operation, timed for 8–10 days after surgery, would reduce formation of adhesions. This, of course, requires a second look. The filmy adhesions encountered at the time of the second operation are broken down bluntly. It is claimed by these fertility specialists that this reduces reformation of adhesions but the authors have no experience with this technique.

Authors' experience

The authors have performed 400 consecutive laparoscopic procedures (Table 12.1). The majority of these patients had laparoscopic cholecystectomy. Sixty-five patients had intra-abdominal adhesions, secondary to previous abdominal surgery (Table 12.2). Forty-two patients had intra-abdominal adhesions but no history of previous surgery (Table 12.3). In 9 patients laparoscopic adhesiolysis was performed for relief of symptoms thought to be caused by adhesions (Table 12.4). In the remainder adhesiolysis was performed to gain access to the chosen operative site.

Table 12.1. 400 laparoscopic procedures–incidence of adhesions (107 patients)

Adhesions–previous abdominal surgery	65
Adhesions–no previous surgery	42

Table 12.2. Adhesions due to previous abdominal surgery (65 patients)

Gastric, colon, small bowel operation	9
Post-appendectomy	17
Post-pelvic surgery (C section, hysterectomy, ovarian surgery)	34
Post-inguinal and ventral hernia repair	5

Table 12.3. Adhesions–no previous abdominal surgery (42 patients)

Acute and chronic gallbladder inflammation (omentum, colon, duodenum)	37
Previous pelvic inflammatory disease (adhesions to liver, diaphragm, gallbladder)	5

Table 12.4. Laparoscopic adhesiolysis for relief of symptoms (9 patients)

1. Post-appendicectomy pain	1
2. Small bowel obstruction (recurrent)	3
3. Pelvic pain	3
4. Endometriosis	2

All of the patients were relieved of symptoms excepting one patient who had Noble's plication. This patient returned in 2 months with recurrent small bowel obstruction and required an open operation. We feel that patients with Noble's plication are not candidates for laparoscopic surgery at present. We have had no complications related to the lysis of adhesions.

Conclusions

1. Monitors and trocar cannulae should be placed in such a way that they allow the operation to proceed rapidly.

2. Electrosurgical generators should be set in the range of 25–30 watts of coagulation.

3. Both cutting and coagulation can be effectively achieved by varying the current density at the point of contact during adhesiolysis.

4. Lasers or electrosurgery are equally effective in adhesiolysis.

5. Sharp dissection preferably with scissors is the preferred method during lysis of adhesions.

6. Minimal serosal trauma should be the goal of the laparoscopist.

7. Laparoscopic adhesiolysis is the preferred method of adhesiolysis in the previously operated abdomen.

8. Goals for adhesiolysis should be set prior to embarking on the operation.

References

1. Hertzler, A.E. (1919). *The Peritoneum.* Mosby, St Louis.

2. Stockel, W. (1947). *Lethrbuch der Gynakologie* (11th edition). Herzel, Leipzig.

3. Raferty, A.T. (1973). Regeneration of parietal and visceral peritoneum. A light microscopial study. *British Journal of Surgery*, **60**, 293–9.

4. Ko, S.T. and Airan, M.C. (1994). Review of 300 consecutive laparoscopic cholecystectomies: development, evolution and results. *Surgical Endoscopy*, in press.

5. Palmer, R. (1948). LaCeolioscopie. *Brux.-med*, **28**, 305.

6. Luciano, A.A., Maier, D.B., Koch, E.I. *et al.* (1989). A comparative study of postoperative adhesions following laser surgery by laparoscopy versus laparotomy in the rabbit model. *Obstetrics and Gynecology*, **74**(2), 220–4.

7. Filmar, S., Gomel, V. and McComb, P. (1986). The effectiveness of CO_2 laser and electro surgery in adhesiolysis–a comparative study. *Fertility, Sterility*, **45**, 407.

8. Jensen, R.P.S. (1988). Early laparoscopy after pelvic operations to prevent adhesions: safety and efficacy. *Fertility, Sterility*, **49**, 26–31.

13

Oesophageal resection

B. Mentges, G. Buess and H.D. Becker

Introduction

The therapy of oesophageal carcinoma still represents a challenge because of the high peri-operative mortality and the poor long-term results. Because the oesophagus lacks a serosal envelope, unlike other gastrointestinal organs, and because of the tight anatomical relations to the neighbouring vital structures, most tumours are well advanced by the time they give rise to symptoms. On the other hand, the high operative mortality has not been reduced in the last decade despite improved pre-operative preparation and peri- and post-operative care of the patient. Because of concomitant risk factors and the great operative trauma, operative mortality is reported on average to be as high as 13% independently of the kind of procedure.[7]

The blunt dissection of the oesophagus was introduced in an attempt to reduce the complication rate by avoiding the thoracic incision. The long-term results do not seem to be worse than those of the abdominothoracic approach, although a radical lymph node dissection is not pursued. In the blind dissection technique the lack of optical control means that important vessels, nerves and other vital structures are at risk of being damaged. A high blood loss, palsy of the recurrent laryngeal nerve, opening of the pleura and so on are frequently reported in the literature.[1,3,4,6,9,10,14,17,18]

The endoscopic microsurgical dissection of the oesophagus (EMDE) is a minimally invasive procedure which avoids the thoracic incision and provides an optimal overview during the operation. After 5 years of development it was introduced in 1989 clinically.[2] Since then 24 patients have been operated upon using this method. In experimental studies on animals comparing abdominothoracic resection, blunt dissection and EMDE in a prospective randomized trial, we have shown that cardiopulmonary parameters were relatively stable using EMDE, and the serum level of certain vasoactive substances and acute phase proteins was only minimally influenced by this procedure.[5]

Materials

Indication

The principal indication for EMDE is histologically proved carcinoma of the oesophagus without distant metastases. The local tumour spread should not exceed the T2 stage. In more advanced tumours palliative procedures should be considered. In many cases, however, pre-operative staging does not reveal the true local spread of the tumour. Therefore tumours which have been understaged pre-operatively might, as T3 or in some cases as T4 tumours, be palliatively resected. Other malignant or benign diseases which require subtotal oesophagectomy, such as strictures after acid or alkali burns, can be included in the indications for this procedure.

Pre-operative diagnostics and preparation

The pre-operative investigation and preparation of the patient do not differ from the normal procedure in oesophageal carcinoma. While computed tomography of the chest is of limited value in evaluating the local tumour spread, endoluminal sonography is becoming the method of choice to assess local invasion. Bronchoscopy with biopsy of suspected areas is also carried out to exclude advanced tumour spread. Because of the cardiopulmonary risk factors the importance of the respective function tests and pre-operative medical therapy and physiotherapy has to be stressed.

Instrumentation

The operating mediastinoscope

The operating mediastinoscope has an obliquely offset eyepiece, a rinsing facility for the optics and a central working channel of 8 × 12 mm diameter. It offers a two- to four-fold enlarged monocular image depending on the distance to the object. In the first prototype the outer metal tube ran into an enlarged olive-shaped tip for mechanical dilatation of the mediastinum (Figure 13.1). To centre the oesophagus as the leading structure of the procedure the dilating cone received a groove and the frontal openings of the aspiration system were moved to the lateral part of the cone in the further development of the instrument (Figure 13.2). The outer tube was designed in a manoeuvrable fashion to be able to rotate it in every position of the mediastinoscope, keeping the oesophagus in a

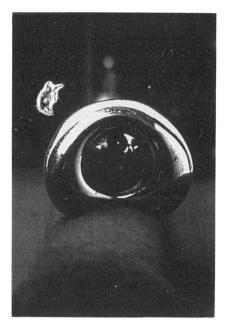

Fig. 13.2

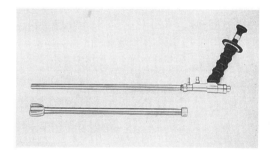

Fig. 13.3

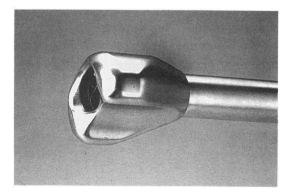

Fig. 13.4

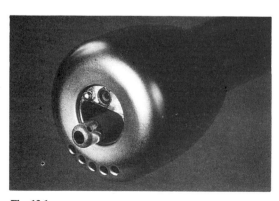

Fig. 13.1

Figs 13.1–13.4. The operating mediastinoscope: different prototypes.

stable position during the dissection (Figure 13.3). In a last step the dilating cone was flattened on the opposite side of the groove to avoid damage of the pars membranacea of the trachea when working on the anterior aspect of the oesophagus (Figure 13.4). The integrated aspiration facility was omitted because the water-consuming technique of 'electrohydrothermonization' was replaced by monopolar coagulation. The suction is now performed by a separate aspiration–coagulation unit which is introduced through the working channel.

The surgical instruments

The first instrument set is shown in Figure 13.5. Blunt dissection of paraoesophageal tissue was performed by an aspirator with a monopolar coagulation facility on the uninsulated tip. After exposure of blood vessels, a bipolar coagulation forceps was used for 'electrohydrothermonization'. The coagulated structures were divided by hooked scissors.

As bipolar coagulation turned out to be ineffective in humans, and the frequent change of the long instruments often led to a loss of view and accumulation of blood, monopolar coagulation was used in a combined device. Figure 13.6 shows the current instrument set. The aspirator with monopolar coagulation facility has an outer diameter of 8 mm. The central channel tapers off to 5 mm at the tip

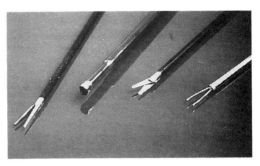

Fig. 13.6. Current instrument set.

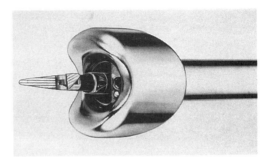

Fig. 13.7. Combined use of aspirator and gripping forceps.

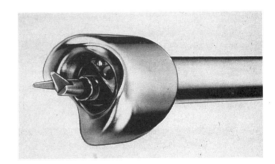

Fig. 13.8. Combined use of aspirator and pair of scissors.

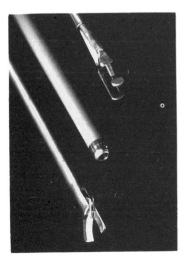

Fig. 13.5. First instrument set.

and contains either a gripping forceps (Figure 13.7), when exact coagulation is required, or a pair of scissors (Figure 13.8). Suction is produced by pulling back the instruments into the working channel, from where they are again advanced into the operation area when necessary. The gripping forceps have a connection for high frequency current at the handle and finely corrugated jaws. This instrument is used both for coagulation and to pull up a nasogastric tube from the abdomen. It is also used to draw the prepared stomach up for anastomosis to the proximal oesophagus.

Operative procedure

The patient is placed in a supine position with the right thorax elevated to allow skin preparation and draping as far as the posterior axillary line (in case emergency thoracotomy is required). The patient's head is rotated to the right and fixed in this position for exposure of the left side of the neck.

At the beginning of the operation a single dose of antibiotic prophylaxis is administered intravenously. A large nasogastric tube (30 French) is placed into the oesophagus to facilitate the manual exposure of the cervical part from the surrounding tissue. The EMDE is a combined procedure with two teams working simultaneously. When the tumour is located in the distal part of the oesophagus, the abdominal team begins a dissection to assess resectability. For a proximal tumour, the mediastinal team clarifies the resectability first before the abdominal team starts. The stomach is prepared in a tube-like fashion as in the normal abdominothoracic approach. The mediastinal part of the operation starts with the exposure of the oesophagus through a left-sided cervical incision along the anterior border of the sternocleidomastoid muscle. After isolation from the surrounding tissue the oesophagus is encircled with a rubber sling. Care is taken not to damage the recurrent laryngeal nerve which should be displayed in this part of the operation. The oesophagus is then dissected further down to its entrance into the mediastinum. Here the endoscopic part of the operation begins. The conventional set of operation instruments is replaced by endoscopic instruments. The exchange of instruments takes place to the right side of the operator, who is now taking a sitting position, the assistant standing next to him. A three chip camera is attached to the eyepiece of the mediastinoscope inside a sterile bag and the operation is followed on the video screen. The surgeon follows the procedure on a monitor which is situated in his direction of view on the left side of the patient. Another video screen is placed on the right side of the patient for the assistant. The endoscopic instruments are connected to the ancillary devices (light source, suction, irrigation).

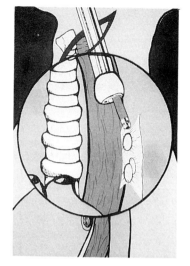

Fig. 13.9. Blunt dissection with the aspirator.

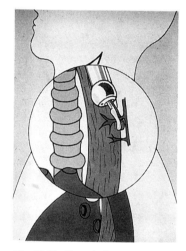

Fig. 13.10. Coagulation of blood vessels with gripping forceps.

The mediastinoscope is then introduced into the mediastinum posterior to the oesophagus with the groove of the outer tube orientated anteriorly to take the posterior aspect of the oesophagus. Blunt dissection is performed by the combination sucker which is used to separate the connective tissue surrounding the oesophagus (Figure 13.9). Remaining blood vessels, if they are bigger than 1 mm in diameter, are coagulated with the aspirator or the gripping forceps (Figure 13.10). Coagulated

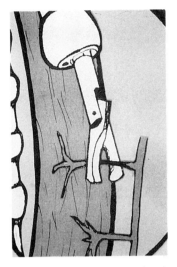

Fig. 13.11. Dividing of coagulated vessels with the scissors.

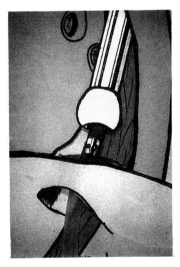

Fig. 13.12. A nasogastric tube is pulled up from the abdomen through the mediastinum.

structures are divided by scissors (Figure 13.11). The assistant operates the diathermy and the irrigation by pressing a foot switch. The dissection of the left side of the oesophagus again starts on the neck with the groove of the dilating cone pointing to the right side to take the left part of the organ. The longitudinal fibres are the best landmark to guide the direction of the dissection. Landmarks on the left side are the aortic arch, the descending thoracic aorta, and, on the anterior aspect of

the oesophagus, the membranaceous part of the trachea. On the right side care should be taken not to display the azygos vein by dissection close to the oesophagus.

Experience has shown that dissection of the tumour-bearing area is more difficult because of hypertrophy of the oesophageal wall and possible infiltration of the surrounding tissue. The plane of dissection should not follow the muscle fibres of the oesophagus in this part of the operation but should be directed more laterally, removing a layer of connective tissue to ensure complete tumour resection. If orientation proves to be too difficult, further dissection should be continued on the non-tumour-bearing part of the organ to establish the plane of dissection distal to the tumour. In the area of the hiatus the finger of the abdominal surgeon facilitates the orientation and helps in blunt dissection. At this level, before entering the abdomen, the oesophagus makes an anterior bend which cannot be followed properly by the rigid instrument, which at this stage has been fully introduced into the mediastinum and is therefore less manoeuvrable.

After completion of the oesophageal dissection, a nasogastric tube is advanced by the abdominal surgeon through the hiatus into the view of the mediastinoscope. The tube is grasped by the gripping forceps (Figure 13.12) and pulled up to the neck by retracting the mediastinoscope. After removal of the large gastric tube (which was in place inside the oesophagus throughout the procedure) the oesophagus is divided using a GIA stapler. The distal stump is sutured to the nasogastric tube, which is then pulled down by the abdominal team. Thus, the distal stump of the organ bends (Figure 13.13) and is drawn through the mediastinum until remaining adhesions, which were left during the dissection, stop this movement. The mediastinoscope follows down and the stretched mediastinal attachments are easily recognized, coagulated and divided. After removal of the oesophagus through the hiatus, the specimen is checked for its integrity, photographed and sent for histological examination (Figure 13.14). The mediastinum is checked for residual bleeding and for integrity of the pleura. The prepared stomach is pulled up to the neck by the gripping forceps. The cervical anastomosis to the proximal oesophagus is done by hand and

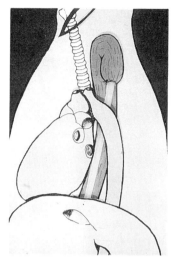

Fig. 13.13. The bending procedure.

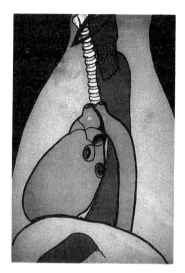

Fig. 13.15. Operation site after completion of the anastomosis.

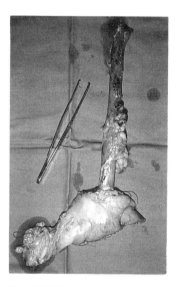

Fig. 13.14. Specimen.

a Penrose drain is placed down to it (Figure 13.15).

Results

Twenty-four patients have been operated on using this technique between September 1989 and June 1991. Only two of the resected tumours were located in the upper third, 14 in the middle third and eight in the distal third of

the oesophagus. Histological examination revealed squamous cell carcinoma in 19 cases, adenocarcinomas in four and a malignant lymphoma in one. The tumour stages were as follows: pT1 (8), pT2 (7), pT3 (7) and pT4 (2). In 9 patients paraoesophageal lymph nodes were removed with the specimen. The average duration of the operation was 3 hours and 20 minutes for the whole procedure and 1 hour and 5 minutes for the endoscopic part. The average blood loss was 1,300 ml for the whole operation with 100 ml for the endoscopic part.

One patient died post-operatively within the first month because of catheter sepsis. The post-mortem examination revealed a septic thrombosis of the inferior vena cava. Further complications were palsy of the recurrent laryngeal nerve in 4 cases, pleural effusions in 9 patients and pneumonia in 3 patients. In 2 patients (not contained in the series of 24) the procedure had to be changed intra-operatively and an emergency thoracotomy performed because of a major haemorrhage.

Discussion

Because of a high rate of pulmonary complications following conventional surgery, blunt dissection of the oesophagus was introduced in the 1970s as the method of choice in many hospitals. The great benefit was considered to be the reduction of the mortality and the complication rate neglecting oncologic radicality. Studies comparing results of oesophagectomy with and without thoracotomy, however, do not suggest an improvement in operative mortality or complications.[11–13,16] Mediastinal trauma is therefore blamed as the cause of the high pulmonary complication rate after blunt dissection. The tearing and blind division of paraoesophageal structures, the introduction of the whole hand of the surgeon into the mediastinum with subsequent compression of the lungs and the heart, the uncontrolled damage to vessels and nerves might be responsible for the high mediastinal blood loss of up to 1,300 ml, the high rate of palsy of the recurrent laryngeal nerve and the frequent entry into the pleural cavity.[1,3,4,6,9,10,14,17,18] The aim of developing the method of EMDE was to avoid the thoracic incision and to minimize the mediastinal trauma. By introducing a mediastinoscope instead of the hand, the mechanical trauma is reduced substantially, and the important structures of the posterior mediastinum can be identified and separated under clear vision. Because of the bad long-term results of oesophageal carcinoma with lymph node involvement, a radical lymph node dissection seems to be of minor relevance, serving only to increase the extent of the procedure.[8,15] According to a recent review of the literature, which included all important publications of the 1980s, there were no differences in operative mortality or 5 year survival between different operations.[7]

The above complications in the first 24 procedures can partly be explained by the high number of advanced tumours. Better patient selection with regard to risk factors and true extent of the tumour stage seems advisable. Furthermore, the transfer of the whole instrumentarium from the animal experiments to humans required some technical changes to facilitate the dissection and avoid complications. Because the paraoesophageal structures of the oesophagus are more dense in humans and spaces are more restricted the dilating cone of the mediastinoscope has had to be changed several times. A groove was added to centre the oesophagus during the dissection, and it was flattened on top to avoid damage to the membraneous part of the trachea. The introduction of combined instruments helped to reduce the frequent change of the long instruments and to save time and maintain the overview.

The appropriate selection of patients and the experience with the new system should further reduce the complication rate.

References

1. Barbier, P.A., Becker, C.D. and Wagner, H.E. (1988). Esophageal carcinoma: patient selection for transhiatal esophagectomy. A prospective analysis of 50 consecutive cases. *World Journal of Surgery*, **12**, 263–9.
2. Buess, G., Becker, H.D., Mentges, B., Teichmann, R. and Lenz, G. (1990). Die endoskopisch-mikrochirurgische Dissektion der Speiseröhre. II. Erste klinische Erfahrungen mit Darstellung der Operationstechnik. *Chirurg*, **61**, 308–11.
3. Finley, R.J., Grace, M. and Duff, J.H. (1985). Esophagogastrectomy without thoracotomy for carcinoma of the cardia and lower part of the esophagus. *Surgical Gynecology and Obstetrics*, **160**, 49–56.
4. Giuli, R. and Sancho-Garnier, H. (1986). Diagnostic, therapeutic, and prognostic features of cancers of the esophagus: results of the international prospective study conducted by the OESO group. *Surgery*, **99**, 614–22.
5. Kipfmüller, K., Buess, G., Naruhn, M., Duda, D., Melzer, A. and Kessler, S. (1990). Die Endoskopisch-Mikrochirurgische Dissektion des Ösophagus (EMDÖ)-tierexperimentelle Ergebnisse. In: *Endoskopie. Von der Diagnostik bis zur neuen Chirurgie* (ed Buess, G.), Deutscher Ärzte-Verlag, Köln, pp. 364–75.
6. Larrieu, H., Millat, B. and Gayral, F. (1985). Oesophagectomies transhiatales. *Chirurgie*, **111**, 835–6.
7. Müller, J.M., Erasmi, H., Stelzner, M., Zieren, U. and Pichlmaier, H. (1990). Surgical therapy of oesophageal carcinoma. *British Journal of Surgery*, **77**, 845–57.
8. Orringer, M.B. (1984). Transhiatal esophagectomy without thoracotomy for carcinoma of the thoracic esophagus. *Annals of Surgery*, **20**, 282–8.
9. Orringer, M.B. (1985). Transhiatal esophagectomy for benign disease. *Journal of Thoracic Cardiovascular Surgery*, **90**, 649–55.
10. Orringer, M.B. (1987). Transhiatal esophagectomy for esophageal carcinoma. In: *Diseases of the Esophagus* (eds Siewert, J.R. and Hölscher, A.H.), Springer, Berlin, Heidelberg, New York, pp. 390–3.
11. Shahian, D.M., Neptune, W.B., Ellis, F.H., Jr. and Watkins, E., Jr. (1980). Transthoracic versus extrathoracic esophagectomy: mortality, morbidity and long-term survival. *Annals of Thoracic Surgery*, **41**, 237–46.
12. Siewert, J.R., Adolf, J., Bartels, H., Hölscher, A.H., Hölscher, M. and Weiser, H.F. (1986). Ösophaguskarzinom: transthorakale Ösophagektomie mit regionaler Lymphadenektomie und Rekonstruktion mit aufgeschobener Dringlichkeit. *Deutsche Medizinische Wochenschrift*, **111**, 647–51.

13. Siewert, J.R., Hölscher, H.A. and Horvath, O.P. (1986). Transmediastinale Oesophagektomie. *Langenbecks Archiv für Chirurgie*, **367**, 203–13.
14. Siewert, J.R. and Roder, J.D. (1987). Chirurgische Therapie des Plattenepithelcarcinoms des Oesophagus-erweiterte Radikalität. *Langenbecks Archiv für Chirurgie*, **372**, 129–39.
15. Skinner, D.B. (1983). En bloc resection of neoplasms of the esophagus and cardia. *Journal of Thoracic Cardiovascular Surgery*, **85**, 59–71.
16. Steiger, Z. and Wilson, R.F. (1981). Comparison of the results of esophagectomy with and without thoracotomy. *Surgical Gynecology and Obstetrics*, **153**, 63–8.
17. Terz, J.J., Beatty, J.D., Kokal, W.A. and Wagman, L.D. (1987). Transhiatal esophagectomy. *American Journal of Surgery*, **154**, 42–8.
18. Ulrich, B., Kasperk, R., Grabitz, K. and Kremer, K. (1985). Die Oesophagusresektion ohne Thoracotomie beim Carcinom. *Chirurg*, **56**, 251–60.

14

Laparoscopic antireflux surgery

Ronald A. Hinder and Charles J. Filipi

In 1935 Winklestein described the condition of hiatal hernia and suggested that the associated oesophagitis was the result of the irritant effect of acid and pepsin on the mucosa.[1] Allison suggested the term 'reflux oesophagitis' for the disorder in 1940.[2] At this time it was generally believed that reflux was synonymous with a hiatal hernia, but with further observation it became apparent that the two disorders can exist independently. Technology capable of allowing study of oesophageal motility became available in the 1950s and the recognition of the lower oesophageal sphincter (LES) that maintains a barrier between the gastric content and the oesophagus gave rise to the finding in the 1960s that many patients with gastro-oesophageal reflux disease (GERD) have a lower resting pressure than that found in the normal population.[3]

Epidemiology of gastro-oesophageal reflux

Heartburn is the most common symptom associated with gastro-oesophageal reflux.[4] A recent Gallup poll reported that 44% of Americans experienced this symptom at least once a month, 18% of these people took some sort of non-prescription medication for this problem at least twice a week. Of those who suffered from heartburn 61% had never discussed this symptom with their doctor.[5] In another study Thompson and Heaton estimated that up to one-third of adults experi-enced heartburn at some time, one-tenth suffered from it weekly and it occurred daily in 1 in 25. This study was conducted on apparently healthy people.[6] A further study has reported that 33% of the population will experience heartburn in a 3 day period.[7] There are, however, problems with investigating the prevalence of this disease simply by reported symptoms. Some patients who report heartburn do not have reflux and conversely there are probably a substantial number of patients who suffer from GERD who are asymptomatic. As witness to this are complications of their disease. This group represents those who are referred for surgical therapy. Finally there are a few patients who will succumb to their disease either by massive upper gastro-intestinal bleeds, though this accounts for only about 6% of such occurrences,[14,15] or those who develop adenocarcinoma in Barrett's oesophagus. The adult annual mortality rate has been estimated to be 0.1 per 100,000 in the years 1957–1961.[16] These figures do not take into account deaths from operative complications or those due to adenocarcinoma.

Medical therapy is aimed at protecting the oesophageal mucosa by decreasing gastric acid secretion, but is flawed in that the basic abnormality of incompetence of the lower oesophageal sphincter is not directly addressed. For this reason, only about 50% of patients show significant healing on H2 blocker therapy. This is increased to 80–90% healing with almost absolute acid reduction using omeprazole. The results of long-term maintenance therapy are disappointing. Only 10% of patients remain healed at 1 year. The risk of severe acid reduction is that persistent alkalinization of the antrum of the stomach results in hypergastrinaemia which is trophic to the gastrointestinal mucosa and potentially may result in tumour formation. Surgical therapy is indicated if there is a poor response to medical therapy or in the presence of complications.

Pre-operative testing

Pre-operative testing involves establishing the:
1. Degree of acid reflux.
2. Amount of mucosal damage.
3. Mechanical competence and relaxation of the lower oesophageal sphincter.
4. Amount of impairment of oesophageal body function.
5. Amount of impairment of gastric function including gastric acid secretion and gastric emptying.

A careful history should be taken to exclude a history of chronic drug ingestion such as non-steroidal anti-inflammatory drugs, iron and vitamin pills which may lodge in the lower oesophagus and produce mucosal damage or stricturing. If surgical treatment is inappropriately aimed at reflux disease in these patients a poor outcome is inevitable. Other conditions such as achalasia, scleroderma and other motility disorders of the oesophageal body and lower oesophageal sphincter may masquerade symptomatically as gastro-oesophageal reflux and these patients would also be poorly served by surgical therapy. The bad perception of surgical therapy held by some gastroenterologists has arisen out of their experience with poorly indicated surgery rather than with appropriately performed surgery.

All patients should have endoscopy with biopsies, a barium swallow preferably with fluoroscopy, 24 hours oesophageal pH studies, oesophageal body and lower oesophageal sphincter manometry, and occasionally gastric secretory or gastric emptying studies. Armed with this information, surgeons should be able to make the decision to operate on patients with troublesome gastro-oesophageal reflux associated with a poorly functioning lower oesophageal sphincter resulting in oesophageal or pulmonary damage. If oesophageal body

function is impaired, a loose or so-called 'floppy' fundoplication must be considered and in those with gastric acid hypersecretion, particularly in the presence of peptic ulceration, a concomitant, highly selective vagotomy may be indicated.

Radiology

Radiology provides very useful information about the disease process and its complications. It is helpful in the pre-operative and post-operative assessment of patients undergoing surgery. Contrast studies can be used to document spontaneous and induced reflux, the presence of a hiatal hernia, oesophageal body dysfunction and the presence of complications such as strictures. It is also useful in assessing the cause of post-operative symptoms.

Spontaneous reflux is demonstrated on barium meal in less than 50% of patients with GERD and therefore is not useful in discriminating these patients from healthy individuals.[17,18] On the other hand, free reflux is a highly specific predictor of reflux detectable by pH monitoring.[19,20] Various manoeuvres used to increase intragastric pressure are often employed. These include applying abdominal compression, the Valsalva manoeuvre, the Trendelenburg position, straight leg raising and turning the patient from side to side.[21] Stress-induced reflux increases the sensitivity of diagnosing GERD but decreases the specificity.[18] Scintigraphy has also been used to diagnose oesophageal reflux but with the development of pH monitoring these techniques are infrequently used to demonstrate reflux.

The radiological criteria for diagnosing hiatal hernia are well established.[22,23] While many patients with GERD have a detectable hiatal hernia, hiatal hernia remains a common finding in healthy subjects and therefore cannot be used as a predictor of oesophagitis.[24,25,26,27] A direct measurement of the internal diameter of the oesophagus generates more useful information.[18,28] By combining the most sensitive radiological test for demonstrating reflux (stress-induced reflux) and the most sensitive double contrast feature (internal diameter measurement) Sellar *et al.* were able to obtain a sensitivity of 85%, an accuracy of 80% with a moderate specificity of 71%.[18]

The advent of double contrast techniques has improved the radiological assessment of oesophagitis. Moderate to severe oesophagitis can be diagnosed fairly reliably by barium studies while mild oesophagitis is often missed.[29] Morphological features include an irregular oesophageal contour due to ulceration, thickened oesophageal folds, a thickened oesophageal wall, or a narrowing of the oesophageal lumen.[30] Oesophageal motor dysfunction results in poor acid clearance, an important mechanism in the development of reflux oesophagitis. Ineffective primary peristalsis is the most important radiological finding in reflux disease because of the associated impairment of oesophageal acid clearance.[31]

Radiology is helpful in the assessment of complicated reflux disease. Peptic strictures and rings are common findings in patients with long-standing GERD. Mild strictures are difficult to visualize on routine barium studies but can be reliably detected by getting the patient to swallow half an unchewed marshmellow with barium.[32] Lower oesophageal rings can be detected but require good oesophageal distension. This can be achieved by performing the study with the patient in the prone position in full inspiration. Barrett's oesophagus is best diagnosed by endoscopy and biopsy, but the finding of a large discrete ulcer by contrast studies supports the diagnosis of Barrett's oesophagus and is an uncommon finding in simple oesophagitis. A lower oesophageal mass on barium studies in a patient with Barrett's oesophagus may indicate the presence of adenocarcinoma which occurs in up to 10% of patients with the condition.

Oesophageal 24 hour pH measurement

This has become the most sensitive measure of abnormal oesophageal acid exposure. During the test the glass or antimony electrode is placed 5 cm above the manometrically determined upper border of the LES.[33] The electrode is connected to a portable datalogger which allows the patient to be ambulant. The datalogger usually records data at a sampling frequency of 4 Hz. Patients are instructed to follow a standardized diet which has a pH > 5, not to smoke and to limit their alcohol intake. Recent reports, however, show that the nature of the diet does not interfere with the results obtained with pH monitoring. Some argue that the diet should not be altered because the

results would then not be an accurate reflection of the patient's individual 24 hour pH profile and also because most reflux symptoms occur postprandially.[34,35] It has also been argued that smoking and alcohol should not be limited. The head of the bed should not be elevated and patients should remain upright until retiring for the night. The period of testing should be in excess of 18 hours. Following the study the data is downloaded from the datalogger to a computer.

Data analysis

Many parameters have been used to discriminate between normals and those that have increased acid exposure. The most important parameter appears to be the total % time pH < 4.[36,37,38,39,40] Johnson and DeMeester devised a discriminant scoring system that uses six parameters for its calculation: total % time pH < 4, % time pH < 4 while upright, % time pH < 4 while supine, number of reflux episodes (pH < 4), number of reflux episodes lasting longer than 5 minutes and the longest reflux episode.[41] This computer-generated scoring system has a sensitivity of 90.3% and a specificity of 90%.

Besides quantifying the amount of acid reflux it is relevant to try to correlate symptoms with acid reflux events. This remains a difficult task. Often the patient will not have symptoms during the study period and the assessment of symptoms itself remains subjective.

Oesophageal manometry

The lower oesophageal sphincter (LES) forms a barrier to acid reflux and should only open following a swallow. A defective sphincter is the cause of increased oesophageal acid exposure in most patients and the cause of a high rate of failed medical therapy.[42] Continual acid reflux eventually leads to oesophageal injury and can result in permanent oesophageal body dysfunction.[43] The competence of the LES depends on the functional integrity of three factors: sphincter pressure, total sphincter length and intra-abdominal length, i.e. that portion of the sphincter that will be exposed to increases in intra-abdominal pressure.[44,45,46] While the most common cause of LES incompetence is inadequate pressure, the additional insult of having inadequate sphincter length, both the total or intra-abdominal component thereof, significantly increases the possibility of acid reflux.[42] The severity of oesophagitis has been shown to be dependent on the number of defective components of the LES.[47]

Manometry is also able to diagnose the presence of hiatal hernia. Hiatal hernia appears to compromise sphincter function during dynamic stresses such as swallowing and abrupt increases in intra-abdominal pressure.[48] This is a reflection of the loss of intra-abdominal length in patients with hiatal hernia. Hiatal hernia also compromises oesophageal acid clearance by impairing oesophageal emptying.[49]

A second component central to the understanding of GERD is acid clearance. Ineffective peristalsis in the oesophageal body is important in the development of GERD in its own right and as a consequence of oesophageal injury due to acid reflux.[50] Oesophageal body dysfunction not initiated by GERD may be related to neuromuscular disorders, metabolic disturbances and especially collagen vascular diseases of which scleroderma, mixed connective tissue disease and dermatomyositis are the most common. In this small group of patients, especially those with scleroderma, GERD may be the result principally of poor body function. A progressive loss of LES function in scleroderma patients compounds the problem. Furthermore, the finding of a short oesophagus on manometry would be an indication for a transthoracic surgical approach which allows for better mobilization of the oesophagus.

Technique for oesophageal manometry

Manometry is performed after an overnight fast using a water-perfused catheter.

The catheter is passed transnasally into the stomach. The baseline gastric pressure pattern should be confirmed before proceeding with the study. The five-channel tracing should show positive fluctuations related to inspiration. The catheter is then withdrawn in a stepwise manner 1 cm at a time. As the catheter is withdrawn the intra-abdominal pattern (positive inspiratory-related excursions) will at some point convert to an intrathoracic pattern (negative inspiratory-related excursions). This point is known as the respiratory inversion point (RIP) and is the point at which the lower oesophageal sphincter pressure can be measured.[51] The upper border of the LES is identified when the pressure drops below gastric baseline to the oesophageal baseline. A pressure tracing is obtained for each port that is slowly pulled through the LES. The radial orientation of the five infusion ports enables any asymmetry in the LES to be noted.[52] The average value of all five tracings are used to describe LES pressure, overall length and intra-abdominal length. Sphincter relaxation is then measured. One port is placed at the sphincter with one port in the stomach and the three remaining ports in the oesophageal body. The patient is asked to swallow a 5 ml bolus of water. The sphincter pressure should drop to gastric baseline if sphincter relaxation is normal. This is repeated 10 times and the average relaxation is calculated.

Hiatal hernia is diagnosed at manometry by the presence of a 'double hump'. The first high pressure zone represents the pressure generated at the RIP by the crura of the diaphragm and any portion of the sphincter still situated at this level. The second high pressure zone is created by the true sphincter that has dislocated into the chest.

In order to assess oesophageal body function the catheter is placed so that the lowest infusion port is 3 cm above the upper border of the LES. The catheter can also be positioned with the uppermost port placed 1 cm below the upper oesophageal sphincter. Ten dry swallows and 10 wet swallows (5 ml water) are then recorded.

Gastric acid analysis

Gastric acid studies involve the collection of gastric juice using a nasogastric tube. Basal samples as well as timed collections following stimulation are collected. Several stimuli can be used: histamine, Histalog (betazole hydrochloride), pentagastrin, and insulin-induced hypoglycaemia. Pentagastrin has the fewest side effects and is most commonly used.

Gastric acid hypersecretion may well be important in GERD but its exact relationship is difficult to establish. In early studies in which varying criteria for GERD were used, gastric acid hypersecretion was shown to be significantly more prevalent in GERD patients than in healthy volunteers.[53] The value of gastric acid analysis in GERD appears to be in the evaluation of patients with high oesophageal acid exposure and normal LES pressure. If these patients have gastric acid hypersecretion, they may be better served by a highly selective vagotomy.

Indications for surgery

Since gastro-oesophageal reflux disease is a common entity and is effectively controlled by medication, patients suitable for surgical therapy should be carefully defined. Gastro-oesophageal reflux disease should be well documented and linked to complaints. Primary GERD due to a mechanically incompetent antireflux barrier should be diagnosed from secondary forms of the disease related to gastric acid hypersecretion, gastroparesis caused by metabolic disorders such as diabetes mellitus, and primary disturbances of oesophageal clearance function as occurs in systemic sclerosis. Since the symptoms of GERD are often non-specific, other functional foregut disorders with similar symptoms should be considered, such as diffuse oesophageal spasm, nutcracker oesophagus, early and vigorous forms of achalasia and duodenogastric reflux. It is important to consider and exclude heart disease.

Surgery is strongly indicated in patients presenting with severe reflux oesophagitis (grades 3 and 4). These patients are at high risk of developing further complications and require long-term therapy. Medical treatment fails in a high proportion of patients with severe reflux oesophagitis as has been demonstrated by Lieberman *et al.*[54] and Spechler *et al.*[55] Mixed reflux episodes of acid or alkali are detected in many of these patients making long-term acid blockade ineffective.

Operative treatment is also advised in patients with low grade reflux oesophagitis (grades 1 and 2) with a mechanically defective sphincter. The latter predisposes to persistent GERD as demonstrated by Zaninotto *et al.*[56] The response to medical treatment over more than a decade is less than satisfactory under these conditions.[54] GERD may present with respiratory symptoms such as chronic laryngitis, pulmonary aspiration with recurrent pneumonia and even asthma. Only about 50%

of these patients have a history of heartburn or show endoscopic evidence of reflux oesophagitis.[57] The causal relationship between the pulmonary symptoms and gastro-oesophageal reflux can be proved by 24 hour pH monitoring. A positive reflux score on 24 hour pH testing with reflux-induced coughing, wheezing or asthma attacks, in addition to a mechanically incompetent sphincter diagnosed by manometry, presents a strong indication for surgical intervention.

Patients without oesophagitis should only be offered surgery if they have symptoms severely affecting their lifestyle. Patients with grade 0 to grade 2 reflux oesophagitis who do not fulfil the above criteria should be thoroughly investigated for other causes of their symptoms and are best treated medically in the first instance. Patients with hiatal hernia presenting with severe dysphagia regardless of whether GERD is present or not should be offered surgery. Kaul *et al.* demonstrated that hiatal hernia may lead to dysphagia.[58] Pathophysiologically, this is caused by trapping of the herniated stomach by the diaphragmatic crura. The degree of dysphagia is directly proportional to the depth of diaphragmatic impression, as seen on contrast radiological studies.

Barrett's oesophagus is usually associated with a mechanically defective sphincter and evidence of acid or alkaline reflux, and therefore warrants surgical therapy. It is not clear if this will lead to an arrest of the progression of Barrett's to malignancy. There are some reports of regression of the extent of Barrett's after antireflux surgery.[59,60]

Patients should be fully involved in the decision for surgical therapy as their co-operation is essential in the post-operative period when symptoms such as sysphagia, satiety after small meals, gas bloat, abdominal distension and diarrhoea may occasionally occur. They should also be made aware of the risks of anaesthesia, the surgical procedure and the risk of unsuspected bowel perforation during the procedure.

The surgical procedure[61]

Surgical therapy is aimed at:
1. Reducing the hiatal hernia which is present in about 50% of patients with gastro-oesophageal reflux disease.

2. Fixation of the lower oesophageal sphincter in the abdomen, allowing it to perform more satisfactorily under the positive intra-abdominal pressure.

3. Narrowing of the crura to hold the lower oesophageal sphincter and stomach in the abdomen and also to act as a pinchcock on the lower oesophagus.

4. Overall lengthening of the lower oesophageal sphincter.

5. Increasing the lower oesophageal sphincter resting pressure.

These objectives must be met without producing undue obstruction to the forward passage of swallowed food.

The laparoscopic procedure is usually carried out under general anaesthesia with the patient in the lithotomy position. It is not usually necessary to have a urinary catheter in the bladder since this is an upper abdominal procedure. A nasogastric tube should be passed and the stomach aspirated of its contents before the tube is removed. The patient is placed in the lithotomy position so that the surgeon may stand between the legs of the patient and be able comfortably to address the upper abdomen without having to twist his or her body during the procedure. Assistants stand on the left and right of the patient. The operating table is placed in the steep reversed Trendelenburg position to allow the stomach and other organs to fall away from the diaphragm to allow good access to the hiatus. This also allows for drainage of blood from this area, which may obscure the surgical field. Meticulous care must be paid in keeping the blood loss to an absolute minimum. The usual blood loss for this procedure is 25–50 ml. The steps of the procedure are:

1. Establishment of the pneumoperitoneum and placement of ports.

2. Exposure of the oesophageal hiatus, oesophagus and stomach.

3. Mobilization of the lower oesophagus and hiatal hernia, should this be present.

4. Closure of the oesophageal hiatus by approximation of the crura behind the oesophagus.

5. Mobilization of the greater curvature of the stomach.

6. Placement and fixation of the fundic wrap around the lower oesophagus.

Following on the creation of a pneumoperitoneum with CO_2 gas using a Veress needle, two 10 mm ports are placed in the midline approximately 2 inches above the umbilicus and 1 inch below the xiphoid. The endoscope is passed through the supraumbilical port. A further 10 mm port is placed in the left subcostal area in the midclavicular line. The upper midline and left subcostal ports are used by the surgeon in a two-handed approach to the oesophageal hiatus. A further 10 mm port is placed in the right subcostal area to allow access for a liver retractor. A final 10 mm port is placed far laterally in the left subcostal area to allow for downward traction of the stomach by the assistant. It is not usually necessary to detach the diaphragmatic connections of the left lobe of the liver. The hook electrocautery is used to elevate small amounts of tissue in the peri-oesophageal area to dissect out the right crus of the diaphragm and the oesophagus. This can best be achieved by dividing the gastrohepatic omentum superior to the hepatic branches of the vagus nerve to allow access to the right side of the oesophagus. Care must be taken to identify and preserve an aberrant left hepatic artery in this area. In most cases the oesophagus can easily be identified to the left of the right crus and cleared of its connections on the anterior and lateral sides (Figure 14.1). The left or anterior vagus nerve is identified and left in contact with the oesophagus. The oesophagus can then be swept upwards and to the left by using the side of a grasper passed through the left lateral port. This is an important manoeuvre which gives excellent access to the area behind the oesophagus (Figure 14.2). The right or posterior vagus nerve is identified and separated from the oesophagus and is placed posterior to the crural repair and wrap. A window is created behind the oesophagus in preparation for the fundoplication. Care must be taken to avoid damage to the oesophagus and stomach. The crura are approximated behind the oesophagus using non-absorbable sutures. A size 58–60 French Maloney bougie should easily be able to be passed into the stomach by the anaesthetist. Attention is then focused on the greater curvature of the stomach where the short gastric vessels should be divided for a distance of approximately 10–15 cm down from the angle of His. This portion of the fundus of the stomach will be used for the fundoplication. Care must be taken at this point to avoid damage to the spleen or stomach. The fundus of the stomach

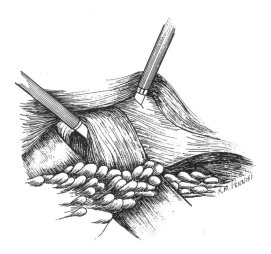

Fig. 14.1. Exposure of oesophagus.

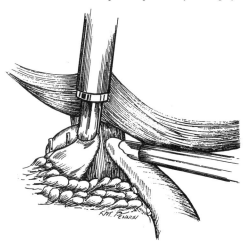

Fig. 14.3. Fundus of stomach brought behind oesophagus.

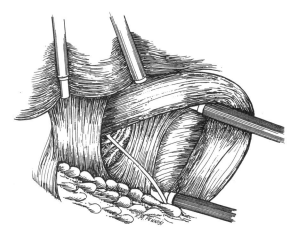

Fig. 14.2. Elevation of oesophagus with identification of posterior vagus nerve.

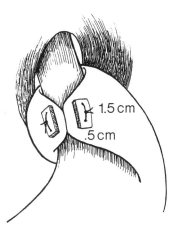

Fig. 14.4. The completed fundoplication.

can easily be brought around behind the oesophagus (Figure 14.3). This can be fixed with a horizontal 'U' stitch held by Teflon® pledgets (Figures 14.4 and 14.5). The exact method of fixation of the fundoplication may be the surgeon's usual choice. Other surgical options include a partial posterior fundoplication (Toupet) or partial anterior fundoplication (Dor). These can both be effectively carried out by the laparoscopic approach.

Blood loss is usually < 50 cc and no patients have required blood transfusion. The operative time is 2–3 hours. The necessity to convert to an open procedure occurred in six of our first 34 cases and was usually precipitated by

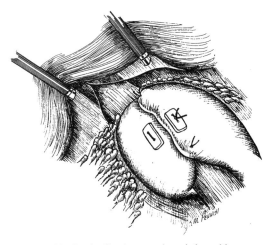

Fig. 14.5. The fundoplication may be reinforced by one or two extra simple sutures as required.

an inability to expose the anatomy to the surgeon's satisfaction, bleeding from a short gastric vessel, severe adhesions from previous operations and perforation of the lower oesophagus or stomach requiring immediate suturing. None of these led to any untoward long-term complications. Only 1 patient in the following 71 cases required conversion to an open procedure due to limitation of endoscopic access caused by peritoneal adhesions. This indicates the lengthy 'learning curve' of this procedure, but once mastered, the procedure can be completed in almost all cases.

Post-operative care

No nasogastric tube is required and patients are encouraged to ambulate on the evening of the operation. The following day a gastro-grafin swallow may be carried out to determine that there is good passage of contrast from the oesophagus into the stomach and to ensure that there is no leakage at the surgical site. Patients are then begun on a liquid diet. They are advanced to a soft diet on the following day, and many patients leave hospital on the second post-operative day. However, if there is any delay in the ability to advance the diet or if there should be any other post-operative concerns the patient is kept in hospital.

Patients are encouraged to exercise frequently within the limits of their abdominal discomfort and ability. They are informed to avoid swallowing chunks of food such as solid meat or dry bread for the first 2 or 3 weeks after surgery. These may occasionally impact in the lower oesophagus due to the presence of oedema around the lower oesophagus and the fundoplication. They are able to stop all antacid medications and can resume a normal diet by the sixth post-operative week.

Post-operative complications

Early complications

Use of the laparoscopic technique has encouraged surgeons to discontinue nasogastric suction early and to start ambulation soon after surgery leading to early discharge from hospital. In patients who have significant nausea, bloating or copious volumes of nasogastric aspirate it may be necessary to leave the nasogastric tube in place for a longer period. Usually 1 day is sufficient but occasionally a longer period is needed. In view of the fact there there is no large abdominal wound and that the small bowel is disturbed less than during open surgery, patients after laparoscopic Nissen fundoplication have less ileus and more rapid return of bowel function. Oedema may be present at the site of the fundoplication and may obstruct the passage of solid food until the oedema settles. It may take up to 6 weeks for normal deglutition to take place and so patients must be warned that they should chew their food well and keep the diet limited to softer foods until that time. It may be necessary to disimpact swallowed solids in the first week or two if there has been injudicious eating of solids by the patient. Whereas patients have naturally in the past limited their food intake because of the prolonged ileus, this does not occur after laparoscopic surgery and may lead to symptoms of bloating and abdominal discomfort in the first weeks. The patient's focus is no longer on the abdominal wound but is now directed at intestinal symptoms.

Wound complications are rare after laparoscopic surgery in view of the small size of the abdominal wounds. Should sepsis occur, this constitutes no problem. In the early post-operative period attention should be focused on the temperature and white blood count which may alert the surgeon to intra-abdominal problems that may have resulted from inadvertent bowel perforation at surgery. Delayed perforation due to ischaemia may potentially occur at the seventh to tenth day after surgery when the patient is at home.

Late complications

Most patients return to normal eating habits with the ability to swallow normally and belch, and are able to relieve gaseous distension or vomit when necessary. As this procedure has only been performed for 3 years at the time of writing, it is not possible to report on late complications beyond this length of follow-up. In view of the fact that the procedure is carried out in exactly the same fashion as with open surgery it is likely that late complications should occur in the same incidence as following open surgery. In a collected series of 1,141 patients after open fundoplication followed up for a period of 1 to 12 years, a good result was reported in 87% of patients.[62] Seven per cent had recurrence reflux and 8% complained of dysphagia. There were 8 patients with the gas bloat syndrome. The mortality in this combined series was 1%. Eighty-two to 96% good results can be expected after the Belsey, Hill, Nissen or Angelchick procedures. The recurrence of reflux should be less than 10% and the incidence of dysphagia should be minimal. Patients should be able to be off all antacid medications and to eat a normal diet. The persistence of nausea, heartburn, regurgitation, dysphagia, chest pain or epigastric pain after an antireflux procedure represents a poor outcome. The incidence of persistent dysphagia, longer than 30 days after surgery, has been reported to be present in 0–21% of patients after Nissen fundoplication. By shortening the wrap to 1.5 cm this has been reduced to 3%.[62]

In a recent retrospective analysis of 63 patients requiring reoperation after a previous antireflux procedure it was found that placement of the wrap around the stomach was the most frequent cause for failure. This is followed by a partial or complete breakdown of the wrap, herniation of the repair into the chest, and construction of a wrap that is too tight or too long. Attention to technical details during construction of the primary procedure would avoid these failures in most cases. Redo surgery will usually require open laparotomy where the customary principles of corrective surgery are applied. The use of Teflon® pledgets in the Nissen fundoplication has resulted in erosion of these pledgets into the oesophagus and stomach with fistula formation and haemorrhage. These can usually be successfully removed endoscopically.

In some patients alkaline gastro-oesophageal reflux may be present. Fundoplication usually controls the oesophageal reflux symptoms but these patients may be left with severe duodenogastric reflux with significant abdominal symptoms and severe gastritis. A small proportion of these patients may have to be considered for subsequent surgical control of duodenogastric reflux by a procedure such as the 'duodenal switch'.[63] Gastric ulceration has been reported after the Nissen fundoplication. This may be due to the dissection at the lesser curvature or may be as a result of duodenogastric reflux.

In the first 100 patients treated by the author, early post-operative symptoms have included bloating, nausea, mild dysphagia and diarrhoea. An elderly patient died of a delayed duodenal perforation resulting in peritoneal sepsis. As with open fundoplication, a dysphagia rate of 30–40% can be expected in the first few weeks after surgery. Follow-up after 4–20 months has shown that 80% are symptom free and that 9% have mild dysphagia, 5% have some chest pain, 3% occasional diarrhoea, 2% heartburn and 2% persistence of asthma. One patient was found to have recurrence of gastro-oesophageal reflux. This patient had gastroenteritis in the early post-operative period with severe vomiting. This presumably resulted in disruption of the fundoplication. Another required reoperation for a stricture at the site of the fundoplication. These results are similar to those obtained after open fundoplication. Otherwise, the patients have been satisfied with the results of the procedure and have had the expected shorter hospital stay and early return to work with good control of symptoms from all medication.

Conclusion

The laparoscopic approach to the oesophageal hiatus requires not only specialized training and skill in laparoscopic surgery but also needs a good knowledge of gastro-oesophageal function to ensure good results. This is a suitable surgical alternative to open fundoplication with all of the advantages of minimally invasive surgery.

References

1. Winklestein, A. (1935). Inflammation of the lower third of the esophagus. *JAMA*, 906–9.
2. Allison, P.R., (1946). Peptic ulcer of the esophagus. *Journal of Thoracic Surgery*, **15**, 308–17.
3. Wankling, W.J., Warrian, W.G. and Kind, J.F. (1965). The gastroesophageal sphincter in hiatus hernia. *Canadian Journal of Surgery*, **8**, 61–7.
4. Jamieson, G.C. and Duranceau, A. (1988). *Gastroesophageal Reflux*, W.B. Saunders, Philadelphia, p. 65.
5. Gallup Survey on Heartburn across America. The Gallup Organization. Princeton, March 28, 1988.

6. Thompson, W.G. and Heaton, K.W. (1982). Heartburn and globus in apparently healthy people. *Journal of the Canadian Medical Association*, **126**, 46–8.

7. Norrelund, N. and Pederson, P.A. (1988). Prevalence of gastro-oesophageal reflux-like dyspepsia. Internation Congress of Gastroenterology, Rome, September, 4–10.

8. Volpcelli, N.A., Bedine, M.S., Hendrix, T.R. *et al.* (1975). Absence of acid sensitivity in patients with benign esophageal strictures. *Gastroenterology*, **68**, 1007.

9. Heading, R.C., Blackwell, J.N. and Cameron, E.W.J. (1981). Longterm management of reflux patients. In: *Cimetidine in the '80's* (ed Baron, J.H.), Churchill Livingstone, New York, pp. 172–80.

10. Kaul, B., Halvorsen, T., Petersen, H. *et al.* (1986). Gastroesophageal reflux disease: scintigraphic, endoscopic and histologic considerations. *Scandinavian Journal of Gastroenterology*, **21**, 134–8.

11. Little, L.G., DeMeester, T.R., Kirchner, P.T. *et al.* (1980). Pathogenesis of esophagitis in patients with gastroesophageal reflux. *Surgery*, **88**, 101–7.

12. de Caestecker, J.S., Blackwell, J.N. and Pryde, A. *et al.* (1987). Daytime gastro-oesophageal reflux is important in oesophagitis. *Gut*, **28**, 519–26.

13. Brand, D.L., Eastwood, V.R., Martin, D. *et al.* (1979). Esophageal symptoms, manometry and histology before and after antireflux surgery. A long term follow-up study. *Gastroenterology*, **76**, 1393–1401.

14. Silverstein, F.E., Gilbert, D.A., Tedesco, F.J. *et al.* (1981). The national ASGE survey on upper gastrointestinal bleeding I. Study design and baseline data. *Gastrointestinal Endoscopy*, **27**, 73–9.

15. Silverstein, F.E., Gilbert, D.A., Tedesco, F.J. *et al.* (1981). The national ASGE survey on upper gastrointestinal bleeding II. Clinical prognostic factors. *Gastrointestinal Endoscopy*, **27**, 80–93.

16. Brunner, P.I., Karmondy, A.M. and Needham, C.D. (1969). Severe peptic oesophagitis. *Gut*, **10**, 831–7.

17. Kaul, B., Petersen, H., Grette, K., Erichsen, H. and Myrvold, H.E. (1985). Scintigraphy, pH measurement and radiography in the evaluation of gastroesophageal reflux. *Scandinavian Journal of Gastroenterology*, **20**, 289–94.

18. Sellar, R.J., De Caestecker, J.S. and Heading, R.C. (1987). Barium radiology: a sensitive test for gastroesophageal reflux. *Clinical Radiology*, **38**, 303–7.

19. Richter, J.E. and Castell, D.O. (1982). Gastroesophageal reflux. Pathogenesis, diagnosis and treatment. *Annals of Internal Medicine*, **97**, 93–103.

20. Pope, C.E. (1976). Pathophysiology and diagnosis of reflux esophagitis. *Gastroenterology*, **70**, 445–54.

21. Fransson, S.-G., Sökjer, H., Johansson, K.-E. and Tibbling, L. (1988). Radiologic diagnosis of gastro-oesophageal reflux by means of graded abdominal compression. *Acta Radiology*, **29**, 45–8.

22. Hameetema, W., Tytgat, G.N.J., Houthoff, H.J. and Van Den Tweel, J.G. (1989). Barrett's esophagus: development of dyspasia and adenocarcinoma. *Gastroenterology*, **96**, 1249–56.

23. Cameron, A.J., Ott, B.J. and Payne, W.S. (1985). The incidence of adenocarcinoma in columnar lined (Barrett's) esophagus. *New England Journal of Medicine*, **313**, 857–9.

24. Dodds, W.J., Hogan, W.J. and Miller, W.N. (1976). Reflux esophagitis. *Digestive Diseases and Sciences*, **21**, 49–67.

25. Ott, D.J., Dodds, W.J., Wu, W.C., Gelfand, D.W., Hogan, W.J. and Stewart, E.T. (1982). Current status of radiology in evaluating for gastroesophageal reflux disease. *Journal of Clinical Gastroenterology*, **4**, 365–75.

26. Ott, D.J., Gelfand, D.W., Chen, Y.M., Wu, W.C. and Munitz, H.A. (1985). Predictive relationship of hiatal hernia to reflux esophagitis. *Gastrointestinal Radiology*, **10**, 317–20.

27. Wright, R.A. and Hurwitz, A.L. (1979). Relationship of hiatal hernia to endoscopically proved reflux esophagitis. *Digestive Diseases and Sciences*, **24**, 311–13.

28. Graziani, L., De Nigris, E., Pesaresi, A., Baldelli, S., Dini, L. and Montesi, A. (1983). Reflux esophagitis: radiologic–endoscopic correlation in 39 symptomatic cases. *Gastrointestinal Radiology*, **8**, 1–6.

29. Ott, D.J., Wu, W.C. and Gelfand, D.W. (1981). Reflux esophagitis revisited: prospective analysis of radiologic accuracy. *Gastrointestinal Radiology*, **6**, 1–7.

30. Dodds, W.J. (1988). The pathogenesis of gastroesophageal reflux disease. *American Journal of Roentgenology*, **151**, 49–56.

31. Stevenson, G.W. (1989). Radiology of gastro-oesophageal reflux. *Clinical Radiology*, **40**, 119–21.

32. Somers, S., Stevenson, G.W. and Thomson, G. (1986). Comparison of endoscopy and barium swallow with marshmellow in dysphagia. *Canadian Association of Radiologists Journal*, **37**, 73–5.

33. Johnson, L.F. and DeMeester, T.R. (1974). Twenty-four-hour pH monitoring of the distal esophagus. A quantitative measure of gastroesophageal reflux. *American Journal of Gastroenterology*, **62**, 325–32.

34. DeCaestecker, J.S., Blackwell, J.N., Pryde, A. and Heading, R.C. (1987). Daytime gastroesophageal reflux is important in oesophagitis. *Gut*, **28**, 519–26.

35. Shaker, R., Helm, J.F., Dodd, W.J. and Hogan, W.J. (1988). Revelations about ambulatory esophageal pH monitoring. *Gastroenterology*, **94**, 421A.

36. Schindlbeck, N.E., Heinrich, C., Konig, A., Dendorfer, A., Pace, F. and Muller-Lissner, S.A. (1987). Optimal thresholds, sensitivity and specificity of long-term pH-metry for the detection of gastroesophageal reflux disease. *Gastroenterology*, **93**, 85–90.

37. Wiener, G.J., Morgan, T.M., Copper, J.B., Wu, W.C., Castell, D.O., Sinclair, J.W. and Richter, J.E. (1988). Ambulatory 24-hour esophageal pH monitoring. Producibility and variability of pH parameters. *Digestive Diseases and Sciences*, **33**, 1127–33.

38. Johnsson, F., Joelsson, B. and Isberg, P.E. (1987).

Ambulatory 24-hour intraesophageal pH monitoring in the diagnosis of gastroesophageal reflux disease. *Gut*, **28**, 1145–50.

39. Irvin, T.T. and Perez-Avila, C. (1978). Diagnosis of symptomatic gastroesophageal reflux by prolonged monitoring of lower esophageal pH. *Scandinavian Journal of Gastroenterology*, **12**, 715–20.

40. Jamieson, J.R., Stein, H.J., DeMeester, T.R., Bonavina, L., Schwizer, W., Hinder, R.A. and Albertucci, M. (1992). Ambulatory 24-H esophageal pH monitoring: normal values, optimal thresholds, specificity, sensitivity, and reproducibility. *American Journal of Gastroenterology*, **87**, 1102–11.

41. Johnson, L.F. and DeMeester, T.R. (1986). Development of the 24-hour intraesophageal pH monitoring composite scoring system. *Journal of Clinical Gastroenterology*, **8** (Suppl. 1), 52–8.

42. Zaninotto, G., DeMeester, T.R., Schwizer, W, Johansson, K.E. and Cheng, S.C. (1988). The lower esophageal sphincter in health and disease. *American Journal of Surgery*, **155**, 104–11.

43. Stein, H.J., Eypasch, E.P., DeMeester, T.R., Smyrk, T.C. and Attwood, S.E. (1990). Circadian esophageal motor function in patients with gastroesophageal reflux disease. *Surgery*, **108**, 769–78.

44. DeMeester, T.R., Wernly, J.A., Bryant, G.H., Little, A.G. and Skinner, D.B. (1979). Clinical and *in vitro* analysis as determinants of gastroesophageal competence: a study of the principles of antireflux surgery. *American Journal of Surgery*, **137**, 39–46.

45. O'Sullivan, G.C., DeMeester, T.R., Joelsson, B.E., Smith, R.B., Blough, R.R., Johnson, L.F. and Skinner, D.B. (1982). The interaction of the lower esophageal sphincter pressure and length of sphincter in the abdomen as determinants of gastroesophageal competence. *American Journal of Surgery*, **143**, 40–7.

46. Bonavina, L., Evander, A., DeMeester, T.R., Walther, B., Cheng, S.C., Palazzo, L. and Concannon, J.L. (1986). Length of the distal esophageal sphincter and competency of the cardia. *American Journal of Surgery*, **151**, 25–34.

47. Rakic, S., Stein, H.J. and DeMeester, T.R. (1990). Standard manometry of the esophageal body. What is normal? Unpublished data.

48. Sloan, S., Rademaker, A.W. and Kahrilas, P.J. (1992). Determinants of gastroesophageal junction incompetence: hiatal hernia, lower esophageal sphincter, or both? *Annals of Internal Medicine*, **117**, 977–82.

49. Sloan, S. and Kahrilas, P.J. (1991). Impairment of esophageal emptying with hiatal hernia. *Gastroenterology*, **100**, 596–605.

50. Joelsson, B.E., DeMeester, T.R., Skinner, D.B., LaFontaine, E., Waters, P.F. and O'Sullivan, G.C. (1982). The role of the esophageal body in the antireflux mechanism. *Surgery*, **92**, 417–24.

51. Winans, C.S. and Harris, L.D. (1967). Quantification of lower esophageal sphincter competence. *Gastroenterology*, **52**, 773–8.

52. Winans, C.S. (1977). Manometric asymmetry of the lower esophageal sphincter. *Digestive Diseases and Sciences*, **22**, 348–54.

53. Winkelstein, A., Wolf, B.S., Som, M.L. and Marshak, R.H. (1954). Peptic esophagitis with duodenal or gastric ulcer. *JAMA*, **154**, 885.

54. Lieberman, D.A. (1987). Medical therapy for chronic reflux esophagitis: long-term follow-up. *Archives of Internal Medicine*, **147**, 1717–20.

55. Spechler, S.J. (1992). VA study group: comparison of medical and surgical therapy for complicated gastroesophageal reflux disease in veterans. *New England Journal of Medicine*, **326**, 786–92.

56. Zaninotto, G., DiMario, F., Costantini, M., Baffa, R., Germanà, B., Dal Santo, P.L., Rugge, M., Bolzan, M., Naccarato, R. and Ancona, E. (1992). Oesophagitis and pH of refluxate: an experimental and clinical study. *British Journal of Surgery*, **79**, 161–4.

57. Pellegrini, C.A., DeMeester, T.R., Johnson, L.F. and Skinner, D.B. (1979). Gastroesophageal reflux and pulmonary aspiration: incidence, functional abnormality, and results of surgical therapy. *Surgery*, **86**, 110–19.

58. Kaul, B.K., DeMeester, T.R., Oka, M., Ball, C.S., Stein, H.J., Kim, C.B. and Cheng, S.C. (1990). The cause of dysphagia in uncomplicated sliding hiatal hernia and its relief by hiatal herniorrhaphy: a roentgenographic, manometric, and clinical study. *Annals of Surgery*, **211**, 406–10.

59. Williamson, W.A., Ellis, F.H., Gibb, S.P., Shahian, D.M. and Aretz, H.T. (1990). Effects of antireflux operation on Barrett's mucosa. *Annals of Thoracic Surgery*, **49**, 537–42.

60. Brand, D.L., Ylvisaker, J.T., Gelfand, M. and Pope, C.E. (1980). Regression of columnar esophageal (Barrett's) epithelium after anti-reflux surgery. *New England Journal of Medicine*, **302**, 844–8.

61. Hinder, R.A. and Filipi, C.J. (1992). The technique of laparoscopic Nissen fundoplication. *Surgical Laparoscopy and Endoscopy*, **2**, 265–72.

62. Stein, H.J., DeMeester, T.R. and Hinder, R.A. (1992). Outpatient physiologic testing and surgical management of foregut motility disorders. *Current Problems in Surgery*, **29**, 415–555.

63. DeMeester, T.R., Fuchs, K.H., Albertucci, M.D. *et al.* (1987). Experimental and clinical results with proximal end-to-end duodenojejunostomy for pathologic duodenogastric reflux. *Annals of Surgery*, **296**, 414–26.

15

Laparoscopic intestinal surgery

John D. Corbitt Jr

Laparoscopic surgery became popular with gynaecologists in the 1960s and early 1970s. It was not until 1989/1990 that it gained popularity with the general surgeon. Interest in laparoscopic procedures rapidly began to increase after laparoscopic cholecystectomy proved that the patient could be discharged from the hospital early with minimal pain and rapidly return to normal activity. Surgeons soon began to consider laparoscopic colon and small bowel resection. Laparoscopic intestinal surgery has been limited, however, because of the lack of appropriate instruments. In 1991 the major manufacturers began to develop laparoscopic intestinal instruments which have now become an important item in the research and development programmes of these major manufacturers. At present intestinal surgery is largely laparoscopic-assisted intestinal surgery, with portions of the procedures being done extra-corporeally using laparoscopic equipment as well as previously available stapling devices. The laparoscopic intestinal procedures described in this chapter probably represent the early beginnings of laparoscopic intestinal surgery which seems likely to be as beneficial for the patient as laparoscopic cholecystectomy.

General preparation of the patient

Patients undergoing any laparoscopic procedure are given appropriate premedication. Patients undergoing surgery of the large intestine are given the same bowel prep as for an open procedure. The most critical portion of the bowel prep is mechanical cleansing of the intestinal tract pre-operatively. Rather than shaving patients for any laparoscopic procedure the author prefers to use a plastic barrier which eliminates uncomfortable post-operative regrowth of hair. A foley catheter is used for most intestinal surgery but may be eliminated in such procedures as gastrostomies, jejunostomies, etc. Post-operatively the patients are allowed to mobilize as soon as possible. Because of the minimal incision required to complete laparoscopic intestinal surgery, patients have decreased pain and early ambulation becomes possible. Generally the patient is allowed an oral intake of fluids on the first or second post-operative day, depending on the return of peristaltic activity. Early experience would indicate that these patients have less post-operative ileus than with the open procedures. Patients undergoing laparoscopic intestinal surgery require approximately 25–50% less hospital time, depending upon the individual patient and the procedure performed. Post-operative antibiotics are administered at the discretion of the surgeon and should not vary because the procedure has been done laparoscopically.

Temporary gastrostomy

Both temporary and permanent gastrostomies may be performed under local anaesthesia, although general anaesthesia is preferred if the patient's general medical status allows. Laparoscopic gastrostomy may be performed on all patients requiring gastrostomy but is particularly indicated in the presence of large head and neck tumours or tumours of the oesophagus, where percutaneous endoscopic gastrostomy (PEG) cannot be performed.

If the patient has not had previous surgery, an umbilical incision is made at the upper portion of the umbilicus and an insufflation needle is used to insufflate the abdominal cavity to 15 mm of mercury (mmHg). If the surgery is being performed under local anaesthesia a lower insufflation limit, e.g. 8–10 mmHg, will suffice. At 10 mmHg the patient is more comfortable and, as a rule, will allow the placement of the temporary gastrostomy or permanent gastrostomy tube.

After insufflation of the abdomen, a 5 mm umbilical trocar is inserted and a 0° 5 mm laparoscope is passed through this port. A second 5 mm port is placed in the midline approximately three fingers' breadth below the xiphoid to assist in the placement of the gastrostomy tube. A small skin incision is made over the body of the stomach. The correct placing of this incision is confirmed by external palpation of the abdominal wall. Through this incision an appropriate gastrostomy tube is placed. The author uses the Russell–Cook gastrostomy tube (Cook Manufacturing, Bloomington, Ind.). This is performed as follows. A spinal needle is placed through the abdominal wall and, under direct vision, into the appropriate place in the body of the stomach. A guide wire is passed through this needle. The needle is then removed from the guide wire and a dilator (contained within the Russell–Cook catheter set) is passed over the guide wire. The stomach puncture is dilated to a sufficient size to allow the 'peel-away sheath' to be passed into the stomach over the dilator. The dilator is withdrawn and an 8 French Foley catheter is passed through this sheath and into the gastric cavity. The 'peel-away sheath' is then removed leaving the Foley catheter in place and the Foley catheter balloon is insufflated. The stomach may now be brought into contact with the abdominal wall by placing tension on the Foley catheter. If the surgeon prefers, the stomach may be sutured under direct vision to the abdominal wall. This is most easily accomplished by

placing a straight needle through the abdominal wall and grasping it with a needle holder through the upper 5 mm port. The stomach is sutured adjacent to the entrance of the gastrostomy tube. The needle is then passed back through the abdominal wall close to its entry site.

The stomach may be approximated to the abdominal wall for a period of 1 week or until adequate adhesions have allowed it to become permanently attached to this area. At the end of 7 days the sutures are removed and the gastrostomy will remain in place. Most surgeons feel that the placement of these gastric/abdominal wall sutures may not be a necessary part of this procedure. The gastrostomy tube may be used immediately.

Permanent Janeway gastrostomy or jejunostomy

Placement of a temporary laparoscopic gastrostomy is quite sufficient for those patients who require a gastrostomy on a short-term basis. A long-term or permanent Janeway gastrostomy or jejunostomy may be performed simply and quickly with the laparoscope. The Janeway gastrostomy allows the patient to remove the feeding tube when not in use and allows more freedom of activity. The decision of a permanent versus a short-term gastrostomy depends upon the individual and his pathology. As with all patients undergoing laparoscopic surgery, the patient must be informed of the possibility of converting from a laparoscopic procedure to an open procedure.

The insufflation needle is placed in the umbilicus and the abdominal cavity is insufflated with CO_2 to a pressure of 15 mmHg or, in the case of local anaesthesia, to 10 mmHg. A 5 mm port is placed in the umbilicus to allow adequate visualization of the stomach area and the establishment of a Janeway gastrostomy. A 0° lens should be used for this procedure. A second 5 mm port is placed two fingers' breadth below the xiphoid process in the midline and angled to the left of the falciform ligament. Through this 5 mm port the stomach is grasped and held as necessary to perform the gastrostomy or jejunostomy. Under direct vision an area of the stomach is located which will allow a satisfactory

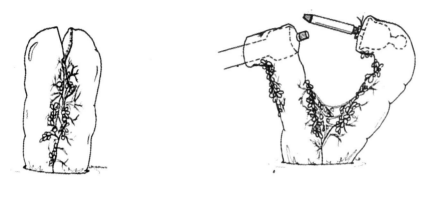

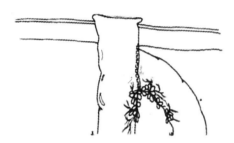

Fig. 15.1   Jejunostomy.

gastrostomy, usually along the greater curvature of the stomach. If a jejunostomy is desired, a loop of jejunum may be brought into a convenient place along the abdominal cavity to complete the jejunostomy. At this exact location a 12 mm port is placed through which the gastrostomy or jejunostomy will ultimately be positioned. The greater curvature of the stomach is brought into view and a small incision is made between the blood supply of the greater curvature of the stomach, or, in the case of the jejunostomy, the antimesenteric border is brought into the operative field. If the blood supply interferes with the formation of the gastrostomy, a vascular Endo GIA (USSC) may be used to divide the blood supply, but this is usually unnecessary. The Endo GIA containing 3.5 mm staples is passed through the 12 mm port and a wedge section of the stomach is stapled so as to form a conical gastrostomy tube (Figures 15.2a,b and c). The same procedure may be performed on a loop of the jejunum by using the Endo GIA to make the same

wedge cut as the stomach on the antimesenteric border of the jejunum. The apex of this conical gastrostomy (jejunostomy) tube is then placed with the grasper through the 12 mm port and is delivered to the skin surface as the port is removed in the same way as the gallbladder is removed after laparoscopic cholecystectomy. The tip of this gastrostomy (jejunostomy) tube is excised and a balloon catheter is placed into the stomach or jejunum. This may be used to place the stomach or jejunum under tension during the healing process until it firmly adheres to the tunnel created by the 12 mm port. The apex of the gastrostomy (jejunostomy) tube may be secured to the skin with interrupted absorbable sutures. The Foley catheter should be left in place for 1 week to assure firm adherence of the gastrostomy (jejunostomy) tube to the abdominal wall.

The placement of a Janeway gastrostomy (jejunostomy) is easily accomplished using two 5 mm ports and a 12 mm port and can be performed under local anaesthesia, if

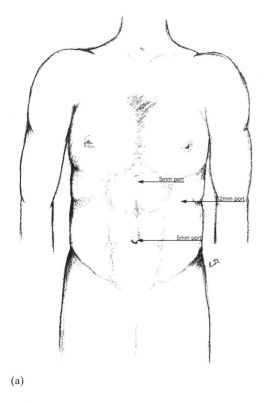

(a)

Fig. 15.2. (a)–(c)

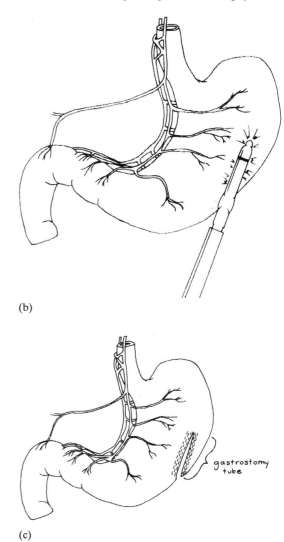

(b)

(c)

necessary. This procedure is done with better visualization through the laparoscope and takes less time than the open method. Because a 12 mm port does not divide the muscular structures a valve effect is produced on the gastrostomy (jejunostomy) tube which tends to reduce the irritation of the abdominal wall caused by secretions when the tube is not in place. After a week the gastrostomy (jejunostomy) should be securely adhered to the 12 mm port track so that the tube may be removed when it is not being used. This allows the patient freedom of activity and less irritation than if the tube is left in permanently.

Roux-en-y cutaneous jejunostomy

In cases where the small intestine is felt to be too small in diameter to create a Janeway type of jejunostomy, a Roux-en-y may be performed in approximately the same way as the Janeway jejunostomy. The procedure is carried out in the same manner as described above for gastrostomies and jejunostomies, except for the final step. In cases where the diameter of the small bowel is too narrow to allow the passage of the Endo GIA, an umbilical tape is passed through the 12 mm port using a reduction sleeve and a 5 mm instrument for the passage of this tape. This allows the pressure of the intra-abdominal CO_2 to be maintained throughout this procedure. The tape is then manipulated under the small bowel so as to be able to bring a loop of jejunum to the entrance of the 12 mm gastrostomy tube. In this case the hole in the abdominal wall created by the insertion of the 12 mm port must be enlarged by placing curved Mayo scissors along the 12 mm port through the abdominal wall and into the intra-abdominal cavity under direct vision. The curved Mayo scissors are used to stretch the fascia and muscle in this area to allow the 12 mm port to be removed with the loop of jejunum in direct contact with the tip of the port. This is done under direct vision and with minimal manipulation the small bowel loop may be removed through this port. After exteriorizing the loop of small bowel, it is then divided and an EEA autostapling device is used to accomplish a Roux-en-y anastomosis. The anvil of the EEA instrument is placed into the open end of the proximal end of the jejunum and a purse-string suture is used to close the jejunum around the anvil (or a purse-string instrument may be used for placement of the purse-string suture prior to insertion of the anvil). The EEA instrument itself is then passed down the distal limb of the small bowel and is placed on the antimesenteric border so as to open the EEA trocar through the antimesenteric border. The anvil is attached to the centre post and an anastomosis is made. This Roux-en-y limb is then replaced into the abdominal cavity and the open jejunum is sutured to the skin. The fascia itself has not been cut and, therefore, will quickly heal around this Roux-en-y jejunostomy limb (Figure 15.1).

Laparoscopic-assisted small bowel surgery

The small bowel is ideally suited for laparoscopic surgery because of its mobility and mobile mesentery. If exploration of the abdominal cavity has revealed a Meckel's diverticulum, this may be treated laparoscopically without difficulty. Usually with abdominal exploration a 5 mm or 10 mm port is placed in the umbilicus after insufflation of the abdominal cavity. This port may be replaced at this time with a 12 mm port to allow the use of

an Endo GIA. An additional 5 mm port is placed under direct vision in the midline above the pubis. A separate 5 mm port is placed in the right upper quadrant in the midclavicular line below the costal margin. Through these two 5 mm ports instruments will be used to manipulate the Meckel's diverticulum into an appropriate area for resection. After freeing adhesions to the Meckel's diverticulum and exposing it to the laparoscopic field, the 10 mm laparoscope is removed from the umbilicus and substituted with a 5 mm 0° scope which is passed through the suprapubic port. The Endo GIA is now passed through the umbilical 12 mm port and using a bowel grasping instrument the diverticulum may be manipulated into the jaws of the Endo GIA which is closed and fired. This instrument fires six rows of titanium staples dividing between the rows so as to leave three rows in place. No further suturing is necessary for removal of this diverticulum. The Endo GIA is then removed through the 12 mm port and grasping forceps are used to grasp the diverticulum and remove it through the 12 mm umbilical port under direct vision. The umbilical incision is easily repaired cosmetically and, because of the lack of musculature in this area, the fascia is easily closed with an interrupted suture, usually No. 1 PDS. Due to decreased innervation in the umbilicus, the pain is minimal. Therefore, the umbilicus is used for the 12 mm port and the 5 mm ports are placed as indicated. The same procedure may be used for the removal of an appendix.

Tumours of the small bowel may be handled in a similar manner. The same port placement is used for the majority of small bowel tumours. If the tumour tends to be more to the left of the patient and cannot be brought into the area on the right, a left midclavicular line port may be substituted for a right midclavicular line port. Excision of a small bowel tumour may be accomplished by locating the tumour and bringing it into the area of the 12 mm umbilical port. The incision is extended superiorly in the midline to allow the delivery of the tumour and portion of small bowel through a small incision. Following this an extracorporeal anastomosis, similar to that described for colon surgery, may be performed. The small bowel is then replaced into the abdominal cavity. The benefit to the patient consists of a thorough exploratory laparotomy through a small incision with a small bowel resection through the same minimal incision.

Intracorporeal laparoscopic small bowel anastomosis may be accomplished by the advanced laparoscopist. Usually resection of the small bowel is performed through the three ports as described above. However, a fourth port for countertraction may be necessary if extensive removal of the small bowel mesentery is to be performed. This fourth port is placed as far away from the other two ports as possible so as to place the mesentery in direct view of the camera which may be placed in any of the 5 mm ports, again using a 0° lens with a 5 mm laparoscope. Through the 12 mm umbilical port the vascular GIA may be used to divide the small bowel mesentery, after appropriate mesenteric 'windows' have been made between vessels with electrosurgical scissors, or dissectors, on the antimesenteric border. After creating a 'V'-shaped incision in the small bowel mesentery, the small bowel is then ready for anastomosis. In a patient with an extremely thin small bowel, both loops of small bowel may simultaneously be placed into the jaws of the 3.5 Endo GIA. When this instrument is fired it closes both loops of small bowel so as to prevent spillage in the abdominal cavity. This looped specimen may later be removed. Anastomosis is accomplished by making a small opening in both loops of small bowel which are stapled together by virtue of the fact they were both placed in the jaws of the same Endo GIA instrument. The Endo GIA is then passed down the antimesenteric openings in each limb of the small bowel and is fired which will, in effect, accomplish a side-to-side anastomosis. At the time of writing the 3 mm Endo GIA was the only instrument available and, therefore, had to be fired twice so as to create an anastomosis which was sufficient in length to prevent an obstruction in this area. Currently being developed is a 6 cm Endo GIA which will be passed through a 15 mm port. After creating a side-to-side anastomosis the defect in the small bowel, through which the shaft of the Endo GIA for this anastomosis has been passed, is then closed with the Endo GIA. The area is inspected to ensure that there are no areas of leakage in this anastomosis. If there is a suspected weakness, or if tension is placed on the small bowel at the level of the anastomosis, a laparoscopic suture may be inserted to correct this. The small

bowel specimen may now be placed into an intra-abdominal laparoscopic retrieving bag to remove the specimen intact. This bag is placed through the 12 mm port. The specimen is then manipulated into the bag and the bag is removed by extending the incision around the 12 mm port as necessary in the midline. The length of the incision necessary to remove the specimen allows an extracorporeal anastomosis of the small bowel to be made more easily and more efficiently so that, at present, extracorporeal anastomosis remains the preferred option.

Laparoscopic colectomy

Laparoscopic colon surgery is at an early stage in development. It has the advantage of more accurately diagnosing associated diseases, such as metastatic disease in the liver. It also allows the surgeon to assess all other areas of the abdomen for metastatic diseases and other pathology. Most significantly, the obvious advantage to laparoscopic colectomy is the lack of pain in the early post-operative period. These patients are able to ambulate, pain free, on their first post-operative day. Post-operative ileus may be shortened, although a few patients have taken a post-operative period which would correspond to an open colectomy before having active bowel sounds. The hospital stay of patients undergoing laparoscopic colectomy has been shortened and has averaged 4 days. In our own small series there have been no complications to date. Laparoscopic colectomy requires the same operative time as open colectomy (60–90 minutes) if extracorporeal anastomosis is carried out.

One of the major problems, especially seen with left colon lesions, is the identification of the pathologic tumour to be resected. If this cannot be identified, obviously the patient must be converted to having an open procedure. To avoid this problem, pre-operative injection with methylene blue through the colonoscope has been carried out with varying success. The 'lost lesion problem' is now avoided by pre-operative placement of metallic clips (Olympus) proximal and distal to the lesion in question via a colonoscope. A pre-operative abdominal X-ray gives the exact location of the lesion. However, if there is any question at the time of surgery, fluoroscopy can be used to identify the lesion. The metallic clips are best placed the day before or on the day of surgery. With right colon lesions, this is usually unnecessary. As an alternative to this procedure, and generally, it is advisable in all colectomies to position the patient so that colonoscopy may be performed under anaesthesia at the time of surgery. This will ensure proper identification of the lesion whether benign or malignant. Carcinomas as well as benign tumours may be removed. In all specimens removed the same number of lymph nodes have been contained within the specimen as with colectomies performed by open laparotomy.

Colectomies with extracorporeal anastomosis (Figure 15.3)

All colectomies are performed in a similar manner. The insufflation needle is inserted into the umbilical area and the abdomen is insufflated to 15 mm of mercury. The 10 mm Surgiport is placed in the umbilicus and a 10 mm 30° laparoscopic camera is used for all colectomies. The 30° lens allows direct visualization of the ureter as well as the ability more efficiently to look into the gutter of the colon being resected. The patient is usually placed in the Trendelenburg position and is rotated to the side opposite the colon to be removed. In patients undergoing a right colectomy, a 5 mm port is placed in the midclavicular line below the costal margin. It is used for upward traction of the right colon and later for dissection of the hepatic flexure. A 10 mm suprapubic port is placed in the midline in both the right and left colectomies. In the left colectomy, a similar midclavicular line port is placed below the left costal margin. All colectomies are done using only three ports. To mobilize the right colon, the bowel grasper is inserted through the upper 5 mm port and is used to reflect the colon superiorly and medially. Through the 10 mm suprapubic port, 5 mm electrosurgical instruments are used to dissect along the white line or avascular peritoneal reflection to mobilize the colon. Then by a combination of sharp and blunt dissection, it is reflected medially as would be done in an open case. Any bleeding encountered may be controlled through this port with the Endoclip (USSC).

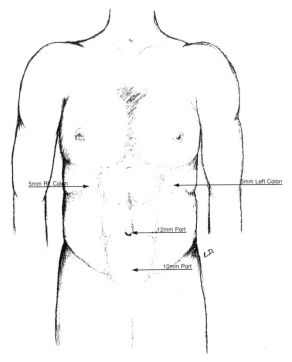

Fig. 15.3. Port placement; right and left colon.

After initial mobilization of the cecum by incising along the white line, the ureter is identified immediately lying medial to the psoas muscle. It is constant in location and is easily identified in the pelvic area. Locating the psoas muscle initially and following it posteriorly is the easiest method of identification of the ureter outside the pelvis. The ureter is located posterior and medial in a 'groove' along the psoas muscle. In the male patient, testicular vessels may sometimes be confused with the ureter but these should be easily identified by tracing them to the internal inguinal ring. Alternatively the ureter may be identified by following the iliac vessels from the pelvis superiorly and identifying it as it crosses over the iliac artery. In thin patients it is seen through the pelvic peritoneum. After identifying the ureter, the dissection can proceed fairly quickly as with open surgery. Following complete mobilization of the right colon up to and including the hepatic flexure, the colon now may be brought superiorly to a position above the umbilicus. The exact location is identified by compressing the abdominal wall and observing this area

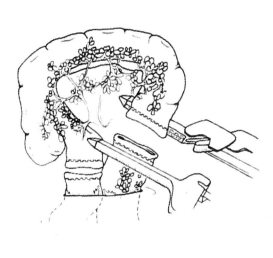

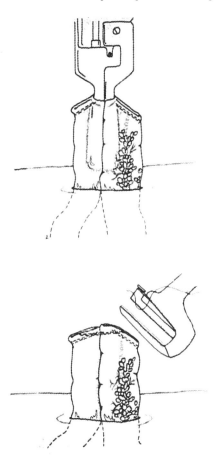

Fig. 15.4. External right colon anastomosis.

laparoscopically. At this point a transverse skin incision is made extending 3–5 cm in length, depending on the size of the lesion. The incision is carried down to the rectus sheath and the rectus muscle is reflected medially without dividing it. The posterior peritoneum is then incised creating loss of pneumoperitoneum. The colon is delivered into this muscle sparing incision and exteriorized through this wound. With minimal traction the blood supply of the colon can be ligated down to the base of the vessels so as to include the entire lymphatic supply. The colon is anastomosed exteriorly and returned to the abdominal cavity (Figure 15.4). This external anastomosis may be performed using a GIA on the antimesenteric surface so as to accomplish a side-to-side anastomosis following which the TA-90 or 90 mm GIA may be used to staple the ends of the side-to-side anastomosis. Peritoneal and fascial layers are closed in separate anatomical layers with a continuous running No. 1 absorbable suture. The pneumoperitoneum is re-established and the anastomosis must be checked to ensure proper alignment of the anastomosis without twisting. Haemostasis is also checked. The same procedure is carried out for the left colon lesion although the left colon is slightly less capable of being mobilized.

The alternative to extracorporeal anastomosis is a complete internal colectomy with internal anastomosis. This will necessitate the placement of another 5 mm port at the level of the umbilicus on the side opposite the colon being resected to manipulate the mesocolon. Instead of a 10 mm port a 12 mm umbilical port is used through which the vascular and 3.5 Endoclip are used. The mesocolon is held by 5 mm dissecting or bowel grasping instruments through two ports and the third port is used to pass a hot dissector or scissors in order to

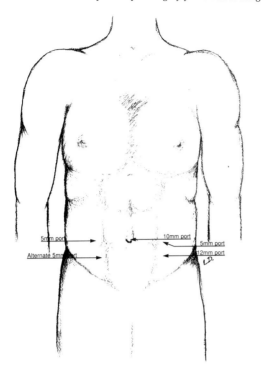

Fig. 15.5. Port placement; low anterior resection.

make windows in the avascular portion of the mesocolon. The mesocolon may then be divided using the vascular Endo GIA taking care to avoid injury to the ureter. After complete division of the mesocolon internal anastomosis may be accomplished as described under small bowel anastomosis or the surgeon may proceed at this time with extracorporeal anastomosis. Division of the mesocolon and internal anastomosis with the Endo GIA is somewhat time consuming, expensive and probably not necessary in view of the necessity of making a substantial 2–5 cm incision to deliver the pathological specimen. A portion of the mesocolon may be divided internally, however, to facilitate mobilization of the colon combined with extracorporeal anastomosis.

Low anterior resection

Performing a low anterior resection requires that the ports be placed lower on the abdominal wall than usual (Figure 15.5). Low anterior resection is formed by placing a 10 mm port in

the umbilicus. A 5 mm port is placed at the level of umbilicus lateral to the rectus sheath on both the right and left side. A 12 mm port is placed in the left lower quadrant, again lateral to the rectus sheath just above the bony pelvis. A 10 mm 30° laparoscope is passed through the umbilical port and is used throughout the procedure. The 5 mm ports lateral to the rectus sheath are used for the manipulation of the colon. Initially, a 5 mm reducing patch is placed over the 12 mm port and this is used in conjunction to other 5 mm ports to visualize the mesocolon. The avascular areas of the mesocolon are opened to allow a vascular Endo GIA to be introduced through the 12 mm port and divide the blood supply to the rectosigmoid area being removed. After dividing the mesocolon the Endo GIA is then used to divide the distal colon, usually two 3.5 Endo GIAs will be required. A small muscle-splitting incision, or an incision similar to that described under right colectomy, is made in the left lower quadrant using the area of the 12 mm port and the specimen is delivered through this incision. The colon is divided and the distal pathologic portion is removed (Figure 15.6).

A purse-string suture is placed in the remaining proximal colon and the anvil of the EEA autostapling instrument is placed in the proximal left colon. This proximal left colon is then replaced into the abdominal cavity and the muscle-splitting or muscle-reflecting incision is closed with a continuous running No. 1 absorbable suture again to make the abdomen airtight for insufflation with CO_2. The abdomen is insufflated and the EEA is passed into the rectum transanally. The EEA is opened to allow the EEA trocar to extend through the rectal stump. A loop-ligature such as an Endoloop (Ethicon) or Surgi-tie (USSC) is placed on this trocar. This ligature is cut long and the trocar is removed from the centre post of the EEA and is placed in the pelvis. At the termination of the procedure, this trocar can be removed when removing the 10 mm umbilical port by grasping the ligature tied to the trocar and manipulating it into the 10 mm port. The proximal colon containing the anvil is then manipulated in place following which the EEA instrument is closed and the anastomosis is accomplished. The transanal EEA is removed and a Foley catheter with a 30 cc balloon is inserted into the rectum and

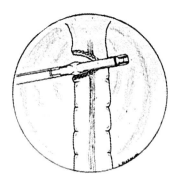

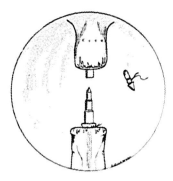

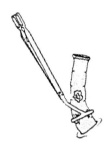

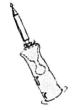

Fig. 15.6. Low anterior resection.

inflated. A saline solution is passed into the rectum through this catheter and the anastomosis is checked for leaks.

Abdominal perineal resection

Abdominal perineal resection fortunately is an extremely rare procedure because of the ability to do extremely low anterior resections with internal anastomoses. The procedure, however, may be more efficiently carried out laparoscopically than with the open method. After insufflation of the abdominal cavity, a 10 mm port is placed in the umbilicus; a 10 mm port is placed in the suprapubic area; and a 5 mm is placed at the level of the umbilicus on the right lateral to the rectus muscle. A 12 mm port is placed at this same level to the left of the rectus muscle. The 30° 10 mm laparoscope is placed in the umbilicus and 5 mm instruments are used through the 10 mm suprapubic port and the right 5 mm and left 12 mm ports to take the colon down from its peritoneal reflection by incising along the white line and reflecting it medially. After complete mobilization of the rectosigmoid area, the ureters are identified and continually observed through the procedure. By manipulation of the mesocolon, incisions may be made in the avascular portion to isolate the blood vessels. The Endo GIA is passed through the 12 mm left port and the mesocolon is divided with vascular staples. The rectosigmoid colon is divided with the Endo GIA through the 12 mm port and will later be pulled through this same port under direct vision to form a colostomy. The 12 mm port incision may have to be stretched with curved Mayo scissors or extended depending upon the size of the sigmoid colon used for the colostomy. This colostomy incision is the only abdominal incision required in an abdominal perineal resection. The peritoneum overlying the pelvis is incised either prior to division of the colon or after the division of the colon, depending upon the ability to manipulate the colon in view of the local area. The pelvic dissection should be completed as much as possible prior to the division of the rectosigmoid colon. The peritoneum is excised along the colon and anteriorly between the bladder and the colon, the same as with an open procedure. The lateral pedicle of the colon may be divided between Endoclips leaving at least two Endoclips in place. If a larger vessel is noted, a pretied ligature such as a Surgi-tie or Endoloop may be used to further secure this vessel. Throughout the procedure of right and left colectomies, care should be taken to maintain meticulous haemostasis in order to optimize the laparoscopic visualization of this area. After sufficient mobilization of the rectum, the colon, if not previously divided, is then divided and placed in the retroperitoneal area. The hernia stapler clip applier (USSC) may now be used to reperitonealize the area, taking care to avoid injury to the ureter. With the peritoneum closed, the specimen may be removed through the perianal incision in the standard manner. Prior to removal of the specimen, the colostomy should be formed. After the perineum is opened the closure of the pelvic peritoneum is insufficient to maintain a pneumoperitoneum and laparoscopic vision will be lost.

Conclusion

Laparoscopic colectomy has now been performed in many patients. The operative time for this approach to colectomy was not significantly longer than normal operating time when extracorporeal anastomoses were performed or when abdominal perineal resections were performed. The pathological specimen removed was equivalent to the same anatomical specimen removed from an open procedure. The margins of the specimens were the same as those from an open procedure and the number of lymph nodes removed in the mesocolon were the same as those patients undergoing standard laparotomy. Post-operative ileus appears to be decreased as does total hospital stay. Perhaps the greatest benefit to the patient is a substantial reduction in post-operative pain. The incision is about the size of an appendicectomy incision and consists of a muscle-splitting or muscle-sparing incision. These factors contribute equally to the lack of post-operative pain. At the time of writing, the division of the blood supply under direct vision using the vascular Endo GIA is being

performed without difficulty. Additionally, internal anastomoses are also being done with the 3.5 Endo GIA in selected cases. It is as yet too early to determine whether this makes a significant difference in the patient's post-operative period. In all cases an additional incision is still required to remove the specimen (except in the abdominal perineal resection). For this reason external anastomosis and division of the mesocolon externally is still preferred at present. When close adherence to surgical principle is carried out, with particular reference to identification of the ureter, there should be no significant complications. New instrumentation is currently under development that may more easily allow complete colectomies laparoscopically with removal of the specimen through laparoscopic ports.

Equipment utilized in laparoscopic intestinal surgery

The majority of the equipment used for laparoscopic intestinal surgery is the same as that for other laparoscopic procedures. A variety of ports, including 5, 10, 12 and 15 mm ports, will be necessary as well as the standard laparoscopic camera, light source and insufflator, etc. Standard equipment such as graspers, scissors and dissectors may be used as in other procedures. Peculiar to colon surgery will be the necessity for a 30° or 45° 5 mm and 10 mm laparoscope. The angle of the lens allows the surgeon better vision of certain areas to be dissected, particularly when doing colon surgery. The laparoscopic clip applier, such as the Endoclip (USSC), is used in vessel ligation. In addition to this instrument, special equipment such as a vascular Endo GIA (USSC) or linear stapler (Ethicon) may be used to divide the mesentery or mesocolon whenever vascular structures need to be controlled. The 3.5 Endo GIA is used to divide the appendix, stomach, intestine, etc. This instrument, which measures 3 cm in length, is passed down a 12 mm port. A 6 cm Endo GIA instrument is placed through a larger 15 mm port. This larger instrument will decrease the number of cartridges used to complete a procedure and should decrease the time necessary to do the procedure. This large Endo GIA (USSC) or linear cutter (Ethicon) will also increase the potential for internal anastomosis. Other instruments are currently being examined to complete the internal anastomosis. Specimen retrieval from a laparoscopic procedure continues to be a concern of laparoscopic surgery but is in the process of being remedied by additional new equipment. Bowel grasping instruments are rapidly being altered and developed to be able to manipulate all portions of the intestine with ease through laparoscopic surgery. Both reusable and disposable instruments, such as Babcock clamps, retractors, and intestinal clamps, are also now available from many manufacturers. With the development of additional instrumentation, laparoscopic intestinal surgery will become a routine procedure.

16

Laparoscopic herniorrhaphy

John D. Corbitt Jr

Introduction

The complete removal of the gallbladder, laparoscopically, was first performed by Philip Mouret in Lyons, France, in 1987.[1] Within a short time this procedure began to gain recognition throughout the world and is progressively becoming the procedure of choice for removal of the diseased gallbladder in the developed world.

In addition to the 500,000 cholecystectomies performed a year, an equal number of inguinal herniorrhaphies are performed in the United States alone.[2] While excellent results have been reported in personal series of inguinal herniorrhaphies, or in series performed by specialists, many reports in the literature still reveal high recurrences of inguinal hernias through a groin approach. It, therefore, seemed reasonable to approach this problem laparoscopically in search of the ideal hernia repair.

Historic prospective of inguinal herniorrhaphies

The groin approach described by Bassini in 1884 placed emphasis on reconstruction of the inguinal floor. In the published literature, this repair has as high as a 10% recurrence rate, thought to be as a result of coapting under tension, which would not normally be in opposition to each other. The recurrence rate has been significantly improved by tension-free repair using prosthetic meshes to reconstruct the floor through a groin approach, such as that originally described by Lichtenstein. His latest personal series of 1,000 patients shows an extremely low recurrence rate approaching 0% (personal communication). A previously reported 1–6 year follow-up of 1,522 patients shows a recurrence rate of 1.3% (2 patients).[3] Stoppa and Warlaumont[4] and Nyhus[5] have reported the preperitoneal approach using prosthetic mesh to cover the floor of the inguinal canal with an extremely low recurrence rate of 1.4–1.7% (572 and 203 repairs). These repairs have utilized the 'giant prosthesis' covering the majority of the floor of the pelvis.

High ligation of the sac and closure of the internal ring, to prevent recurrences, was first emphasized by Henry Marcy[6–9] and later modified by LaRoque[10] who performed over 1,700 of these procedures. Unfortunately, the information regarding the first reported 'transabdominal' approaches to inguinal hernia repair is scanty.

Early approaches to laparoscopic herniorrhaphy

L.W. Popp[11] in 1990 was the first to publish a report of a laparoscopic repair in which case a dehydrated piece of dura mater was secured with catgut endo-sutures tied extracorporeally over the internal ring. Dr Ralph Ger[12,13] reported a series of 13 patients whose hernias were repaired during laparotomy using a Kocher clamp and Michel clips to close the peritoneal opening of the inguinal hernia. The sac was left in place in these patients (and later, experimentally, in a study using dogs, also published by Ger). The patients whose hernias were repaired by Ger during laparotomy have been followed for more than 5 years with only one recurrence. The thirteenth herniorrhaphy reported by Dr Ger in his clinical series was performed using a special instrument, the herniastat, laparoscopically guided and used to close the internal ring. Dr Ger[14] continues to use this same technique of laparoscopic closure of the peritoneal opening (internal ring) without removing the hernia sac. This procedure is mainly limited to small hernias in women and young men. In the larger hernias and direct hernias he inserts mesh directly into the distal sac, and staples it in place when closing the peritoneal defect or internal ring. Unfortunately, after two and a half years he reports an overall recurrence rate of about 30% in a series of 30 patients (personal communication). These recurrences were mainly due to complications or failure of the original herniastat, small staples, or other technical problems which are currently being addressed by Dr Ger.

Utilizing the concept of a tension-free repair, Leonard Schultz (Minneapolis, Minnesota, personal communication) began one of the first series of laparoscopic herniorrhaphies in 1989, by placing a Marlex plug in the inguinal canal and a patch over the internal ring, the latter of which was covered by peritoneum at the termination of the procedure. Large, direct hernias were repaired by Dr Schultz by stuffing as much mesh as necessary into the defect to fill the hernia so the intestines could not later protrude into the hernia space. Schultz has performed this procedure in more than 100 patients. Using experience gained from the work of Marcy and LaRoque, Corbitt[15] added, to Schultz's repair, ligation of the sac in the indirect inguinal hernia using Endoloops initially, and later the Endo GIA (USSC). This also took advantage of a tension-free repair and added high ligation of the sac. The patients were allowed to return to normal activity in both series immediately. After a 2 year follow-up using a plug and patch graft with or without closure of the sac, a depressing recurrence rate in excess

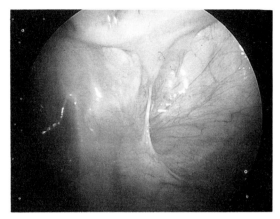

Fig. 16.1   Indirect inguinal hernia with colon attached

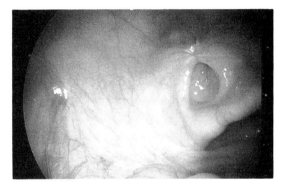

Fig. 16.2   Recurrent direct hernia

of 25% has been observed (Corbitt and Schultz). Both surgeons noted that occasionally if an indirect hernia was repaired, the recurrence may be found in the direct space and vice versa. A further cause of recurrence was a small patch slipping off the hernia defect. The conclusion by both surgeons was that a large piece of mesh covering the entire inguinal floor, fixed in place by sutures or staples, similar to a Stoppa repair, should be performed. Of greatest benefit in the early laparoscopic herniorrhaphy was the observation that a tension-free, painless repair could be performed allowing the patient to return to normal activity the following day. The debilitating complications associated with a groin approach, such as haematomas, spermatic cord injuries, ischaemic orchitis, neuralgias, extreme post-operative discomfort, prolonged recovery period and the lack of ability to rapidly return to normal activities, were much less frequent in the laparoscopic hernia repair.

Indications for laparoscopic herniorrhaphy

At present, the major indication for laparoscopic herniorrhaphy is bilateral hernia because of the lack of post-operative pain and the recurrent hernia because of the lack of distortion of the anatomy. Patients who wish an early return to work are also requesting laparoscopic repair.

Laparoscopic herniorrhaphy also provides the surgeon with the ability more clearly to diagnose a hernia in question as well as an unsuspected hernia on the contralateral side. If an unsuspected contralateral hernia is found this can be repaired more efficiently and quickly laparoscopically.

New approaches in laparoscopic hernia repair

Modified plug and patch repair

As a result of the benefits of laparoscopic herniorrhaphy, and the encouraging results obtained in the tension-free and preperitoneal repair, a new prospective on laparoscopic herniorrhaphy is presently in progress.

Dr Leonard Schultz (personal communication) initially continued to use the plug and patch method by making an incision across the superior aspect of the hernia defect whether it was direct or indirect. He then reduced the sac into the abdominal cavity and placed the plug into the space where the sac had been. A large patch was then positioned over the floor of the canal so as to cover most of the inguinal region. These preperitoneal patches were then covered with peritoneum to prevent intestinal adhesions to the prosthetic mesh. Schultz did not staple the polypropylene mesh in place, but rather allowed the intra-abdominal pressure against the peritoneum to control migration of the mesh until it adhered to the abdominal wall, which usually takes only 24 hours. The plug used in this repair was usually approximately 3–5 cm in length. The floor of the canal was usually covered by a portion of mesh 6 × 8 cm. After early recurrences,

Schultz has now increased the size of the mesh which he currently staples in place. The plug has also been eliminated because of the ability of the patient to palpate it. Dr Schultz now performs a preperitoneal repair which will be described in detail. Independently, Corbitt developed the same preperitoneal approach but eliminated the plug and fixed the mesh in place.

Intraperitoneal 'onlay' mesh repair

Fitzgibbons *et al.*[16] (personal communication) first reported experimental repair of hernias in animals by placing a piece of Marlex or Goretex mesh in the intra-abdominal cavity over the indirect hernia, leaving the distal sac in place. This mesh was tacked to the peritoneum and covered with Interceed (Johnson & Johnson) to protect the mesh from internal adhesions to the small bowel. While early results were promising it became apparent that this was not the ultimate hernia repair, especially for the direct hernia. This was because Interceed did not offer a significant adhesive barrier, and Gor-tex did not allow significant fibrous ingrowth unlike Marlex. It is believed that this fibrous ingrowth is responsible for the permanent hernia repair and Fitzgibbons has therefore discontinued the use of Gore-tex. The early animal experience also indicated that when the indirect inguinal hernia was repaired by the onlay technique using Marlex and leaving the distal sac in place, the distal sac was obliterated in approximately 6 weeks and the repair succeeded. There was an acceptably low recurrence rate in animal hernias repaired in this way and Fitzgibbons continues to repair indirect hernias using Marlex mesh as an onlay graft tacked directly to the peritoneum. In summary, a rectangular polypropylene mesh is placed over the internal inguinal ring defect and the sac of the larger indirect hernia is left in place. The indirect sac in a large defect is incised circumferentially around the neck and the distal portion is left intact. The polypropylene mesh is then tacked to the peritoneum to cover completely the indirect defect.

Using the same procedure on direct hernias, Fitzgibbons found early recurrences due to the herniation of the mesh together with the peritoneum into the direct defect. The conclusion was that a properitoneal approach (see below) to the direct hernia would give improved results. Fitzgibbons, therefore, continued to repair only indirect hernias with this technique. Follow-up of the onlay technique revealed an acceptable 2% recurrence rate in over 500 cases followed up for as long as 2 years. Unfortunately, significant complications resulted from adhesions to the exposed graft and as a result Fitzgibbons suggests close observation in a controlled setting until results of further follow-up are available.

Other advocates of a laparoscopic onlay peritoneal approach by placing such prosthetic materials as Gor-tex (PTFE) over the defect, both direct and indirect, include Toy and Smoot[17] and Spaw. Both these groups suture or tack the prosthesis directly onto the peritoneal surface to cover either the direct or indirect space. In Toy and Smoot's original series the indirect sac was inverted into the abdominal cavity and ligated with a pretied laparoscopic suture (Endoloop, Ethicon) or a laparoscopic stapling device (Endo GIA, USSC). The large pseudo-sac in the direct hernia was treated in a similar manner. Smaller, direct sacs were left in place. After the first year there was a 30% recurrence rate if a small patch was tacked to the peritoneum (Toy, personal communication). There was also a significant number of cord injuries with inversion of the sac. Toy and Smoot have now changed their procedure so that a large prosthesis covers both the direct and indirect space. Cooper's ligament and the inguinal ligament are exposed to allow fixation of the graft medially. The graft is stapled laterally through the peritoneum to the deep fascia. In order to avoid cord injuries the distal sac is now left in place. Spaw also exposes Cooper's ligament and inguinal ligament medially and staples to the deep structures laterally using the onlay or intraperitoneal procedure. The graft is exposed to the abdominal contents which allows possible post-operative adhesion.

The tendency in the onlay technique is to expose more of the preperitoneal space which is a shift toward the preperitoneal or extraperitoneal approach. Ligation of the large sac is also giving way to amputation of the sac at its neck and leaving the distal sac in place. In a Nyhus Type I indirect hernia, Spaw places sutures between the transversalis fascia and the iliopubic tract to close the defect without inversions or ligation of the sac and without placement of the Gor-tex graft.

The tension-free preperitoneal approach

Using a preperitoneal tension-free repair all hernias, whether primary or recurrent, direct, indirect or femoral, can be repaired. The development of the Endo-hernia stapler by USSC and a similar stapler by Ethicon have made the preperitoneal approach an efficient and reasonable repair in terms of time. This approach is also supported anatomically and historically.

Pre-operatively appropriate premedication is used. The author favours a scopolamine patch placed behind the ear of the patient the night prior to surgery to prevent post-operative nausea and vomiting. An appropriate prophylactic long-acting antibiotic is administered pre-operatively. The patient is not shaved for this procedure but a protective barrier, such as Steri-drape, is used. Initially when the procedure requires excessive time for the surgeon to perform laparoscopic herniorrhaphy, a Foley catheter is put into place. However, as more experience is gained and the operative time is reduced, the catheter may be eliminated so long as the surgeon has been assured that the patient has voided pre-operatively. All laparoscopic herniorrhaphies are performed under general anaesthesia with the patient placed in the Trendelenburg position.

A 12 mm incision is made in the umbilicus and a Veress needle is used to insufflate the abdominal cavity with CO_2 to 15 mm of mercury. A 12 mm port is inserted through the umbilical incision and a 10 mm laparoscopic camera with a 0° or, preferably, 30° lens is used to observe direct placement of two additional secondary ports. These ports are placed at or below the level of the umbilicus, lateral to the rectus sheath. Secondary 5 mm ports may be used as these minimize the patient's post-operative pain and give a better cosmetic result. Routinely, however, the secondary ports are 10 mm. The 12 mm port is placed in the umbilicus for cosmetic reasons and because of the need to close the fascia at all 12 mm port sites. Of greatest importance, however, is the ability to repair a hernia on either side using the hernia stapler (requiring the 12 mm port) through this centrally located umbilical port. Using the two secondary ports

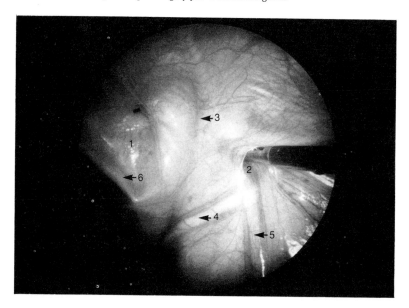

Fig. 16.3 (a) 1. Recurrent direct inguinal hernia 2. small indirect defect, 3. inferior epigastric vessels, 4. vas, 5. testicular vessels, 6. umbilical ligament.

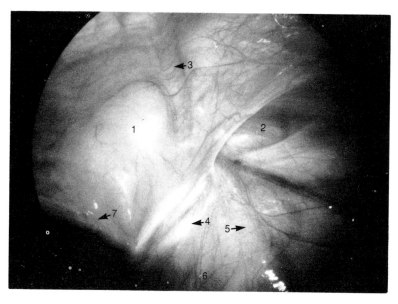

Fig. 16.3 (b) 1. Direct defect, 2. indirect defect, 3. inferior epigastric vessels, 4. vas, 5. testicular vessels, 6. iliac vessels, 7. umbilical ligament.

the surgeon standing on the opposite side of the hernia may now incise the peritoneum transversely superior to the hernia defect creating a transverse incision, bounded medically by the area of the umbilical ligament, and laterally by the edge of the indirect defect or the approximate area of the anterior superior iliac spine. Initially, dissection of the pelvis is easier from the side opposite the hernia. After minimal experience, however, a left-handed surgeon may stand on

the right side of the table and a right-handed surgeon on the left side of the table. The camera operator standing on the side opposite the hernia will operate the camera and hold portions of the peritoneum as indicated throughout the procedure. In large indirect inguinal hernias as well as some (usually recurrent) large direct hernias, the distal sac is left in place by extending the transverse incision 360° circumferentially around the neck of the sac (making sure the incision is made inside

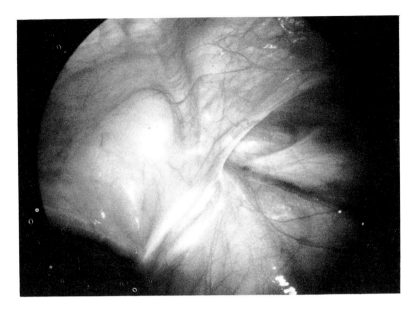

Fig. 16.4 Boundaries of the transverse incision across direct and indirect defect with 360° incision around internal ring of the indirect defect

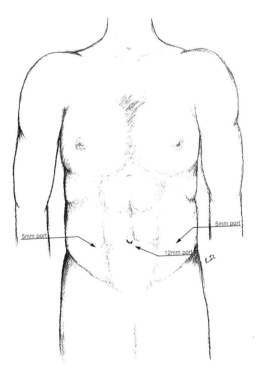

Fig. 16.5 Hernia; port placement

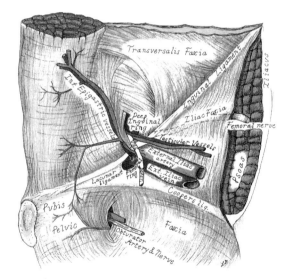

Fig. 16.6 Schematic of pelvic floor

Leaving the distal sac in place is not likely to produce a hydrocele. The sac obliterates in approximately 6 weeks. By avoiding unnecessary dissection of the distal sac, haematomas and injuries to cord structures and the genitofemoral nerve are avoided. When continuing the circumferential incision around the cord structures posteriorly in the indirect defect, care should be taken to avoid injury to

the neck of the sac rather than flush with the peritoneal cavity). This allows for the future closure of the peritoneum preventing a hole where this circumferential incision was made.

these structures. Most direct hernias are reduced into the abdominal cavity and the fatty contents removed. If the direct hernia is extremely large or has a narrow neck, it is excised as with the indirect hernia. The posterior dissection of the flap in the area of an indirect inguinal hernia is the most critical part of the peritoneal dissection. In this area the vas deferens, the testicular vessels and below the inguinal ligament, the iliac vessels are located. A 10 mm laparoscope with a 30° or 0° lens remains in the umbilical port for this incision in the peritoneum and for further dissection.

The flaps of the peritoneum are firstly developed posteriorly, then anteriorly to expose the entire floor of the inguinal canal. Dissection is begun posteriorly to prevent the anterior flap from occluding the field by hanging in front of the laparoscope. Anteriorly the inferior epigastric vessels are left attached to the anterior abdominal wall, and the peritoneum is removed from them. Dissection is extended posteriorly below the level of the inguinal ligament or iliopubic tract which comprises the posterior portion of the internal ring (Figure 16.1). Caution is observed while dissecting posterior to the iliopubic tract especially in the area of the internal ring because of the location of the testicular vessels and, slightly more posteriorly, the iliac vessels. This area forms a triangle (the 'triangle of doom'). After exposing the entire floor, the 10 mm laparoscope is removed and the prosthesis is pushed into the abdominal cavity through the 12 mm port, if the secondary ports are 5 mm. If 10 mm secondary ports are used, the prosthesis may be pushed through either of these. Originally Marlex mesh was used for this procedure but a newly developed mesh, SurgiPro (USSC), is now being used. SurgiPro, like Marlex, is a polypropylene material. The size of each prosthesis differs depending upon the size of the patient, but a mesh measuring 3 × 5 inches (7.5 × 12.5 cm) will be sufficient in 95% of cases. A horizontal line the length of the mesh and two vertical lines are inked on either end of the mesh approximately 2 cm from the margins forming an 'H' on the mesh. This will facilitate proper orientation of the mesh in the pelvis so it is not stapled at an angle which prevents coverage of the entire floor. It also allows the surgeon to identify the important structures obscured by the mesh by

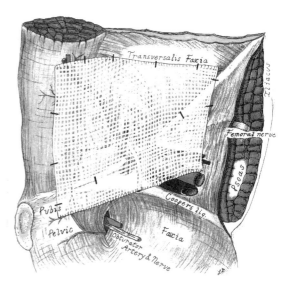

Fig. 16.7 Schematic of mesh covering pelvic floor

lifting a corner of the prosthesis and orienting the structure to the lines drawn on the mesh. The 10 mm laparoscope remains in the 12 mm port. The graft which has been placed blindly into the abdominal cavity is easily found in the pelvis and is then placed across the entire floor of the pelvis to cover the area of both the indirect and direct inguinal hernias in the preperitoneal area. Fixation of the anterior portion of the mesh is usually done first and assisted by external compression of the abdominal wall when firing the staple. This external compression of the abdominal wall allows counterpressure which allows the staple to be properly seated into the fascia. The mesh is placed over the epigastric vessels and it is important to avoid stapling these. After placing the anterior staples, the mesh may be stapled either laterally or medially. Medially the mesh is stapled into the area of the pubic tubercle. If the staples appear to bend or will not penetrate the area, the stapler should be moved slightly to one side or the other to penetrate periosteal tissue or the inguinal ligament as it joins the pubic tubercle. New, shorter, 4 mm staples (USSC) will penetrate the periosteum of the pubic tubercle on Cooper's ligament without difficulty. Laterally the mesh extends to the area of the anterior superior iliac spine. Below the ileopubic tract laterally branches of the femoral nerve extend

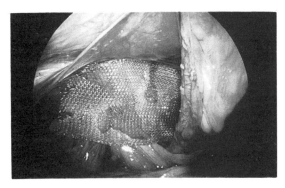

Fig. 16.8   Mesh in place

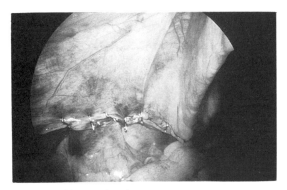

Fig. 16.9   Closure of peritoneum

circumferential incision made around the sac to provide some redundant peritoneum for future closure. In this case, as well as in the large indirect inguinal hernia, the distal portion of the sac is left intact, so as to reduce injury to the cord structures and genitofemoral nerve. Leaving the distal sac in place will not cause formation of a hydrocele. If a lipoma is encountered in this dissection, it is removed. It is, however, not necessary to remove all fatty tissue in the preperitoneal area prior to stapling the mesh in place.

The extraperitoneal approach

The extraperitoneal approach has been independently described by McKernan and Phillips. McKernan places a Hassan trocar via the umbilicus directly into the extraperitoneal space. The abdominal cavity is not entered. The extraperitoneal space is insufflated to 8 mm of mercury to allow the peritoneum to drop away from the anterior abdominal wall. Using a balloon dissector a large extraperitoneal space is created and additional ports are placed on either side of the umbilical port to allow the stapling device and laparoscopic instruments into the extraperitoneal space for dissection and attachment of the prosthesis. Areolar tissue in this area is bluntly dissected to expose the iliopubic tract, Cooper's ligament, the iliac and gonadal vessels. The dissection extends as previously described in the preperitoneal approach. Minimal bleeding is encountered during this procedure. A 12 × 6 cm piece of mesh is put into this space with a notch cut posteriorly for the cord structures. The mesh is attached to the same area as described in the preperitoneal approach. This procedure is used for both inguinal hernias and femoral hernias. The indirect hernia sac is divided at the internal ring, as previously described, and the distal sac is left in place. In patients over 50 years of age both sides are repaired. Phillips uses a similar approach except that the laparoscope is initially inserted into the cavity for abdominal exploration and later for conformation of an adequate hernia repair. Phillips insufflates the extraperitoneal space with a Veress needle under direct vision. In older patients he also repairs both sides even though an identifiable hernia is present only on one side. Bilateral extraperitoneal

into the leg, and to avoid these nerves staples are not placed below the iliopubic tract. By compression of the abdomen externally, the tract is identified. Below the iliopubic tract the leg will not allow indentation of the abdominal wall. Posteriorly and medially the mesh is allowed to 'drape' over the iliac vessels without being tacked in this 'triangle of doom'. The number of staples used varies from 20–30 to 30–40 per case. It is only necessary to hold the graft in place for 24–48 hours after which it becomes 'fixed' by fibrosis. After stapling the prosthesis in place, the peritoneum is replaced over the prosthesis by reducing the insufflation pressure to 8 mm of mercury pressure with evacuation of a corresponding amount of CO_2 from the abdominal cavity. This allows relaxation of the peritoneum, which is now clipped together using the hernia stapler. The peritoneum should not be stapled to the mesh.

In cases where extremely large direct pseudo-sacs exist, the transverse incision is carried across the mid-portion of the sac and a repairs are preferred in this approach because once the extraperitoneal area has been insufflated future access is extremely difficult. Early reports indicate that 10% of extraperitoneal repairs cannot be completed because of confusion of the anatomy and must be converted to another approach until appropriate expertise is achieved.

Recurrent hernias and femoral hernias

Recurrent hernias may be repaired as described above. If, however, they only represent a small defect in the fascia, they may be repaired by the plug method similar to that described below for femoral hernia repairs. As these small, recurrent, direct hernias are very rare, the entire floor is usually repaired.

Femoral hernias and selected small recurrent hernias may be repaired by reducing the sac of the hernia into the abdominal cavity. A transverse incision is then made along the superior aspect of the peritoneal surface of the sac and a cone-shaped polypropylene plug may be inserted into the defect. This plug should not be palpable exteriorly by the patient. A palpable plug may be as much of a concern and discomfort to the patient as the hernia itself. A small patch is placed over this plug, or defect, and both are tacked with a hernia stapler to hold them in place. Femoral hernia repair staples are placed along the inguinal ligament, pubic tubercle, and Cooper's ligament. Staples are not placed laterally but rather the mesh is allowed to drape over the femoral vessels similar to the posterior 'triangle of doom' in an inguinal hernia repair.

Complications

Laparoscopic herniorrhaphy has resulted in minimal complications using any of the procedures described above. Dissection in the area of the iliac vessels could possibly result in severe complications, the greatest being haemorrhage which could be fatal. Cautious dissection in the 'triangle of doom' will prevent injury to the structures contained in this space. A less severe complication of injury to the femoral nerve or its branches such as the lateral cutaneous nerve of the thigh results in numbness and paraesthesia along the lateral

aspect of the thigh. This complication is usually transient but may be prolonged and associated with atrophy of leg muscles. This injury is due to dissection in the area of the anterior superior iliac spine posterior to the iliopubic tract. Staples in the area of anterior superior iliac spine posterior to the iliopubic tract area are to be avoided. Injury in this area to the femoral nerve trunk may cause muscle weakness and atrophy in the thigh. Injury to the genital branch of the genitofemoral nerve may occur if the sac is dissected free from the cord structures. If the distal sac is dissected from the inguinal canal additional complications of oedema and haematomas in the area of the cord and/or testicle are possible. This complication is avoided by leaving the distal sac in place, which should not result in a hydrocele at a further date and will prevent early post-operative problems. Injury to the bladder with resultant intravesical mesh has been reported but is rare. Bladder injuries are a result of dissecting far more medially than the umbilical ligament or failure to recognize when the bladder has been incorporated into the hernia defect. To avoid bladder damage the medial aspect of the dissection is limited by the umbilical ligament. More minor complications of scrotal insufflation of CO_2 and subcutaneous crepitus are transient and usually resolved by gentle compression of the scrotal sac with the patient still under anaesthesia. If the distal sac is left in place, these minor complications will be greatly reduced. Subcutaneous emphysema is more common with the extraperitoneal approach but does not appear to be of significance even when apparently extensive. Studies have been performed which have indicated some transient rise in blood CO_2 content and/or change in pH but these changes have not been clinically significant. Infection or rejection of mesh placed in the preperitoneal or abdominal area have not yet been reported. Intra-abdominal adhesions to mesh which is placed on the peritoneal surface, or where the preperitoneal mesh has not be reperitonealized, have been reported. It is as yet too early to assess the significance of this. Fitzgibbons has reported complications associated with adhesions to the prosthesis using the onlay technique. He has suggested close observation of these patients and recommends that this approach should be discontinued pending further evaluation. Wound haematomas, intraperitoneal bleeding from trocar sites, and trocar wound infections can be avoided by close attention to basic laparoscopic principles. So too can major intra-abdominal injuries such as injury to bowel or great vessels as a result of laparoscopy itself and these must be taken into consideration when recommending a laparoscopic herniorrhaphy. General anaesthesia is a requirement for laparoscopic hernia repair although in recent years general anaesthesia has improved to the extent that it is almost as safe as local anaesthesia. Any contraindication to general anaesthesia is a contraindication to laparoscopic herniorrhaphy.

Equipment used in laparoscopic herniorrhaphy

Equipment used for laparoscopic herniorrhaphy is essentially the same as that for other laparoscopic procedures. Additional equipment includes standard graspers, dissectors, and an extremely sharp pair of scissors. The laser may be used if the operator is trained to use laser in other procedures. A 30° or 45° angled lens allows the surgeon better visualization of the inguinal area and the structures that are being dissected. It is of some importance that the surgeon learns to use these laparoscopes as well as the 0° lens. These laparoscopes also allow exact placement of sutures or staples when fixing the mesh into place. The hernia stapler (disposable or reusable) is a special instrument which has been developed by USSC and Ethicon. The USSC instrument now produced is a disposable multifiring reloadable instrument which fires a 'B' type of staple while the similar single use and multiple use Ethicon stapler uses a 'box' staple. These instruments have the ability to rotate 360° and the distal end can be flexed 30–60°. Also peculiar to hernia repairs are the polypropylene (Prolene, Marlex, SurgiPro and Mersilene) and polytetrafluoroethylene (Gortex) meshes. SurgiPro mesh differs from the other polypropylene or screen-like meshes in that it appears to be a solid cloth-like mesh similar to Gor-tex. It, however, has the quality like all polypropylene meshes of allowing rapid fibrous infiltration into it, unlike Gor-tex. Unlike the other polypropylene meshes SurgiPro does not have a memory and is therefore more easily manipulated into the area of the hernia repair. This semi-transparent mesh adheres to the area on which it has been placed until it is tacked or sutured in place. In order to keep all meshes orientated properly, a transverse or horizontal line and two vertical lines on either end of the mesh are drawn with a surgical marker prior to their placement into the abdominal cavity. Which mesh is best for hernia repair is still under consideration and will not be known until adequate time has been allowed for evaluation of results of current repairs. Currently under investigation by many companies is a mesh which will allow fibrous ingrowth on one side and has an adhesive barrier on the opposite side making it unnecessary to cover the mesh with peritoneum to prevent post-operative adhesions. Balloon expanders are currently being manufactured for extraperitoneal dissection.

Diagnostic hernia laparoscopy

The surgeon is sometimes confronted with a patient who complains of inguinal pain but in whom a hernia cannot be demonstrated at the initial visit. These patients are usually asked to return for review. Some return free of their pain while in others pain persists. Particular difficulties may be caused by the 'compensation patient' or the patient who is unable to obtain a particular occupation because of the stigma of hernia being diagnosed by an examining physician which cannot subsequently be confirmed or excluded by the surgeon. In these cases a diagnostic laparoscopy using a 5 mm port through the umbilicus is of great diagnostic value. It gives the surgeon the opportunity to examine better the pelvic wall and to establish definitively the presence or absence of a hernia both in the indirect, direct and femoral areas. It then can be conclusively said whether or not the patient has a hernia or simply a lipoma. If no hernia is found, no further surgical procedure is necessary and the patient is reassured. If, however, a hernia is demonstrated, it can then be repaired laparoscopically or, if the patient has refused laparoscopic repair, a groin approach may be used to treat the hernia.

On many occasions bilateral hernias are found at laparoscopy when only one was suspected pre-operatively. Both hernias may be repaired by the port placement previously described resulting in a pain-free repair which is one of the major indications for laparoscopic herniorrhaphy.

Results

At the present time laparoscopic herniorrhaphies are being used to repair direct, indirect, femoral and recurrent hernias. Size is no longer a limiting factor. Bilateral herniorrhaphies are performed because they are tension-free, painless repairs and bilateral repair does not significantly add to the trauma of the procedure. The age of the patient has not been of significance, although it is obvious that a paediatric herniorrhaphy can be performed through a groin approach with minimal scarring and pain and, therefore laparoscopic hernia repair is not indicated in this age group. The age of the patient is of consideration only when associated with coexisting illnesses, and the patient's fitness for general anaesthesia.

Currently, preperitoneal and onlay laparoscopic herniorrhaphies have been successfully completed with limited significant complications. Early studies may indicate that the onlay technique of laying a prosthetic mesh over the hernia defect, especially in the direct defect, and securing it only to the peritoneum, results in a high rate of recurrences which will consist of a peritoneum covered with mesh found in the recurrent hernia. Fitzgibbons, Spaw, Toy and Smoot, however, report good results in the repair of the indirect defect using an onlay graft, especially if the graft is stapled to the inguinal ligament and Cooper's ligament medially. The original onlay technique of stapling only to the peritoneum has a high recurrence rate and is no longer being performed.

The preperitoneal tension-free repair originally was very time consuming because of the slow process of laparoscopic suturing. The time necessary for these repairs has greatly been reduced by the development of multifire hernia staplers (USSC and Ethicon). Time required for this procedure is now about 30–45 minutes after very little experience. Postoperatively the patients may be discharged on the day of surgery and the result is an almost pain-free repair. Cosmetically the incisions are almost completely hidden by either the umbili-cus or plastic skin closures. It appears that all patients, including those with direct, indirect, femoral, sliding and large scrotal hernias, may be successfully treated by a laparoscopic approach.

Follow-up at this time is too short to evaluate fully the recurrence rate. However, current follow-up indicates a recurrence rate of less than 1% using the preperitoneal or extraperitoneal approach and 2% using the modified onlay approach for indirect hernias. Many of these repairs have now been followed over 48 months. A significant number of patients have been followed in excess of 3 to 4 years with a constant recurrence rate of 1%, which seems to have stabilized.

References

1. Dubois, F., Berthelot, G. and Levard, H. (1991). Laparoscopic cholecystectomy: historic perspective and personal experience. *Surgical Laparoscopy and Gastroscopy*, **1**(1), 52–7.
2. Selected data on hospital and use of services (1989). In: *Socio-economic Factbook for Surgery* (eds Pollister, P. and Cunico, E.), American College of Surgeons, Chicago, Ill., pp. 25–42.
3. Lichtenstein, I.L. (1990). Scientific exhibit ACS meeting, San Francisco, CA, October. Personal communication.
4. Stoppa, R.E. and Warlaumont, C.R. (1989). The preperitoneal approach and prosthetic repair of groin hernia. In: *Hernia* (eds Nyhus, L.M. and Condon, R.E.), J.P. Lippincott Co., Philadelphia, PA, pp. 199–225.
5. Nyhus, L.M., Pollak, R., Bombeck, T.C. and Donahue, P.E. (1988). The preperitoneal approach and prosthetic buttress repair for recurrent hernia. *Annals of Surgery*, **208**, 733–7.
6. Marcy, H.O. (1871). A new use of carbolized catgut ligatures. *Boston Medical Surgical Journal*, **85**, 315–16.
7. Griffith, C.A. (1989). The Marcy repair of indirect inguinal hernias: 1870 to present. In: *Hernia* (eds Nyhus, L.M. and Condon, R.D.), J.P. Lippincott Co., Philadelphia, PA, pp. 106–18.
8. Marcy, H.O. (1887). The cure of hernia. *JAMA*, **8**, 589–92.
9. Marcy, H.O. (1892). *Hernia*. Appleton Press, New York.
10. LaRoque, G.P. (1932). The intra-abdominal method of removing inguinal and femoral hernia. *Archives of Surgery*, **24**, 189–203.
11. Popp, L.W. (1990). Endoscopic patch repair of inguinal hernia in a female patient. *Surgical Endoscopy*, **4**, 12–20.
12. Ger, R. (1982). The management of certain abdominal

hernias by intra-abdominal closure of the neck. *Annals of the Royal College of Surgeons of England*, **64**, 342–4.

13. Ger, R., Monroe, K., Duvivier, R., Mishrick, A. (1990). Management of indirect inguinal hernias by laparoscopic closure of the neck of the sac. *American Journal of Surgery*, **159**, 371–3.

14. Ger, R. (1991). The laparoscopic management of groin hernias. *Contemporary Surgery*, **39**, 15–19.

15. Corbitt, J.D. Jr. (1991). Laparoscopic herniorrhaphy. *Surgical Laparoscopy and Endoscopy*, **1**(1), 23–5.

16. Salerno, G.M., Fitzgibbons, R.J. Jr. and Filipi, C.J. (1991). *Surgical Laparoscopy*. Quality Medical Publishing Inc., St Louis, MO, pp. 281–93.

17. Toy, F.K. and Smoot, R.J. Jr. (1991). Toy–Smoot laparoscopic hernioplasty. *Surgical Laparoscopy and Endoscopy*, **1**(3), 151–5.

17

Pulmonary surgery

R.J. Donnelly

Thoracoscopy has been used in clinical practice for many years since it was first described by Jacobeus early this century.[1] Before the advent of effective antituberculous chemotherapy, it found widespread use for the division of apical pleural adhesions in collapse therapy for pulmonary tuberculosis.[2] In recent years it has been used mainly for taking biopsies of the pleura, lung and mediastinum[3] but other procedures have been described including pleurodesis,[4,5] the sealing of air leaks[6] and bronchopleural fistula,[7] and removal of foreign bodies from the chest.[8]

Stapling instruments have become progressively more sophisticated in recent years and their safety and efficiency in pulmonary surgery is well established. They have been used for a variety of procedures on the lung including open lung biopsy, wedge resection, lobectomy, pneumonectomy, blebectomy and bullectomy.

Following the recent upsurge of interest in laparoscopic cholecystectomy and other intra-abdominal endoscopic procedures, thoracic surgeons have looked at the potential for the application of some of these new techniques inside the chest, based upon their long experience of diagnostic thoracoscopy. The stapling technology has, however, lagged behind that of the optical instrumentation and it was only in 1991 that the first stapler suitable for use endoscopically inside the chest became generally available. Before this, several endoscopic-assisted procedures were carried out using conventional stapling instruments and the first endoscopic-assisted resection of a lung carcinoma at the Cardiothoracic Centre, Liverpool, was carried out on 2 April 1991. Since then a number of other endoscopic-assisted and truly endoscopic operations have been performed and the experience is described below.

Technique

All procedures were carried out under general anaesthesia and a double lumen endotracheal tube was used to allow single lung ventilation and collapse of the ipsilateral lung. The patient was placed in a full thoracotomy position and prepared and draped for immediate thoracotomy in case of complications or if the procedure proved to be impossible endoscopically.

The endoscope used was a 10 mm laparoscope with a wide view and 90° field (GU Manufacturing Co. Ltd). Attached to this was a high resolution camera and this was connected to a 21 inch television monitor from which the operation inside the chest was viewed and performed. Included within the system was a video recorder for recording of relevant parts of the procedure.

The site for insertion of the endoscope varied with the intended procedure and might be changed during the course of the operation. The usual first port of entry was in the 6th space in the posterior axillary line from which a good general view of the lung, pleura, diaphragm and mediastinum could usually be obtained. Because of the possibility of adhesions between the lung and chest wall, a short skin incision was made and the muscles of the chest wall separated with a large artery forceps until the pleura was exposed. This was then opened under direct vision and, if there were no adhesions, a large metal conventional trocar and cannula were inserted into the thoracic cavity. The trocar was removed and the endoscope passed through the cannula.

There is no need to maintain an air seal within the chest during endoscopic procedures and, in fact, it is the entry of air and subsequent collapse of the lung which allows adequate visualization of the lung and other intrathoracic structures. The presence of extensive adhesions can make the operation very difficult and even impossible, but localized adhesions can be divided endoscopically.

One or two additional ports were made for insertion of dissecting and stapling instruments but all entry sites were interchangeable for instruments and the endoscope. Incisions of 1.8 cm were usually adequate except when conventional staplers, e.g. RLH30 (Ethicon Ltd), were used when a slightly larger opening was made to allow manipulation of the instrument into the chest.

Lung biopsy

The endoscope was inserted as described and the most abnormal part of the lung identified. Through an anterior incision, usually in the same space, an RLH30 instrument or, more recently, an Endo GIA (USSC) was inserted and applied to the lung which was manipulated into the jaws of the stapler using grasping forceps inserted alongside the endoscope. When the RLH30 was used, a pair of scissors was inserted alongside to cut the piece of lung before removal of the stapler. The Endo GIA cuts and staples simultaneously and has the added advantage of being small enough to be inserted through a cannula. The lung biopsy is simply extracted through one of the entry ports.

Wedge resection

The procedure is very similar to that described for lung biopsy but several applications of the stapler are required and the lesion to be excised must be identifiable and this usually means that it involves the pleural surface or

can be readily 'palpated' with a long artery forceps or other instrument.

Three sites of entry are made, one for the endoscope and two for instrumentation.

Extraction of the resected lesion can be difficult and it may be necessary to enlarge the incision a little. The limiting factor, however, is usually the size of the rib space and a very limited thoracotomy may be required until technology advances sufficiently to achieve morcellation of the specimen prior to extraction.

Pneumothorax

One patient in this series was a young woman with cystic fibrosis and a persistent pneumothorax who had been in hospital for 13 weeks. She was taken to theatre and the endoscope inserted into the pleural space to identify the site of the air leak in the upper lobe. Through a separate 2 cm incision a long conventional needle holder with a Mersilene suture attached was used to stitch the hole in the lung. The patient was discharged from hospital 6 days later.

Pleurectomy

Three sites of entry are made in the 6th rib space and each was interchangeable for endoscope and instruments. The pleura is exposed for the first incision by separation of the fibres in the muscles of the chest wall. The trocars are inserted at the other sites through short skin incisions after identifying endoscopically that the lung is free at those points and that it is safe to do so.

Under endoscopic vision the parietal pleura is completely separated from the chest wall using a long Roberts artery forceps, sometimes with a small gauze peanut attached. If a peanut is used in this way it is important to transfix it with a strong suture which is secured outside the chest. By a combination of this technique together with cutting, pulling and stripping the pleura, the whole parietal pleura can be excised from the apex of the thorax to the diaphragm and from the aorta posteriorly to the mediastinum anteriorly.

The lung is examined for blebs or bullae which can be stapled with the Endo GIA. Two of the entry ports are used for the placement of intercostal tubes and the third closed with sutures.

Results

Twenty-five patients have undergone conventional thoracic surgical operations using endoscopic techniques at the Cardiothoracic Centre, Liverpool. Eight were for resection of pulmonary masses, 6 for pneumothorax, 9 for lung biopsy, 1 for resection of an oesophageal duplication cyst and 1 pericardial window for malignant pericardial effusion. Two of the patients with recurrent pneumothorax underwent one-stage bilateral endoscopic pleurectomy and these patients would normally have undergone sternotomy or bilateral-staged thoracotomies.

Of the solid lung masses removed, four were reported as primary adenocarcinoma, one as a primary squamous carcinoma, two as metastases (one seminoma, one adenocarcinoma) and one as Wegener's granuloma.

A clear diagnosis was made on all patients undergoing endoscopic lung biopsy. There were 4 patients with cryptogenic fibrosing alveolitis, 3 with sarcoidosis and 1 with non-Hodgkin's lymphoma.

The patient with a duplication cyst of the oesophagus had presented with significant dysphagia which was completely relieved after surgery.

In this series there has been only one complication and that was in the first patient on whom endoscopic pleurectomy was attempted. He was readmitted soon after discharge with a further pneumothorax and was submitted to formal thoracotomy and stapling of blebs. The pleurectomy appeared complete. Following this second operation he had a prolonged air leak which delayed his further discharge from hospital.

Post-operative pain was much reduced compared with conventional thoracotomy and mobilization, and recovery from operation was more rapid.

Discharge from hospital was early in all cases, most commonly being 2 days after lung biopsy, 4 days after wedge resection and up to 6 days following pleurectomy.

Discussion

There is no doubt that a new era of thoracic surgery has begun based upon many years of experience with thoracoscopy and, more recently, stapling instruments. The advantages to the patient are clear and have already been demonstrated in abdominal surgery. These include a reduction in post-operative pain, rapid mobilization and return to normal activity, an improved cosmetic result and early discharge from hospital.

It is not unreasonable also to expect to be able to demonstrate a reduction in post-operative morbidity, particularly in pulmonary infection since the reduced pain should allow improved breathing, coughing and co-operation with physiotherapy. It is likely that some patients who would not tolerate conventional thoracotomy because of poor pulmonary function may be able to withstand intrathoracic procedures using endoscopic techniques.

Lung biopsy is now an established and simple procedure, as is wedge resection of small peripheral lung masses, although its application at this stage to lung carcinoma should be restricted to patients with poor pulmonary function who would be poor risks for thoracotomy or those in whom biopsy excision is appropriate. The lesion, of course, must be identifiable endoscopically, i.e. it must extend to the pleural surface or be palpable subpleurally with an instrument inserted through one of the ports in the chest wall. The position of the lesion in the lung is determined by the pre-operative CT scan and the entry ports planned on this basis.

Pleurectomy is not a difficult endoscopic procedure and pleurodesis even easier. The ability to staple, sew or laser small bullae and close air leaks will find widespread application in the management of pneumothorax.

Our experience has been confined so far to relatively straightforward procedures. More extensive operations, such as lobectomy or pneumonectomy, are technically feasible in selected cases with current technology but the problem of getting the lung out of the chest has not yet been solved. The development of bags into which the lung can first be manipulated and then emulsified or broken up before being extracted through one of the ports in the chest wall may overcome this problem.

Other thoracic operations which are possible include bullectomy, plication of the paralysed hemi-diaphragm, and various oesophageal procedures such as myotomy for achalasia or diffuse spasm, hiatus hernia repair, oesophagectomy and excision of leiomyosarcoma. It is likely that, before long, the ingenuity of surgeons and engineers working together will solve the technical problems which currently prevent the application of endoscopic techniques to some of those major thoracic surgical procedures which presently require formal thoracotomy.

References

1. Jacobeus, H.C. (1910). Ueber die moglichkeit die Zystoskopie bie Untersuchung serosen hohlungen anzuwenden. *Munchen Med. Wochenschrift*, **57**, 2090–2.
2. Jacobeus, H.C. (1921). The practical importance of thoracoscopy in surgery of the chest. *Surgery, Gynecology and Obstetrics*, **32**, 493.
3. Page, R.D., Jeffrey, R.R. and Donnelly, R.J. (1989). Thoracoscopy: a review of 121 consecutive procedures. *Annals of Thoracic Surgery*, **48**, 66–8.
4. Boutin, C., Astoul, P. and Seitz, P. (1990). The role of thoracoscopy in the evaluation and management of pleural effusions. *Lung*, **168** (Supp.), 1113–21.
5. Daniel, T.M., Tribble, C.G. and Rodgers, B.M. (1990). Thoracoscopy and talc poudage for pneumothoraces and effusions. *Annals of Thoracic Surgery*, **50**(2), 186–9.
6. Wakabayashi, A., Brenner, M., Wilson, A.F., Tadir, Y. and Barns, M. (1990). Thoracoscopic treatment of spontaneous pneumothorax using carbon dioxide laser. *Annals of Thoracic Surgery*, **50**(5), 786–9.
7. Tschopp, J.M., Evequoz, D., Karrer, W., Aymon, E. and Naef, A.P. (1990). Successful closure of chronic BPF by thoracoscopy after failure of endoscopic pleural glue application and thoracoplasty. *Chest*, **97**(3), 745–6.
8. Oakes, D.D., Sherck, J.P. and Brodsky, J.B. (1984). Therapeutic thoracoscopy. *Journal of Thoracic and Cardiovascular Surgery*, **87**, 269–73.

18

Endoscopic sympathectomy

J.G. Geraghty and W.A. Tanner

Introduction

Hyperhidrosis is a condition characterized by sweating which occurs in excess of that required for thermoregulation. This condition most commonly affects the palms and axillae but may also occur in the feet, face, groin and legs. No large epidemiological studies have been carried out, but one source has put the incidence of hyperhidrosis at 0.6–1%.[1] Hyperhidrosis may be classified as primary in which there is no obvious underlying cause, or secondary to conditions such as phaeochromocytoma or thyrotoxicosis. This condition most commonly affects young women and is often a source of intense social embarrassment.

Hyperhidrosis may be managed by medical or surgical means. Medical treatment of hyperhidrosis is generally ineffective. Biofeedback techniques have been used with very limited success,[2] while iontophoresis gives only short-term relief of symptoms. A variety of surgical techniques have been described in the management of hyperhidrosis. The sweat glands in the axillae may be excised if the disease is confined to the axilla alone.[3] However, over 65% of patients with hyperhidrosis have involvement of the hands alone or the hands and axillae. The majority of patients therefore require a surgical procedure to control sweating to both of these regions. The mainstay of surgical treatment for hyperhidrosis of the upper limb consists of ablation of the sympathetic chain using an open technique.

A variety of approaches have been used to identify the sympathetic chain including cervical and supraclavicular approaches,[4] the transaxillary approach,[5] or the posterior approach.[6] There are well-recognized complications associated with each of these approaches. Given that cosmetic embarrassment is one of the major symptoms of patients with hyperhidrosis it is important that the surgical procedure itself should give a good cosmetic result. The cosmetic result associated with open procedures, however, has been very variable.[7]

Endoscopic ablation of the thoracic sympathetic chain is an attractive alternative to open surgery for hyperhidrosis. It permits easy visualization of the sympathetic chain and gives an excellent cosmetic result.

Transthoracic endoscopic ablation of the sympathetic chain was first described by Kux[8] in 1978. This technique is now the procedure of choice for upper limb hyperhidrosis in some centres but has not yet gained widespread acceptance. The evidence suggests, however, that this technique gives a physiological result as good as open techniques and most importantly provides an excellent cosmetic result.

Technique of transthoracic endoscopic sympathectomy

Patients

Transthoracic endoscopic sympathectomy may be carried out as an inpatient or as a day case procedure. It is important that patients are fully informed of the nature of the procedure, and of complications such as post-operative chest pain, pneumothorax and compensatory hyperhidrosis. A chest X-ray is always performed pre-operatively and the presence of lung pathology or pleural thickening are contraindications to sympathectomy using this endoscopic technique. The patient is intubated using a double lumen endotracheal tube to enable deflation of the lung on the side requiring surgery. The patient is placed supine on the table with the arms extended on arm boards to enable access to the lateral chest wall. The patient's blood pressure, pulse and in particular oxygen saturation are monitored continuously during the procedure.

Operative technique

The patient is draped to enable access to the 3rd and 4th intercostal spaces along the midaxillary line. After the lung on the appropriate side is deflated, a Veress needle is passed through a stab incision in the 3rd interspace into the pleural cavity. An artificial pneumothorax is created by insufflating 1 litre of carbon dioxide into the pleural cavity. The needle is removed and the skin incision enlarged to allow a 5 mm disposable port to be inserted into the pleural cavity via the 3rd intercostal space (Figure 18.1). A laparoscope is then inserted and the carbon dioxide line is connected to an automatic insufflator. The maximum intrathoracic pressure should not exceed 10 cm of water. A 5 mm port is inserted in a similar fashion into the pleural cavity via the 4th intercostal space in the midaxillary line (Figure 18.1). Alternative sites have been used for the positioning of this port, the most common of which is the 2nd intercostal space in the midclavicular line. It is occasionally necessary to divide adhesions in the upper chest with diathermy scissors and occasionally dense pleural thickening in the region of the sympathetic chain makes it impossible to continue with the procedure.

It is important to identify the vital structures in the region of the thoracic sympathetic chain before proceeding with the sympathectomy. These structures are detailed in Figure 18.2. The stellate ganglion cannot be seen with the laparoscope as it is covered with a characteristic pad of fat. The sympathetic chain is seen to

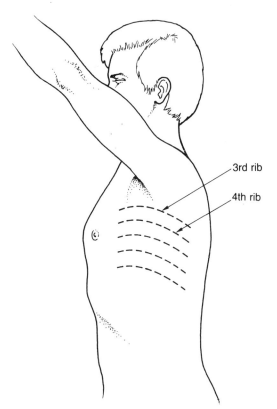

Fig. 18.1. The Veress needle is introduced into the 3rd interspace. A 10 mm port is then inserted through the space. A 5 mm port for insertion of the diathermy forceps is placed in the 4th interspace.

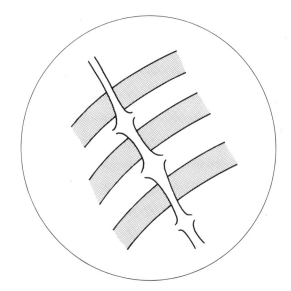

Fig. 18.2. Diagrammatic representation of the structures adjacent to the left sympathetic chain.

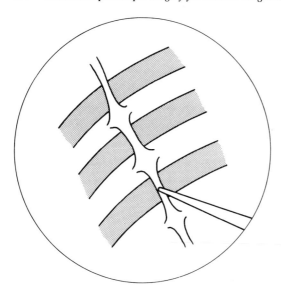

Fig. 18.3. The diathermy forceps is placed in contact with the sympathetic chain as it passes over the 2nd, 3rd and 4th ribs.

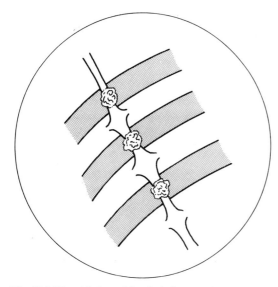

Fig. 18.4. The ablation of the chain is recognized by a charred appearance after diathermy.

run over the necks of the 2nd, 3rd, 4th and 5th ribs. Although visualization of the sympathetic chain is important, it is equally important to identify the site of the sympathetic chain by tactile sensation as it runs over the ribs. This is done by passing the diathermy forceps into the

pleural cavity via the 5 mm port and gently rolling the chain as it passes over the ribs. Ablation of the chain is carried out by placing the diathermy probe in contact with the chain as it passes over the neck of the ribs (Figure 18.3). The diathermy is adjusted to the coagulation setting of 5 and as the current is passed the chain is ablated by electrocautery. This procedure is repeated over the necks of the 3rd and 4th ribs such that the 2nd, 3rd and 4th thoracic ganglia and intervening chain are electrocoagulated. It is particularly important to ablate the 4th and possibly 5th thoracic ganglion if axillary hyperhidrosis is the predominant symptom. Adequacy of ablation is confirmed by the presence of a charred appearance of the chain at the site of diathermy (Figure 18.4).

The chain should not be ablated with diathermy in the intercostal spaces as the intercostal veins may be damaged. The area is checked for haemostasis and the diathermy forceps withdrawn. Once the procedure is finished the carbon dioxide line is disconnected and the lung is reinflated. The port containing the laparoscope is gradually withdrawn and this enables completeness of lung insufflation to be assessed under direct vision. Once this has occurred the anaesthetist is asked to perform a maximum inspiratory manoeuvre during which the laparoscope and port are withdrawn. The incisions are closed with absorbable subcuticular sutures. If indicated, the same procedure can be carried out on the opposite side during the same anaesthetic. No chest drain is inserted and a chest X-ray is carried out in the recovery room to ensure there is no pneumothorax present.

Complications

Compensatory hyperhidrosis

Compensatory hyperhidrosis is the most common complication of transthoracic endoscopic sympathectomy. It is defined as the presence of excessive sweating at sites other than the upper limb and axilla. The most common site for compensatory hyperhidrosis is the chest and back, although it may also occur in the feet, head and neck, legs, thighs and groin. Byrne *et al.*[9] found that 64% of their patients developed some degree of compensatory hyperhidrosis. Precipitating causes include heat, food, exertion, stress and hypothermia. In many cases, however, there is no identifiable precipitating cause of compensatory hyperhidrosis. This complication is not unique to transthoracic endoscopic sympathectomy and similar incidences have previously been reported.[1,7,8,10] The cause of compensatory sweating following sympathectomy is unclear. The most popular theory is that this excessive sweating is due to loss of upper limb sweat gland function. It has been calculated that up to 40% of total body sweat gland function is lost after bilateral cervical sympathectomy and that compensatory sweating at other sites will occur as a thermoregulatory response. Gustatory sweating is another type of compensatory hyperhidrosis which can also be a troublesome complication after transthoracic endoscopic sympathectomy. It should be stressed, however, that compensatory hyperhidrosis is a minor inconvenience only and that at most 5% of patients will require medical therapy.

Failure of treatment

Once a successful transthoracic endoscopic sympathectomy has been carried out, the immediate post-operative response is invariably good. Byrne *et al.*[9] showed that all but one of 85 patients had dry hands and/or axilla on returning from the operating theatre. Failure to identify the sympathetic chain is invariably due to intrathoracic pathology. Milewski[11] was unable to see the chain in 5% of patients and this was due to the presence of apical pleural adhesions. It is often possible to divide pleural adhesions to enable an adequate view of the sympathetic chain. Such dissection runs the risk of damaging the visceral pleura resulting in post-operative pneumothorax.

Late failures can also occur but two retrospective questionnaire studies have shown that at least 80% of patients remain dry. A further 15% have some return of symptoms but still remain better when compared to the time of initial presentation. An important distinction needs to be made between the results of transthoracic endoscopic sympathectomy for hyperhidrosis and for Raynaud's disease. Despite the good results of thoracic sympathectomy for upper limb and/or axillary hyper-

hidrosis, the results for Raynaud's disease are less impressive. Milewski[11] showed that 11 out of 12 sympathectomies were associated with good immediate results. Fifty per cent of these patients, however, had a poor result when reviewed at 26 months. These findings were similar to those of Campbell[12] who found that recurring upper limb hyperhidrosis occurred in 15 out of 24 patients when followed up at 31 months. These results therefore show that transthoracic endoscopic sympathectomy has excellent immediate results in both upper limb hyperhidrosis and Raynaud's disease, but that the long-term results are poor for the latter condition. Transthoracic endoscopic sympathectomy is therefore of dubious value in the treatment of Raynaud's disease.

Horner's syndrome

Horner's syndrome results from damage to the stellate ganglion during the procedure of thoracic sympathectomy. Permanent Horner's syndrome has been shown to occur in 4% of patients after cervical sympathectomy.[13] In theory this complication should not occur as a permanent feature after transthoracic endoscopic sympathectomy. This is because the stellate ganglion is not visible during transthoracic endoscopy as it is covered by a fat pad. If the sympathetic chain is ablated over the necks of the 2nd or 3rd ribs, permanent Horner's syndrome should not occur. No permanent case of Horner's syndrome has been reported in the literature after transthoracic endoscopic sympathectomy. Malone[14] reported that 1 of 14 patients undergoing transthoracic endoscopic sympathectomy developed temporary Horner's syndrome which resolved within 48 hours. Byrne *et al.*[9] found that 3 out of 85 patients undergoing this procedure developed temporary Horner's syndrome. This complaint resolved completely in 6 weeks in 2 patients and in 6 months in the third patient. Although the cause of temporary Horner's syndrome following transthoracic endoscopic sympathectomy is not clear, it is most likely due to transmitted heat to the stellate ganglion at the time of diathermy of the sympathetic chain. Care should be taken therefore not to use excessive diathermy when ablating the uppermost thoracic ganglion.

Bleeding and pneumothorax

Bleeding after transthoracic endoscopic sympathectomy is rare. Byrne *et al.*[9] had no case of intrathoracic bleeding in 85 patients undergoing bilateral endoscopic sympathectomy. Claes and Gothberg[15] reported that 1 patient in a series of 100 consecutive sympathectomies developed an intrathoracic bleed which required a chest drain 2 days post-operatively. No further treatment was necessary in this case. The intercostal veins are at greatest risk of damage at the time of endoscopic sympathectomy. This complication should not occur if the principle of ablating the chain using diathermy only over the ribs is adhered to.

Pneumothorax requiring a chest drain post-operatively is also a rare complication of transthoracic endoscopic sympathectomy. It is not uncommon to find a small apical pneumothorax due to retained carbon dioxide in the immediate post-operative chest film. This pneumothorax should be distinguished from the expanding type which is due to damage to visceral pleura. Malone *et al.*[14] reported visceral pleural rupture in one of 13 cases requiring a chest drain for 24 hours. Byrne *et al.*[9] also had one case of pneumothorax requiring a chest drain in their series of 85 patients. These complications, although rare, raise the issue of timing of discharge following transthoracic endoscopic sympathectomy. In the early learning experience, it is safer to keep these patients for up to 1–2 days post-operatively to check for these complications. Bleeding should be recognized at the time of surgery and a tension pneumothorax should not occur unless the visceral pleura has been damaged. If one is sure that neither of these intra-operative complications has occurred, then it is feasible to perform this procedure as a day case.

Post-operative pain

As with any thoracic procedure, chest pain and/or back pain can occur with transthoracic endoscopic sympathectomy. Claes and Gottenberg[15] report that 15% of their patients developed troublesome back pain. This symptom resolved within 3 to 6 months. Similarly, Byrne *et al.*[9] showed in their series of 85 bilateral sympathectomies that 4 patients developed back pain, 8 patients chest pain, and a further 5 had parasthesia in the distal upper limbs. All of these complications were transient and had disappeared completely by 6 months. Weale[16] suggested that the use of a laparoscope with its own diathermy channel obviated the use of a second port, resulting in a reduced incidence of post-operative chest pain. In our experience, however, the intercostal spaces easily admit a 5 mm port, and it is unlikely that this incision will result in significant chest pain.

Other complications

Surgical emphysema will occur in a small number of patients due to escape of carbon dioxide into the subcutaneous tissues. We have found that direct visualization of the lung as it expands at the end of the procedure together with the performance of a maximum inspiratory manoeuvre minimizes the chance of this complication occurring. Byrne *et al.*[9] reported that 4 of 85 patients developed post-operative temporary Raynaud's phenomenon which settled within 3 months. Finally, complications such as wound sepsis can occur with this procedure as with any skin incision.

Discussion

Transthoracic endoscopic sympathectomy is a simple, safe and effective means of treating patients with upper limb hyperhidrosis. All reported series show that the immediate outcome after endoscopic sympathectomy is comparable to that using standard open techniques. Furthermore, patient satisfaction at follow-up with this procedure is as good as that with open techniques using the cervical and transaxillary approaches. These results indicate that diathermy ablation of the thoracic sympathetic chain achieves the same physiological response as division of the chain using other techniques. The compensatory physiological responses after transthoracic endoscopic sympathectomy are also similar to those reported in patients treated by open sympathectomy. Adar *et al.*[1] reported that 63% of their patients experienced some degree of compensatory hyperhidrosis which is similar to that reported following endoscopic sympathectomy. Open and endoscopic techniques also have a similar incidence of gustatory sweating and a similar incidence of recurrent sweating at long-term follow-up. Although the mechanism of recurrent sweating is unclear, Haxton[17] has shown that nerve regeneration occurs in histological specimens obtained at the time of resympathectomy. It is clear therefore that transthoracic endoscopic sympathectomy should not be judged on the basis of adequacy of sympathectomy but on its safety compared to other techniques.

Thoracic sympathectomy using a cervical approach is still the most common way of treating patients with upper limb hyperhidrosis. This procedure is technically difficult and injury to the phrenic nerve, apical pleura, subclavian artery and brachial plexus are well-recognized hazards of this procedure. Transthoracic endoscopic sympathectomy allows ablation of thoracic ganglia under direct vision and injuries to the aforementioned structures have not been reported using this technique. Transthoracic endoscopic sympathectomy has two further important advantages over cervical sympathectomy. It allows easy access to the 4th and 5th thoracic ganglia while access to this section of the thoracic chain is extremely difficult using the cervical approach. For this reason, transthoracic endoscopic sympathectomy is superior to cervical sympathectomy in treating patients with axillary hyperhidrosis. The second major advantage of endoscopic sympathectomy over cervical sympathectomy is that Horner's syndrome is a rare permanent complication. Adar et al.[1] showed that 43% of their patient population developed Horner's syndrome after cervical sympathectomy and 8% were left with a permanent Horner's syndrome. The cause of temporary Horner's syndrome after this procedure is not clear, but is most likely due to the fact that the ciliospinal centre is not sharply confined to the 1st thoracic ganglion, but it may extend as low as the 5th ganglion.[18]

The major advantage of transthoracic endoscopic sympathectomy is that it is easy to perform and is simple to learn. The renewed interest in this technique in recent years parallels the advent of minimally invasive surgical techniques. It is likely that the reluctance to perform this technique previously was predominantly due to a lack of familiarity with endoscopic techniques. Most surgeons who now perform laparoscopic cholecystectomy will find the technique of transthoracic endoscopic sympathectomy comparatively simple. This also has important implications in the field of surgical training. The demonstration of the thoracic sympathetic chain at transthoracic endoscopy is a far better way to train the technique of thoracic sympathectomy compared to the limited view and technically more hazardous technique of cervical sympathectomy.

Conclusion

Transthoracic endoscopic sympathectomy is a minimally invasive technique which achieves an equally good result with a lesser complication rate than conventional techniques. It should be considered the treatment of choice in patients who have palmar and axillary hyperhidrosis.

References

1. Adar, R., Kurchin, A., Zweig, A. *et al.* (1977). Palmar hyperhidrosis and its surgical treatment. *Annals of Surgery*, **186**, 34–41.
2. Duller, H., Doyle-Gentry, W. (1980). Use of biofeedback in treating chronic hyperhidrosis; a preliminary report. *British Journal of Dermatology*, **103**, 143.
3. Keaveny, T.V., Fitzgerald, P.A.M., Donnelly, C. *et al.* (1977). Surgical management of hyperhidrosis. *British Journal of Surgery*, **64**, 570–7.
4. Telford, E.D. (1935). The technique of sympathectomy. *British Journal of Surgery*, **23**, 448–50.
5. Atkins, H.J.B. (1949). Peraxillary approach to the stellate and upper thoracic sympathetic ganglion. *Lancet*, **2**, 1152.
6. Adson, A.W. and Brown, G.E. (1932). Extreme hyperhidrosis of the hands and feet treated by sympathetic ganglionectomy. *Mayo Clinical Proceedings*, **7**, 394.
7. Sternberg, M.O., Bakkman, S., Kott, J. *et al.* (1982). Transaxillary thoracic sympathectomy for primary hyperhidrosis of the upper limbs. *World Journal of Surgery*, **6**, 458–63.
8. Kux, N. (1978). Thoracic endoscopic sympathectomy in palmar and axillary hyperhidrosis. *Archives of Surgery*, **113**, 264–6.
9. Byrne, J., Walsh, T.N. and Hederman, W.P. (1990). Endoscopic transthoracic electrocautery of the sympathetic chain for palmar and axillary hyperhidrosis. *British Journal of Surgery*, **77**, 1046–9.
10. Bogokowsky, H., Slutzki, S., Bacahi, L. *et al.* (1983). The surgical treatment of primary hyperhidrosis. *Archives of Surgery*, **118**, 1065–7.
11. Milewski, P.J., Hodgson, S.P. and Highman, A. (1985). Transthoracic endoscopic sympathectomy. *Journal of the Royal College of Surgeons of Edinburgh*, **30**, 221–3.

12. Campbell, W.B., Cooper, M.J., Sponsel, W.E. *et al.* (1982). Transaxillary sympathectomy; is a one-stage bilateral procedure safe? *British Journal of Surgery*, **69**, S29–S31.

13. Greenhalgh, R.M., Rosengarten, D.S. and Martin, P. (1971). The role of sympathectomy for hyperhidrosis. *British Journal of Surgery*, **1**, 332–4.

14. Malone, P.S., Cameron, A.E.P. and Rennie, J.A. (1986). Endoscopic thoracic sympathectomy in the treatment of upper limb hyperhidrosis. *Annals of the Royal College of Surgeons of England*, **68**, 161–4.

15. Claes, G. and Gothberg, G. (1991). Endoscopic transthoracic electrocautery of the sympathetic chain for palmer and axillary hyperhidrosis. *British Journal of Surgery*, **78**, 760.

16. Weale, F.E. (1972). Upper thoracic sympathectomy by transthoracic electrocoagulation. *British Journal of Surgery*, **67**, 71–2.

17. Haxton, H.A. (1971). Upper limb re-sympathectomy. *British Journal of Surgery*, **57**, 106–9.

18. Warwick, R. and Williams, P.L. (1973). *Grays Anatomy* (35th ed.), Longman, Edinburgh.

19

Pelvic lymphadenectomy

J. Fowler

Curative treatment for carcinoma of the genitourinary organs, notably prostate, bladder and cervix, depends upon the disease being organ confined. Early metastases may occur by lymphatic or blood spread. Conventional imaging will detect early bony metastasis, or where there is doubt, define the area to be biopsied. Lymphatic metastases on the other hand may exist in anatomically normal tissues as seen on computed tomography. The potential for lymphatic metastasis increases with the degree of dedifferentiation, size and extent of the carcinoma. This is especially so in prostatic carcinoma. The propensity to metastasize, however, cannot be predicted by these parameters alone (McLaughlin et al. 1976). The general feeling among urological surgeons that low grade, early stage prostatic carcinoma is not associated with lymphatic metastasis has increasingly been challenged (Wilson et al. 1983).

In the United States where radical prostatectomy has been the cornerstone of curative treatment for carcinoma prostate, much information about nodal spread with relation to grade and stage has been obtained. This has shown the necessity for nodal staging where curative treatment of prostatic carcinoma is considered. This applies also to bladder and cervical carcinomas where closed treatment (i.e. radiotherapy) is to be used.

Open lymphadenectomy is not without postoperative complications, especially when it is combined with immediate further treatment (McLaughlin et al. 1976; McCulloch et al.

1977). Minimally invasive assessment of enlarged pelvic nodal tissue can be carried out by ultrasonically guided fine needle aspiration (Bellinson 1981).

In 1969 Bartell reported examination of the retroperitoneum using the mediastinoscope. This was followed by the development of the pelviscope by Hald and Rasmussen in 1980. In 1985 Fuerst reported the use of a laparoscope in the visualization and biopsy of pelvic lymph nodes in dogs and in 1991 several series of laparoscopic pelvic lymphadenectomy, as an adjunctive treatment planning for pelvic neoplasms, were reported (Schueller et al. 1991; Querlev et al. 1991).

Laparoscopic lymphadenectomy, a much lesser procedure in terms of general morbidity and hospital stay, can reduce time from lymphadenectomy to treatment. Furthermore, where positive nodes are found then the potentially harmful effects of radiotherapy may be avoided.

Extent of lymphadenectomy

Lymphadenectomy may be radical, confined to first tier of nodes (obturator), or confined to the appropriate side of the organ (sampling).

Most studies have shown that in prostatic carcinoma, if lymph node metastases have occurred, then they will invariably affect the obturator groups (Grossman et al. 1980).

Where a cure is sought and an attempt is made to remove the nodes to ensure removal of nodal micrometastasis then a radical bilateral operation should be undertaken.

The patient lies supine in the Trendelenburg position. The pneumoperitoneum is induced in the standard manner and the 10 mm port then introduced in the subumbilical position and the camera introduced. The right (12 mm) and left (5 mm) ports are then inserted in position Right 1 and Left 1. One or two further ports may be introduced either in the midline (C2) or left (L2) or right (R2) where further retraction of colon, peritoneal flap or medial aspect of great vessels is required. The surgeon stands on the side opposite the dissection and the assistant on the ipsilateral side. A second assistant holding the camera is positioned towards the head of the patient and the VDU screen situated conveniently at the foot of the table.

Dissection for right sided pelvic lymphadenectomy

The patient (having been catheterized with a fine urethral catheter) is in the Trendelenburg position with the right side elevated to allow the bowel to fall away from the pelvic wall. Once the camera is introduced time should be taken to become orientated within the pelvis identifying the sigmoid colon, the bladder and the rectum and small bowel. Thereafter the following landmarks are identified: the obliterated umbilical artery as it runs in the peritoneal fold to the bladder; the vas as it crosses the great vessels of the pelvic brim and passes to the internal inguinal ring; the great vessels as they run along the brim of the pelvis or, if there is too much extra peritoneal fat, the pulsation of the vessels; and where possible the common iliac artery and its bifurcation.

Where all landmarks have as far as possible been identified the dissection is started at the level of the obliterated umbilical artery distally. The umbilical artery is held in grasping forceps and elevated, the assistant grasping the peritoneum immediately lateral to it and the operator incising the peritoneum. This is an avascular area and there is little danger of injuring the external iliac vessels in this position. The pubis can be felt through the fat at this point. After elevating and retracting the medial leaf of the peritoneum medially and the

lateral leaf laterally, the incision is deepened by blunt dissection to identify the external iliac artery and vein. The incision is then carried proximally as far as the bifurcation of the common iliac artery. The vas will be encountered as the dissection proceeds proximally and will serve as a useful landmark. The vas may be either left as a landmark or alternatively clipped and divided as it is encountered.

Having identified the proximal and distal extent of the dissection, the lateral boundary, the genital branch of the genitofemoral nerve may be identified by blunt dissection, care being taken as the lateral peritoneal leaf is retracted that the genital vessels are not injured.

Starting anteriorly the fat and nodal tissue may be gently elevated using grasping forceps and teased off the anterior surface of the artery. As this tissue is retracted medially the medial margin of the vein should be clearly identified. The nodal tissue and fat should be removed from the medial margin of the vein by a mixture of blunt and sharp dissection. The tissue should be cleared from the femoral canal proximally along the whole of the length of the external iliac vein. During this dissection care must be taken to clearly identify the medial margin of the vein. This may be difficult if the vein is collapsed because of the pneumoperitoneum or by pressure from the assistant's grasping forceps or tension on the tissue.

Once the nodal tissue has been dissected free from the vein, the obturator fossa is entered. The fat and nodal tissues should be displaced en bloc medially by blunt dissection until the obturator nerve is clearly identified in the depths of the obturator fossa. This defines the deep limit of the dissection. The nerve should be followed along its length and cleared of the fat and nodes.

Attention may now be turned to the femoral canal and the nodes either removed or the chain divided at this point. It is important to look for the abnormal obturator vessels and the circumflex vein. The inevitable bleeding which occurs when the nodal tissue is divided should be anticipated, by diathermy of the tissue prior to dissection or clipping before division of the tissue. The free nodal tissue is grasped by grasping forceps or sponge holding forceps and withdrawn medially and towards the sacrum. The peritoneal leaf is retracted medially by the assistant. The full length of the obturator nerve should be clearly seen as the nodal tissue is dissected proximally by blunt and sharp dissection. In practice the medial external iliac chain and the obturator nodes are removed together. The nodal tissue is followed back to the point where it disappears deep behind the internal iliac vein. At this point it may be divided and removed.

While in the line of the obturator nerve, within the obturator fossa, care should be taken to identify the ureter as it runs along the lateral surface of the medial leaf of the peritoneum. It is important not to mistake the ureter for the obturator nerve. Attention is then turned to the external iliac chain. Here the limits of dissection are the inguinal ligament distally, the bifurcation of the common iliac artery proximally and laterally the genital branch of the genitofemoral nerve. The nodal tissue can be removed without undue difficulty as far as the iliac bifurcation.

Having cleared the nodal tissue from the vessels it is possible gently to displace the vessels medially and to look into the obturator fossa from above. This helps in the removal of nodal tissue lying behind the division of the common iliac veins.

Removal of nodal tissue

The removal of nodal tissue, especially when en bloc, may be difficult because of its bulky nature. It is helpful to have two large ports, one 10 mm, the other 12 mm. The tissue may then be grasped by sponge holding forceps or crocodile forceps. Once grasped it should be rotated and be followed into the port under direct vision through the camera. The tissue may be so bulky as to need to be divided before it can be removed. Having entered the port is may impact at the exit and the assistant should be ready to 'vent' the port and so blow the nodal tissue out.

Dissection of the left pelvic nodes

The lateral tilt is reversed. This usually has to be preceded by freeing the sigmoid mesocolon from the lateral pelvic wall. This is accomplished by sharp dissection. The mesocolon should be elevated and cleared so that the common iliac artery and the bifurcation of the iliac vessels may be clearly seen. It will otherwise be impossible to delineate the obturator fossa and the proximal boundaries of dissection. The Trendelenburg tilt, which is acceptable for a right-sided dissection, will have to be increased as may the lateral elevation of the left side. The colon will require to be held medially and proximally by atraumatic forceps. The dissection then proceeds as for the right side.

The obese patient

It may be impossible to identify the landmarks due to extra peritoneal fat in the obese patient. In this case the pulsation of the external iliac artery should be sought over the pelvic brim. When the pulsation has been identified the peritoneum overlying the pulsation should be elevated as far as possible and incised over a centimetre in the line of the artery. By blunt dissection the incision should be deepened and the artery identified. Once the artery is identified it should be followed proximally and distally. As the dissection proceeds the vas deferens will be identified giving a useful landmark. The vas may then be elevated and divided to allow further exposure of the iliac vein. Care should be taken in the obese patient not to injure the spermatic vessels laterally. The landmarks and extent of dissection should be clearly identified before the obturator fossa is entered.

When introducing the lower R2 or C2 ports it is important that the anterior abdominal wall is clearly illuminated by the camera internally so that the inferior epigastric vessels may be avoided.

Post-operative complications

The complications reported following laparoscopic pelvic lymphadenectomy have been minimal and markedly less than those following open lymphadenectomy (Meeney *et al.* 1991; Bouller *et al.* 1991). There have been no significant post-operative complications in the author's personal experience.

Pneumoscrotum is the most striking finding. It is of no significance and quickly resolves as CO_2 is rapidly absorbed into the bloodstream within a few hours. Despite retroperitoneal dissection, ileus has not been a problem. Bleeding is the greatest risk but other than injury to the inferior epigastric vessels as reported by Winfield *et al.* (1991) this remains theoretical. In the author's experience post-operative stay ranges from 24 hours to day case surgery as described by Schueller *et al.* (1991). There has been no evidence of deep vein thrombosis immediately following the procedure. Two patients, however, developed deep venous thromboses in the ileofemoral segment following definitive treatment; 1 patient received radiotherapy to the prostate a week after adenectomy, and 6 weeks later developed pulmonary emboli. One patient developed ileofemoral thrombosis following radical penectomy and bilateral inguinal open lymphadenectomy. He had suspicious internal iliac glands and had undergone laparoscopic lymphadenectomy a week before. It seems that while the primary procedure carries minimal risk, if prompt treatment is to be carried out then prophylactic anticoagulation should be employed.

Staging pelvic laparoscopic lymphadenectomy may be accomplished with little direct morbidity and minimal hospital stay. It opens the way to accurate staging not only in the genitourinary carcinomas, but also carcinomas of the external genitalia, perianal area and lower limbs.

References

Bartel, M. (1969). Die retroperitoneoscopy method, fur inspection und bioptician unterzum des retroperitoneum romers. *Zentralblat Chirurgie*, **94**, 377.

Belinson, J.L. (1981). Fine needle aspiration cytology in the management of gynaecological cancer. *American Journal of Obstetrics and Gynaecology*, **139**, 131–48.

Bouller, J.A., Andres, C.A. and Barrer, P. (1991). Staging laparoscopic pelvic lymph node dissection. Initial report. *Journal of Urology*, **1454**, 423A.

Curlew, D., Leblanc, E. and Casteling, B. (1991). Laparoscopic pelvic lymphadenectomy in the staging of early carcinoma of the cervix. *American Journal of Obstetrics and Gynaecology*, **161**(2), 579–81.

Feverst, D. (1985). Laparoscopic examination of pelvic lymph nodes. *Urology*, **XXVI**, 5.

Grossman, I.C., Carpinello, V., Greenburg, S., Malloy, T. and Wynne, A. (1980). Staging pelvic lymphadenectomy for carcinoma of the prostate. Review of 91 cases. *Journal of Urology*, **124**, 632–4.

Hald, T. and Rasmussen, F. (1980). Extra peritoneal pelvioscopy. A new aid in staging of lower urinary tract tumours. *Journal of Urology*, **124**, 245.

McCulloch, D.L., McLaughlin, A.P. and Gittes, R.F. (1977). Morbidity of pelvic lymphadenectomy and radical prostatectomy for prostatic cancer. *Journal of Urology*, **117**, 206–7.

McLaughlin, A.P., Salts, S.L., McCulloch, D.L. and Gittes, R.F. (1976). Prostatic carcinoma; incidence and location of unsuspected lymphatic metastasis. *Journal of Urology*, **115**, 89–93.

Meeney, J.T., Schueller, W.H., van Kale, Th. and Griffiths, D.P. (1991). Initial results of endoscopic pelvic lymph node dissection as compared with open pelvic lymph node dissection. *Journal of Urology*, **145**, 422A.

Querleu, D., LeBlanc, E. and Castelain, B. (1991). Laparoscopic pelvic lymphadenectomy in the staging of early carcinoma of the cervix. *American Journal of Obstetrics and Gynaecology*, **164**, 579–81.

Schueller, W.W., van Kaley, T.G., Reich, H. and Griffiths, D.P. (1991). Transperitoneal endosurgical lymphadenectomy in patients with localised prostatic cancer. *Journal of Urology*, **145**, 988–91.

Wilson, J.W.L., Morrales, A. and Bruce, A.W. (1983). The prognostic significance of histological grading, a pathological staging in carcinoma of the prostate. *Journal of Urology*, **130**, 481–2.

Winfield, H.N., Donovan, J.F., See, W.A., Loening, S.A. and Williams, R.D. (1991). *Journal of Urology*, **146**, 941–8.

20

Endoanal surgery – principles, techniques and results

B. Mentges and G. Buess

Transanal endoscopic microsurgery (TEM) was one of the earliest minimally invasive procedures in general surgery. It was initially introduced in 1983 to remove adenomas from the rectum.[1] Later the indication was extended to include the local resection of low risk carcinomas and to the palliative treatment of more advanced rectal cancer.[2] Since 1989 patients with rectal prolapse have been treated using the same equipment as for TEM.[10] It is expected that the procedure will become more widespread and will soon establish itself as a routine method. The advantages include: precise excision made possible by a magnified, stereoscopic image and constant gas dilation of the rectum; minimal postoperative pain; short hospitalization and rehabilitation; good cosmetic results; and low complication and recurrence rates.

Indications

The indications for TEM are:

- Histologically confirmed adenomas in the rectum and lower sigmoid colon up to a height of 25 cm from the anal verge.
- Well and moderately differentiated rectal carcinoma, stage CS I or uT1.
- Well and moderately differentiated carcinoma of the preoperative stage CS II or uT2 in patients over 70 years or younger patients with risk factors.
- Palliative excision of pT3 carcinomas.

- Less common tumours and lesions are carcinoid, solitary rectal ulcer syndrome etc.
- 2nd and 3rd degree rectal prolapse.

Instruments

The main component of the instrument set is the operating rectoscope (Fig. 20.1) with an external diameter of 40 mm and a length of 12 cm, or alternatively, 20 cm. The tube and the handle of the rectoscope are connected by a bayonet mechanism. The free end of the tube is slanted at the same angle as the tip of the telescope thus preventing it from being covered and soiled by the rectal wall (Fig. 20.2). The rectoscope can be attached to the operating table by a double ball and socket

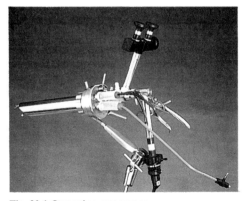

Fig. 20.1 Operating rectoscope.

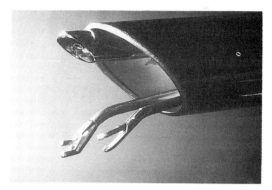

Fig. 20.2 Angulation of the rectoscope tube, the telescope and of the tip of the instruments.

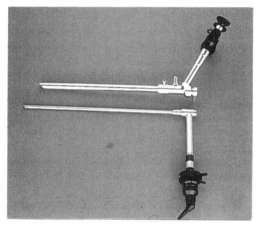

Fig. 20.3 Stereoscopic telescope with a third eyepiece for the connection with the camera.

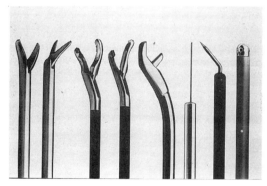

Fig. 20.4 Instrument set.

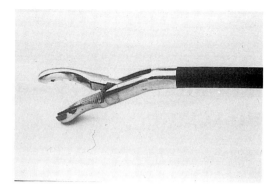

Fig. 20.5 Jaws of the forceps with teeth at the front and fine grooves at the back.

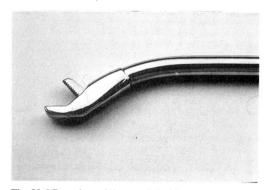

Fig. 20.6 Branches of the needleholder.

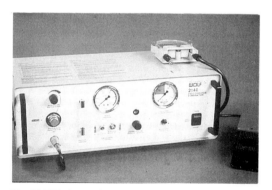

Fig. 20.7 Endo-surgical-unit.

joint and locked in any suitable position. Four instruments up to 47 cm in length can be inserted through the instrument channels simultaneously. A further channel is reserved for the stereoscopic telescope which provides a three-dimensional image and up to six-fold magnification. A third rigid eyepiece is angled to the bottom for the connection to the video system (Fig. 20.3). The instrument set includes the following: a needle holder, forceps and scissors curved both to the left and right, a high-frequency knife, a clip applicator and an aspirator (Fig. 20.4).

The HF-knife, the forceps and the needleholder are angled inferiorly at their ends so as to reach the operating area. This lengthens the distance between the tips of the instruments and the telescope which improves the overview. The jaws of the forceps have teeth at the front for grasping tissue and fine grooves at the back for holding the needle (Fig. 20.5). The jaws of the needleholder are designed to ensure that the needle sits at the correct angle (Fig. 20.6). The needleholder can be locked at the handle which makes it easier to hold the needle in the correct working position during suturing. The shaft of the aspirator is angled several times so as not to interfere with the other instruments which are kept parallel to each other within a tight range.

The combined endo-surgical unit (Fig. 20.7) has four functions: CO_2 insufflation to dilate the rectum, endoluminal pressure measurement, rinsing of the telescope, and aspiration. The aspiration is performed by a roller pump which can be adjusted. The rate of CO_2 insufflation exceeds that of aspiration even on a high working level, so that dilatation of the rectum is always maintained.

Preoperative diagnosis and preparation of the patient

As part of the investigation of the patient, diagnostic examination of the whole colon is recommended. Today, an endorectal ultrasound procedure is the most sensitive method of establishing the depth of infiltration of the tumour and should play a part in planning the operation. The operator should perform a rectoscopy with the rigid instrument to localize the tumour exactly before deciding on the positioning of the patient. On the day before the operation, orthograde lavage of the colon is performed with 10 litres of lactated Ringer's solution. At the beginning of the operation the patient is given a single dose of combined antibiotic prophylaxis.

Surgical procedure

Rectal tumours

Although recently epidural anaesthesia has been used increasingly, general anaesthesia should be performed when the patient is positioned prone and when the operation is expected to take a long time.

The patient is positioned on the table so that the tumour is situated at the bottom of the operating field. After the operating rectoscope has been inserted the obturator is replaced by the viewing window, and the area to be excised is exposed while air is manually insufflated and the rectoscope is fixed in this position. The viewing window is now replaced by the working insert through which the stereoscopic telescope and the instruments with their sealing sleeves are inserted. The sealing sleeves are fitted with different coloured caps with openings to match the instruments inserted through them. This allows the operation to be performed under gas-tight conditions. A lubricant makes it easier to introduce the instruments and prevents the caps from tearing. The tube connections from the combined endosurgical unit to the rectoscope and the aspirator are now established. They are clearly identified to prevent incorrect connections being made. The water for the rinsing of the telescope and the gas for the dilatation of the rectal cavity are delivered through separate channels inside the telescope. A bottle of saline solution is attached to the right side of the endosurgical unit. When the unit is switched on, the saline comes under pressure from CO_2 delivered from the back of the unit. Water can be taken out of the bottle by a long needle connected to a hose. This hose runs through a lock, which itself works as an electromagnetic piston. The lock is activated by a foot switch which also triggers the rinsing mechanism. The three chip camera of the video system is connected to the third eyepiece of the stereoscopic telescope.

The area to be excised is first marked out by setting coagulation points with the HF-knife. This is helpful for orientation during the actual excision. As a safety margin we recommend 0.5 cm for adenomas and 1 cm for carcinomas. Arterial haemorrhage often occurs when the muscularis is divided. This can be coagulated by the aspirator or a forceps which both have a connection for high frequency current. When the HF-knife is being used or during active rinsing and bleeding, the aspirator should be set to a high working level to clear the operation site from smoke, water and blood. After cutting the rectal wall the specimen is lifted, separated from the pararectal tissue and removed. The remaining defect is checked for bleeding and cleaned by rinsing and suction. It is closed with a 3-0 monofilament thread using the transverse continuous technique and beginning at the right-hand edge of the wound. A silver clip is used instead of a knot. During the procedure, the position of the rectoscope has to be adjusted several times because the optimal working position is in the middle of the range of vision.

Dissecting techniques

A mucosectomy is the simplest dissecting technique in which the mucosa with the polyp is separated from the inner circular layer of the muscularis. This method is now only used in small polyps, since malignant change not discovered preoperatively can be expected in a high proportion of polyps larger than 3 cm. In the extraperitoneal part of the rectum we normally perform the full-thickness technique, whereas in the intraperitoneal part we restrict ourselves to the partial-wall excision because of the risk of opening the peritoneum. In this technique the circular layer of the muscularis is separated from the outer longitudinal part. This method can also be used after snare polypectomy since, because of scarring, the anatomical layers cannot be distinguished adequately for mucosectomy. If the lesion is known to be a carcinoma preoperatively and local excision is indicated, pararectal fatty tissue with lymph nodes can also be removed when performing the full thickness technique. If, however, the tumour is located on the anterior wall, caution is advised because of the close proximity of the vagina (risking rectovaginal fistula) or the prostate (risking haemorrhage). In cases of circular growing adenomas, segmental resection can be performed in the extraperitoneal part of the rectum followed by end-to-end anastomosis.

Rectal prolapse

A rectopexy in cases of rectal prolapse can also be performed with the TEM instrument set. The posterior wall of the rectum is incised in a transverse direction 10 cm above the anal canal. It is then mobilised proximally and the fascia of Waldeyer is exposed (Fig. 20.8). This mobilised part of the posterior wall is fixed to the fascia using several 2-0 sutures. The sutures are inserted from the

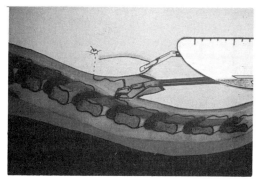

Fig. 20.8 Mobilisation of the posterior wall of the rectum in rectopexy.

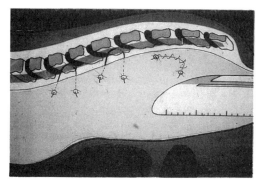

Fig. 20.9 Operation site after completion of rectopexy.

lumen through the rectal wall, through the fascia and back towards the lumen. The fixation sutures are secured by silver clips. Following this, the transverse defect is closed again using the continuous suture technique (Fig. 20.9). The retrorectal scarring anchors the rectum to the sacrum, while the fixation suture holds the rectum in place during the healing process.

Handling of the specimen

Immediately after its removal, the specimen is cleaned and pinned to a cork plate with a 1 cm grid for documentation and the further histological workup (Fig. 20.10). A pathologist then examines the specimen, slicing it in sections to determine the depth of infiltration and to assess whether the tumour is high or low risk according to the Hermanek criteria.[7]

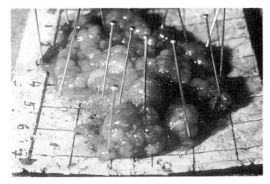

Fig. 20.10 Preparation of the tumour for documentation and histological workup.

Postoperative treatment

If no complications occur, the patient can resume food intake on the first postoperative day after mucosectomy, on the second day after partial wall excision and on the third day after full-thickness excision. Because most of the patients come to our hospital from some distance away they normally stay in the clinic until the final histology is established. This might entail a radical procedure according to oncologic principles.

Follow-up

Follow-up examinations are performed 3 months postoperatively and then at 12-monthly intervals after removal of adenomas, and on a 3-monthly basis after local excision of carcinomas during the first two postoperative years. Thereafter, patients are reviewed every 6 months to the end of the fifth year and finally every year.

Patients

The patients in our series were operated upon using TEM techniques at the University clinics of Cologne, Mainz and Tübingen. Because the concept of local excision of early carcinoma is of particular interest, all patients with locally resected rectal cancer were followed-up. In the period from July 1983 to June 1991, 88 carcinomas were locally excised. For the adenomas the results reported here come from the Mainz

and Tübingen period, when 229 patients with adenomas were operated upon between January 1986 and June 1991. There were 183 males and 134 females, with an average age of 63.5 years (62.7 years for women and 64.1 for men).

Results

The majority of the tumours were localised in the middle third of the rectum. In the patients with adenomas, 71 of the 229 tumours were located in the lower third of the rectum, 116 in the middle third, 29 in the upper third, and 13 between 17 and 24 cm above the anal verge. 21 of the 88 carcinomas were localised in the lower third of the rectum, 47 in the middle third, 17 in the upper third, and 3 between 17 and 24 cm above the anal verge.

40% of the patients with adenomas had already undergone one or more operations using the snare technique. In 9%, polyps had been treated surgically. 29% of the patients with carcinomas had already been treated with the electro-snare and 6% surgically.

Of the patients with adenomas, 158 were symptomatic at the time of diagnosis. 98 patients complained of rectal bleeding and 42 patients had mucous discharge. Diarrhoea was present in 35 cases, 19 patients reported pain and 14 constipation. In the carcinoma patients, a high proportion complained of pain (46 of 88). The overall symptoms, however, were not significantly different from those of the adenoma patients.

The mucosectomy technique was performed to remove adenomas in 26 cases; in 42 patients a partial wall excision was used, and in 161 patients a full thickness excision. In 10 cases, retrorectal fatty tissue was also removed. In 74 of the 88 patients with carcinomas the full thickness technique (on 20 occasions with retrorectal fat) was employed. Ten tumours were removed using the partial wall excision, and in 4 patients the tumour was excised by primary mucosectomy.

The operation time was related to the type of excision. While mucosectomy took an average of one hour, segmental resections required twice as long. The average duration of the operation was 85 minutes, the minimum time 20 minutes and the maximum 240 minutes.

Complications

Adenomas

One patient died of recurrent pulmonary embolism. An anterior resection was necessary in one case because of an extensive opening of the peritoneum during the removal of an intraperitoneal tumour. Dehiscence of a suture was observed 3 times and treated conservatively. One fistula between the rectum and small intestine was discovered during a contrast enema performed as a part of the follow-up in an asymptomatic patient. Since the patient had no discomfort, he rejected therapy. Brief postoperative retention of urine lasting more than 24 hours was encountered relatively often and possibly resulted from compression of the urethra by the operating rectoscope. In 8 cases, catheterisation was necessary. Postoperative stenoses were successfully treated with a bougie in all 5 cases.

Carcinomas

Inadequate sutures were observed twice, one was treated conservatively and another required a colostomy. Rectovaginal fistulas were also encountered in two cases. In one case, histological examination revealed a pT2 carcinoma, and abdominoperineal resection of the rectum was performed subsequently. In a further case, healing was achieved after establishing a defunctioning colostomy. One patient suffered a cerebrovascular event postoperatively.

Incontinence

Thirteen of the 321 patients developed postoperative incontinence for gas ($n = 1$), liquid ($n = 9$) or solid stools ($n = 3$). This incontinence receded in 12 patients during the first 5 postoperative months, and in only one case stool incontinence remained permanently.

Histology

The largest specimen removed had an area of 140 cm^2. The average area of the specimen was 19.7 cm^2 and the size of the tumours was 16.7 cm^2.

The adenomas showed atypia grade I in 27 cases, atypia grade II in 151 cases and grade III

in 51 cases. 61 of the 88 carcinomas were classified as pT1 tumours and only 3 of them as high risk cases. pT2 tumours were found in 21 cases, among them one high risk carcinoma. pT3 carcinomas were observed 6 times.

Recurrence rate

Adenomas

Seven recurrent adenomas were diagnosed during the follow-up. Five of them were removed with the snare or by hot biopsy. One female patient not only developed a recurrent adenoma but also had polycystic ovaries and a laparotomy with resection of the rectum was performed. A TEM procedure was repeated in only one case. 13 new polyps were found in areas not related to the site of the former operation. 12 of these were removed by snare or hot biopsy. An intervention with TEM was only necessary in one case. Thus surgical intervention because of recurrent or newly formed polyps was only necessary in three cases (1%) during the follow-up.

Carcinomas

Of the 44 patients with pT1 low risk carcinomas and local resection alone, only one has so far developed a recurrent tumour. Review of the histology of the original specimen showed (in contrast to the original report) that the edges of the resection were not free of tumour tissue. Recurrences were diagnosed in 2 of the 3 patients with pT1 high-risk tumours.

Discussion

The TEM instrumentation was developed for the removal of sessile polyps from the rectal cavity. The observation that in approximately 20% of larger polyps the final histology reported an invasive carcinoma raises the question of whether a second resection according to radical oncological criteria is necessary. In the first 8 cases involving a second resection of pT1 carcinomas following local resection of an adenoma, neither remnants of the tumour nor metastatic involvement of the lymph nodes were found, two patients developed suture dehiscence, and one patient died as a result of ARDS. We therefore decided not to reoperate in cases of low-risk pT1 carcinomas provided the tumour was resected in healthy tissue. Gall and Hermanek[4] report that second resection in patients following polypectomy of pT1 low-risk carcinomas revealed lymph node metastases in 5% of cases. In an analysis of the literature[9] the proportion of affected lymph nodes is reported as being from 9% to as high as 29% regardless of the differentiation with an average rate of 11.5%. The authors themselves report a rate of 3.1%. In the latest analysis of his case material,[8] Hermanek found a recurrence rate of 3% after local resection of pT1 low risk carcinomas.

If preoperative endorectal ultrasound and histology indicate the presence of such a carcinoma, we only perform a local excision. According to the literature, the chances of a curative operation for a recurrent tumour after local excision are as high as 50%.[5] On the other hand, the recurrence rate in the presence of lymph node metastases, despite a radical primary operation, must be considered extremely high,[11] so that the concept of local removal of early, low-risk tumours should be retained until sufficient comparative statistics are available.

Approximately two-thirds of the adenomas are found in the rectosigmoid region. Access to the rectal cavity can be achieved transanally (Parks), posteriorly (Mason, Kraske) or anteriorly with anterior resection of the rectum. In the anterior procedure, a large abdominal incision is necessary, in the posterior procedures, important functional structures must be divided before the site of the tumour is accessible. Exact dissection is possible with the Parks method up to 10 cm above the anal verge, with the York Mason method in the middle-third and with the Kraske procedure in the upper-third of the rectum. Transanal endoscopic microsurgery with its constant gas dilation of the rectum and magnified stereoscopic view allows dissection up to a height of 25 cm. The low complication and recurrence rates, the possibility of accurate dissection, the wide range of application and the transanal approach recommend this system for the removal of rectosigmoid neoplasms.

Schildberg and Wenk[13] report 22.2% wound infection, 18.8% fistulas and a mortality of 1.7% using Kraske's method and 2.2% infection, 7.4% fistulas, 3% incontinence and a mortality of 1.3% after York Mason's transsphincteric approach.

Recurrence rates of 20% following the Parks method were reported by Schiessel and Wunderlich[12] and 17.3% by Häring *et al.*[6] Following the York Mason method, rates of 3.3% and following the Kraske procedure, 5.5% have been reported. According to Gall and Hermanek[3] a complication rate of 33% and a mortality rate of 4.8% can be expected following anterior resection of the rectum. Compared with these figures, TEM demonstrates a recurrence rate of 5% after polypectomy and a complication rate of 6.5%. The advantaqge of TEM compared with the Parks method is the low rate of recurrence, compared with the other methods reduced invasiveness and a lower complication rate.

References

1. Buess G., Hutterer F., Theiss J., Böbel M., Isselhard W. and Pichlmaier H. (1984) Das System für die transanale endoskopische Rectumoperation. *Chirurg*, **55**, 677–80.
2. Buess G., Kipfmüller K., Hack D., Grüssner R., Heintz A. and Junginger T. (1988) Technique of transanal endoscopic microsurgery. *Surgical Endoscopy*, **2**, 71–5.
3. Gall F.P. and Hermanek P. (1988) Die erweiterte Lymph-knotendissektion beim Magen- und colorektalen Karzinom. *Chirurg*, **59**, 202–10.
4. Gall F.P. and Hermanek P. (1988) Cancer of the rectum-local excision. *Surgical Clinics of North America*, **68**, 1353–65.
5. Graham R.A., Garnsey L. and Jessup J.M. (1990) Local excision of rectal carcinoma. *American Journal of Surgery*, **160**, 306–12.
6. Häring R., Karavias Th. and Konradt J. (1978) Die posteriore Proktorektotomie. *Chirurg*, **49**, 265–71.
7. Hermanek P. (1977) On the diagnosis of colorectal polyps. *Beitrage Path.* **161**, 203–5.
8. Hermanek P. (1990) Behandlung colorectaler Carcinome durch endoskopische Polypektomie. Vortrag Symposium der CAO Heidelberg 1990.
9. Hermanek P. and Gall F.P. (1986) Early microinvasive colorectal carcinoma. *International Journal of Colorectal Disease*, **1**, 79–84.
10. Melzer A., Buess G., Kipfmüller K., Mentges B. and Naruhn N. (1990) *Transanale Endoskopische-Mikrochirurgische Rectopexie*, Häring R. *et al.* (Hrsg), Chirurgisches Forum, pp. 523–527.

11. Mentges B., Mentges W., Grüssner R. and Brückner R. (1988) Art und Prognose des lokoregionären Rezdives beim Rektumkarzinom. *Deutsche Medizinische Wochenschrift*, **113**, 806–10.

12. Schiessel R., Wunderlich M. and Karner-Hanusch J. (1986) Transanale Excision und Anastomosentechnik *Chirug*, **57**, 773–8.

13. Schildberg F.W. and Wenk H. (1986) Der posteriore Zugang zum Rektum. *Chirurg*, **57**, 779–91.

Index